METACOGNITIVE THERAPY
FOR ANXIETY AND DEPRESSION

Metacognitive Therapy for
Anxiety and Depression

||||||||||||||||||||||||

Adrian Wells

THE GUILFORD PRESS
New York   London

© 2009 The Guilford Press
A Division of Guilford Publications, Inc.
72 Spring Street, New York, NY 10012
www.guilford.com

Printed in the United States of America

This book is printed on acid-free paper.

Last digit is print number: 9   8   7   6   5   4   3   2   1

Library of Congress Cataloging-in-Publication Data

Wells, Adrian.
    Metacognitive therapy for anxiety and depression / Adrian Wells.
       p. ; cm.
    Includes bibliographical references and index.
    ISBN 978-1-59385-994-7 (hardcover: alk. paper)
    1. Metacognitive therapy.   2. Anxiety disorders—Treatment.   3. Depression,
Mental—Treatment.   I. Title.
    [DNLM: 1. Cognitive Therapy.   2. Anxiety Disorders—therapy.
 3. Depressive Disorder—therapy.   WM 425.5.C6 W453m 2008]
    RC489.M46W45 2009
    616.85′220651—dc22

                                                                                    2008029157

About the Author

Adrian Wells, PhD, is Professor of Clinical and Experimental Psychopathology at the University of Manchester, United Kingdom, and Professor II in Clinical Psychology at the Norwegian University of Science and Technology, Trondheim, Norway. He is internationally known for his contributions to understanding psychopathological mechanisms and advancing cognitive-behavioral therapy, particularly for anxiety disorders. The originator of metacognitive therapy, Dr. Wells has published over 130 scientific papers, chapters, and books. He is Associate Editor of the journals *Behavioural and Cognitive Psychotherapy* and *Cognitive Behaviour Therapy,* and is a Founding Fellow of the Academy of Cognitive Therapy.

Preface

Cognitions count. By now it is well established that thoughts have a strong impact on emotional and psychological well-being. But consider the following: You had thousands of thoughts yesterday. Some were pleasant and some were less so. Where did all those thoughts go?

Thoughts appear and disappear. A central premise of the approach described in this book is that psychological disorder is the extent to which some thoughts are extended and recycled and some are simply let go. This is a process of selection and control of thinking styles, which depends on metacognition. It is also a matter of how we relate to our own inner experiences.

In cognitive-behavioral theories the content of thought has been given great importance as determining the presence of disorder. But how we think about an event, or how we think about a constellation of conversations, ourselves, and the world around us, is the more profound effect. In fact, how we respond to thoughts can, and all too frequently does, lead to emotional suffering.

Over the past 40 years the cognitive-behavioral model has provided a robust understanding of the impact of cognition on psychological well-being, and led to techniques for treating anxiety, mood, and other disorders. Like this model, metacognitive therapy (MCT) assumes that psychological disorder results from biased thinking; however, it provides a different account of its nature and causes. Earlier approaches have said surprisingly little about the issue of what gives rise to unhelpful thinking patterns. It is incomplete to attribute such patterns to the presence of underlying beliefs about the self and world, such as "I'm vulnerable" or

"I'm a failure." A negative belief, such as "I'm a failure," can be the impetus for a range of responses, such as the deployment of strategies for becoming a success that might include learning from mistakes, working harder, developing new skills, or dismissing the belief as simply a thought that is irrelevant.

Negative beliefs do not necessarily lead to disturbed thinking patterns and prolonged emotional suffering. Metacognitive theory proposes that disturbances in thinking and emotion emerge from metacognitions that are separate from these other thoughts and beliefs emphasized in cognitive-behavioral therapy (CBT).

There is something significant about the pattern of thinking seen in psychological disorder. It has a repetitive, recyclic, brooding quality that is difficult to bring under control. Earlier theories have tended to say little or nothing of such qualities and instead have preferred to focus on the content of thoughts. Earlier approaches have focused on specific irrational beliefs or shorthand negative automatic thoughts, but this is only a small feature of cognition and might be of limited importance. For instance, most patients report long chains of uncontrollable cognitive activity that hardly fits the description of automatic thoughts. It is control of mental processes and selection of some ideas for sustained thinking that is at the heart of emotional suffering. Rather than identifying emotional problems with automatic thoughts, MCT views troublesome internal states as closely related to unhelpful processes of worry, rumination, and strategies of mental control.

At the beginning of my journey leading to MCT, which has taken over 20 years, it seemed that what might be needed to advance the field was an account of the factors that control thinking and cause distressing thoughts to be enriched and extended. I believed that this would depend on extending the concept of metacognition and its assessment and using this to formulate the control of attention and mental processes in psychological disorder.

Metacognition refers to the internal cognitive factors that control, monitor, and appraise thinking. It can be subdivided into metacognitive knowledge (e.g., "I must worry in order to cope"), experiences (e.g., a feeling of knowing), and strategies (e.g., ways of controlling thoughts and protecting beliefs).*

---

*I should like to point out that there are important issues of cognitive architecture, the relative effects of levels of control of attention, and cognitive resource issues that are taken account of in the theory and are described elsewhere (Wells & Matthews, 1994, 1996). The metacognitive model assimilates theory and research in these important areas and offers an explanation of bias and attention effects on task performance. However, this will be of peripheral interest to most practitioners of MCT, and it is therefore not considered in detail in this book.

A central idea is that metacognitive factors are crucial in determining the unhelpful thinking styles seen in psychological disorder that give rise to the persistence of negative emotions. In its "hard" form, the metacognitive theory suggests that the irrational beliefs or schemas emphasized by Albert Ellis and Aaron T. Beck in their respective cognitive theories—or at least, their persistence and influence—are the products of metacognitions.

Metacognitions direct attention, determine the style of thinking, and direct coping responses in a way that repeatedly gives rise to dysfunctional knowledge. This is a dynamic view of beliefs as created by more stable metacognitions. This view implies that metacognitions, and not their consequences, should be modified in treatment.

In a "soft" form the theory suggests that metacognitive beliefs exist alongside other stored beliefs about the self and world, but as separate entities that are responsible for controlling cognition and making use of other more general beliefs and knowledge. In this form treatment might retain a component of challenging traditional beliefs, but it must also deal with the coexistent metacognitions.

In both its hard and soft forms, the metacognitive approach has profound implications for treatment. It guides us toward strategies that enable patients to develop new relationships with their thoughts and beliefs. Rather than questioning the validity of thoughts and beliefs as in traditional CBT, it directs the therapist toward changing the metacognitions that give rise to maladaptive styles of difficult-to-control repetitive negative thinking. For example, the metacognitive approach to treating trauma assumes that metacognitive beliefs and control strategies that disrupt in-built self-regulation are the reasons symptoms do not naturally subside. The tendency to worry or ruminate, lock attention onto threat, and cope by avoiding thoughts interferes with a normal adaptation process and leads to sustained thinking about danger and a persistence of symptoms.

It follows from this that treatment should consist of removing worry and rumination, abandoning attentional strategies of threat monitoring, and helping individuals to experience intrusive thoughts without avoiding or reacting to them with unhelpful suppression, or with ruminative or extended thinking strategies. This treatment differs from standard CBT in that it does not involve challenging thoughts or beliefs about trauma, or prolonged and repeated exposure to trauma memories. Instead, it consists of relating to thoughts in a different way, banning resistance or elaborate conceptual analysis, and suspending maladaptive thinking styles of worry, rumination, and inflexible threat monitoring. In MCT, beliefs *are* challenged—but the focus is on the person's beliefs about cognition itself.

In treating depression, MCT targets the process of rumination rather than the content of a range of negative automatic thoughts. Treatment consists of the attention training technique to interrupt repetitive styles of negative thought and regain flexible control over thinking styles. This is coupled with challenging negative metacognitive beliefs about the uncontrollability of depressive thinking, and challenging positive beliefs about the need to ruminate as a means of coping and finding answers to sadness.

Inevitably, each person who approaches this book will have his or her own goals in reading it, and his or her own style of processing the material contained within. The book is a detailed treatment manual and is replete with therapy techniques grounded in theory. The reader will find interview schedules for developing case formulations, treatment plans, and measures to assist in assessment. Many of the ideas will be new, and it is likely to require experience in applying them to fully appreciate the nature of MCT. I have tried to omit as much technical terminology as possible, I hope without losing the scientific and conceptual integrity of the MCT approach.

Acknowledgments

The journey culminating in the work presented in this book began more than 20 years ago. I have worked with many people during that time, both colleagues and students. My doctoral research addressed self-attentional processes in anxiety. My supervisor was D. Roy Davies, an important influence and mentor. Later I was fortunate to be joined by Gerald Matthews in coauthoring the book *Attention and Emotion: A Clinical Perspective*, which provided the early theoretical grounding for MCT. I worked with Aaron T. Beck in Philadelphia, where I received training in cognitive therapy. In the early to mid-1990s I collaborated with David M. Clark and colleagues at Oxford, where we developed a cognitive model and treatment of social phobia drawing on my earlier metacognition work. At that time I was developing both cognitive therapy and MCT in parallel. This is evident in my book *Cognitive Therapy of Anxiety Disorders: A Practice Manual and Conceptual Guide*.

After moving to the University of Manchester I continued to develop and evaluate MCT and authored the first book devoted completely to MCT, *Emotional Disorders and Metacognition: Innovative Cognitive Therapy*. I was not courageous enough to lose "cognitive therapy" completely from the title of that work, as MCT was proving to be controversial. However, many colleagues are involved in MCT today. I am particularly grateful to my academic colleagues in Trondheim—Hans Nordahl, Tore Styles, and Patrick Vogel—who are undertaking MCT research. I am also grateful to Chris Brewin for our recent collaborations on a project funded by the Medical Research Council involving MCT for depression.

One of my PhD students, Costas Papageorgiou, has been a long-standing collaborator; our work on depression can be found in our edited book, *Depressive Rumination: Nature, Theory and Treatment*. My secretary, Joyce

Russell, has been a great support throughout. Sundeep Sembi was involved in the early evaluation of MCT for posttraumatic stress disorder, Peter Fisher has been involved in the early evaluation of MCT for obsessive–compulsive disorder, and Marcantonio Spada worked on addictions. Karin Carter played an important role in early work on attention training and research on GAD and made helpful suggestions on how to improve the manuscript. I am very grateful to each of these people and to the many others with whom I have worked over the years.

ADRIAN WELLS

Contents

Appendices   259

References   293

Index   303

METACOGNITIVE THERAPY
FOR ANXIETY AND DEPRESSION

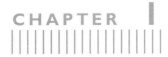

Theory and Nature
of Metacognitive Therapy

Thoughts don't matter but your response to them does.

Everyone has negative thoughts and everyone believes their negative thoughts sometimes. But not everyone develops sustained anxiety, depression, or emotional suffering. An important question is: What is it that controls thoughts and determines whether one can dismiss them or whether one sinks into prolonged and deeper distress?

This book offers an answer to this question. It proposes that metacognitions are responsible for healthy and unhealthy control of the mind. Furthermore, it is based on the principle that it is not merely *what* a person thinks but *how* he or she thinks that determines emotions and the control one has over them.

Thinking can be likened to the activity of a large orchestra involving many players and instruments. To produce an acceptable overture there must be a music score and a conductor. Metacognition is the score and the conductor behind thinking. Metacognition is cognition applied to cognition. It monitors, controls, and appraises the products and process of awareness.

For most of us, emotional discomfort is transitory because we learn ways of flexibly dealing with the negative ideas (i.e., thoughts and beliefs) that our minds construct. The metacognitive approach is based on the idea that people become trapped in emotional disturbance because their metacognitions cause a particular pattern of responding to inner experiences that maintains emotion and strengthens negative ideas. The pattern in question is called the cognitive attentional syndrome (CAS) which consists of worry, rumination, fixated attention, and unhelpful self-regulatory strategies or coping behaviors.

A hint of this toxic pattern can be seen in the response of a recent patient. I asked this person, "What is the main thing you have learned during metacognitive therapy for your depression?" She replied, "The problem isn't really that I have negative thoughts about myself, it's how I've been reacting to them. I've discovered that I've been pouring coal on the fire. I just didn't see that process before." This patient discovered that her responses to negative thoughts had inadvertently developed into an unhelpful thinking style that reinforced her negative self-view. We will return to the nature of this process later in this chapter.

Metacognitive therapy (MCT) is based on the principle that metacognition is vitally important in understanding how cognition operates and how it generates the conscious experiences that we have of ourselves and the world around us. Metacognition shapes what we pay attention to and the factors that enter consciousness. It also shapes appraisals and influences the types of strategies that we use to regulate thoughts and feelings. The argument developed and illustrated throughout this book proposes metacognition as a crucial influence on what we believe and think and as the basis of normal and abnormal emotional and conscious experiences.

A basic premise of traditional cognitive-behavioral therapy (CBT), such as Beck's schema theory (e.g., Beck, 1967, 1976) and Ellis's rational-emotive behavior therapy (REBT; Ellis, 1962; Ellis & Harper, 1961) is that disturbances or biases in thinking cause psychological disorder. Both of these approaches give a central role to dysfunctional beliefs. MCT is in agreement with this view as a general principle, making it a type of cognitive therapy. Where it differs from previous approaches is in identifying a particular style of thinking and types of beliefs not emphasized by these other theories as the cause of disorder. The style of thinking emphasized is not about cognitive distortions such as absolutistic standards or black-and-white thinking. The style of interest in MCT is the CAS, which is marked by engaging in excessive amounts of sustained verbal thinking and dwelling in the form of worry and rumination. This is accompanied by a specific attentional bias in which attention is locked onto threat. The beliefs of importance in MCT are not the ordinary cognitions of CBT and REBT concerning the world and the social and physical self, but are beliefs about thinking (metacognitive beliefs).

The traditional CBT approach to psychological disorder asserts that it is not events themselves that cause psychological problems but the way those events are interpreted. CBT deals with the meanings that people give to their experiences. It assumes that the problem rests with erroneous and distorted views of the self and the world. It deals with changing this thought content and the person's belief in the validity of that content. In contrast, MCT deals with the way that people think and it assumes the problem rests with inflexible and recurrent styles of thinking in response to negative thoughts, feelings, and beliefs. It focuses on removing unhelpful processing styles. It proposes that any challenges to cognitive themes (content) occur exclusively at the metacognitive level. For instance, if we consider the case of a depressed patient who believes "I'm worthless," the CBT therapist tackles the problem by asking, "What is your evidence?" In contrast, the MCT therapist asks, "What is the point in evaluating your worth?"

In both the CBT and the MCT approaches, the content of beliefs and thoughts determines the type of disorder experienced. Thoughts about danger give rise to anxiety; thoughts about loss and self-devaluation give rise to sadness. MCT posits that this content does not cause disorder because most people have these thoughts and for most the emotion is transitory. Emotional disorder is a problem of being trapped in a state of distress. It is chronic or recurrent. Emotional disorder is caused by the metacognitions that give rise to thinking styles that lock the individual into prolonged and recurrent states of negative self-relevant processing. In essence, MCT is about the factors that lead to sustained thinking and misdirected coping.

In CBT erroneous interpretations of events that cause psychological disorder are assumed to emanate from beliefs, but the beliefs emphasized are in the ordinary cognitive domain. These are beliefs such as "The world is dangerous" and "I'm inadequate." In MCT these beliefs can be seen as the products of metacognitions that give rise to patterns of attention and thinking that repeatedly generate or lock onto these ideas. The implication is that metacognition and patterns of thinking should be modified in treatment because these are the cause of stable negative beliefs or "ordinary cognitions." The beliefs or schemas of CBT are not seen by the MCT practitioner as stable entities that should be erased but instead are seen as the products of thinking processes.

It is clear from the foregoing introduction that MCT introduces an important distinction between cognition and metacognition, with therapeutic work focused primarily on the latter domain. There is no clear differentiation between cognition and metacognition in earlier cognitive therapies. This is exemplified in an extract taken from Beck's influential writing: "Through interviewing this depressed mother, I discovered that her thinking was controlled by erroneous ideas about herself and her world. Despite contrary evidence, she believed she had been a failure as a mother" (Beck, 1976, p. 16).

Here, it is apparent that depressive thinking is attributed to the presence of negative beliefs about being a "failure." Beck assumes that the patient's thinking is controlled by her erroneous ideas about being a failure.

However, it does not invariably follow that believing that one is a failure will control one's thinking. If we take all of the individuals who believe this, will they all become depressed? According to cognitive theory they should, but this is unlikely to be true. MCT views this situation differently. It assumes that most people will have thoughts or beliefs about being a failure, but that individuals will respond to these thoughts in different ways depending on their metacognitions. So it is metacognitive knowledge or beliefs that control subsequent thinking, not the ordinary cognitions that do so.

Let's look at this in more detail. Most people will believe that they are a "failure" at some time in their lives, but for some this belief is followed by renewed efforts to succeed, while for others it is followed by chains of negative thoughts consisting of brooding on personal failings and weaknesses. What is needed is a mechanism that accounts for the existence of these different cognitive and emotional response patterns. I have proposed that the mechanism is metacognition, that aspect of cognition that controls the way a person thinks and behaves in response to a thought, belief, or feeling.

In the case of the depressed mother Beck describes, we might assume that her thinking is controlled by metacognitive beliefs, perhaps something resembling the following: "If I think about my failings and analyze why they occurred, I will be a better mother." Unfortunately, the thinking process of rumination that results from this metacognitive belief is unlikely to lead to satisfactory answers, and the patient will persist in thinking about being a failure.

In the remainder of this chapter, I describe in greater depth the basic principles of MCT theory and treatment. A basic implication of metacognition as a central driver of psychological disorder is that treatment should not invest effort in interrogating and reality testing the person's individual thoughts and beliefs but should focus on changing *how* a person responds to these ideas. The focus of intervention shifts to cognitive processes and the metacognitions giving rise to them and away from evaluating the evidence for and against the cognitive products (e.g., "I'm a failure"). The only exception occurs when the products themselves are metacognitions, as in the form of worry about worry (e.g., "Worrying will harm me").

Having built an argument for metacognition so far in this chapter, now I will explore this construct in greater detail before presenting the complete metacognitive model of disorder.

THE NATURE OF METACOGNITION

The study of metacognition emerged in the area of developmental psychology and subsequently in the psychology of memory, ageing, and neuropsychology (Brown, 1978; Flavell, 1979; Metcalfe & Shimamura, 1994). Only recently has metacognition been examined as a fundamental basis for most or all psychological disturbances (Wells & Matthews, 1994; Wells, 1995, 2000).

Metacognition describes a range of interrelated factors comprised of any knowledge or cognitive process that is involved in the interpretation, monitoring, or control of cognition. It can be usefully divided into knowledge, experiences, and strategies (e.g., Flavell, 1979; Nelson, Stuart, Howard, & Crawley, 1999; Wells, 1995).

Knowledge and Beliefs

"Metacognitive knowledge" refers to the beliefs and theories that people have about their own thinking. For example, this knowledge consists of the beliefs that are held about particular types of thoughts as well as beliefs about the efficiency of one's memory or powers of concentration. An individual may believe that some thoughts are harmful. A religious person may believe that experiencing certain thoughts is sinful and will lead to punishment. These are examples of metacognitive beliefs about the importance of thoughts. Holding such beliefs has implications for how a person responds to his or her thoughts and how he or she orchestrates his or her thinking.

According to the metacognitive theory of psychological disorder, there are two types of metacognitive knowledge (Wells & Matthews, 1994; Wells, 2000): (1) explicit (declarative) beliefs and (2) implicit (procedural) beliefs.

Explicit knowledge is that which can be verbally expressed. Examples include "Worrying can cause a heart attack"; "Having bad thoughts means I'm mentally defective"; and "If I focus on danger I'll avoid harm."

Implicit knowledge is not directly verbally penetrable. It can be thought of as the rules or programs that guide thinking, such as the factors controlling the allocation of attention, memory search, and use of heuristics in forming judgments. The plan or program for processing can be indirectly inferred from assessment strategies such as metacognitive profiling (Wells & Matthews, 1994). Implicit or procedural knowledge represent the "thinking skills" that individuals have.

In addition to these two types of metacognitive knowledge, there are two broad-content domains in MCT. Individual disorders show some content-specificity within these domains. The broad domains are positive and negative metacognitive beliefs. *Positive metacognitive beliefs* are concerned with the benefits or advantages of engaging in cognitive activities that constitute the CAS. Examples of positive metacognitive beliefs include "It is useful to focus attention on threat," and "Worrying about the future means I can avoid danger."

Negative metacognitive beliefs are beliefs concerning the uncontrollability, meaning, importance, and dangerousness of thoughts and cognitive experiences. Examples of such beliefs include "I have no control over my thoughts"; "I could damage my mind by worrying"; "If I have violent thoughts I will act on them against my will"; and "Being unable to remember names is a sign of a brain tumor."

In MCT metacognitive beliefs are a key influence on the way individuals respond to negative thoughts, beliefs, symptoms, and emotions. They are a driving force behind the toxic thinking style that leads to prolonged emotional suffering.

Experiences

Metacognitive experiences are the situational appraisals and feelings that individuals have of their mental status. For example, the negative interpretations that obsessional patients make of their intrusive thoughts are metacognitive experiences. The worry about worry that is a feature of generalized anxiety is an example of a metacognitive experience. The misinterpretations of cognitive events made by patients with panic disorder when they believe they are about to lose control of their behavior or lose their mind is a further example.

Experiences also include subjective feelings. A familiar and normal metacognitive feeling state is the *tip-of-the-tongue* effect, where individuals have a strong sense that an item of information is stored in memory even though it is currently not retrievable. There are similar experiences such as "feeling of knowing" and judgments of learning that have been examined in experimental work on metamemory and judgments (e.g., Nelson, Gerler, & Narens, 1984; Nelson & Dunlosky, 1991). These subjective experiences influence behavior such as retrieval efforts and learning strategies.

In MCT, negative appraisals of feelings and thoughts contribute to perceived threat and motivate attempts to control thinking. Subjective feeling states and appraisals of cognition can be used as information for influencing judgments about threat and coping. Often these experiences are not fit for purpose. For example, a man suffering from obsessional thoughts that he might have committed a murder focused on the completeness of his memory for a period of time to decide whether or not he had committed murder. Any blanks in his memory were interpreted as possible times during which he could have committed the act. In this example his strategies and his appraisals of his memory status (meta-experiences) were unhelpful and maintained his anxiety.

Strategies

Metacognitive strategies are the responses made to control and alter thinking in the service of emotional and cognitive self-regulation. The strategies selected may intensify, suppress, or change the nature of cognitive activities. Some of them are aimed at reducing thoughts or negative emotions by altering aspects of cognition. For example, an individual may turn his or her attention toward threat in an attempt to be prepared, or he or she may try to suppress distressing thoughts, use positive thinking, or distract from emotion.

In psychological disorders, the patient's subjective experience is one of being *out of control*. Strategies often consist of attempts to control the nature of thinking. These attempts tend to be counterproductive in the long term. They include attempts to suppress certain thoughts, to analyze experiences to find answers, or to try and predict what might happen in the future so as to avoid problems. In anxiety disorders, individuals often negatively interpret the occurrence of thoughts and their strategies often involve attempts to suppress them. In disorders such as hypochondriasis and generalized anxiety a strategy consists of focusing on particular negative stimuli and worrying about them. For example, a hypochondriacal patient explained how he analyzed possible *harmful causes* for his muscle weakness to be sure that he did not miss anything that could be important. The problem with this strategy, as with most strategies used by our patients, is that it maintained his sense of threat.

In another case, a depressed woman receiving MCT described dealing with her feelings of sadness by dwelling (ruminating) on her inadequacies and mistakes. Her goal was to make herself feel worse so that she was "forced to snap out of it."

Clearly, strategies are dependent on the metacognitive knowledge and internal models that individuals have concerning how their cognition and emotion operates. Metacognitive knowledge (beliefs), experiences, and strategies are interdependent and function together in psychological disorder.

In the metacognitive theory of psychological disorder, maladaption in knowledge, experiences, and strategies combine to give rise to an unhelpful pattern of thinking that leads to psychological disturbance. However, before describing that pattern in detail, I would like to turn attention to an aspect of metacognitive experiences that plays an important role in MCT. The fact that humans have the capacity to engage in ordinary cognition and also to think about thinking means that there are two ways of experiencing thoughts. Previously I have called these "modes" (Wells, 2000).

TWO WAYS OF EXPERIENCING: MODES

It is not typical to experience thoughts or beliefs as events in the mind, that is, to objectify them. They are usually experienced directly, like perceptions, in the same way that a person experiences the sound of a ticking clock or the sight of snowflakes falling on the rooftops. However, cognitions can be experienced in different ways such as a thought or a feeling and not as the actual world itself.

We do not normally see our thoughts or beliefs as inner events: we fuse them with reality. It's as if we see through them at the outside world and ourselves and yet they act as the filter coloring our model of everything. We fail to see our thoughts as inner representations or constructions independent of the actual self or world. I have termed this usual type of experiencing the *object mode,* in which thoughts or beliefs are not distinguished from direct experiences of the self or the world. We normally experience an undifferentiated consciousness, making no distinction between inner and outer events and thoughts and perceptions.

The object mode can be contrasted with the *metacognitive mode* of experiencing, in which thoughts can be consciously observed as separate events from the self and the world. These events are simply some form of representation that has a varying degree of accuracy. In this mode the individual's relationship to thoughts is one of standing back and observing them as part of a greater multifaceted landscape of conscious experience.

The metacognitive mode is not the same as identifying and challenging negative thoughts in CBT. In CBT the therapist challenges the patient's belief in the degree of accuracy of a thought, but this challenge may not shift the way that thought is experienced. To experience the metacognitive mode takes practice in shifting and experiencing that mode. It is a skill of relating to inner experiences in an alternative way irrespective of the accuracy of thought. This skill is acquired through practice. By approximating and experiencing the metacognitive mode the necessary metacognitive mechanisms and processes to support this type of processing are strengthened and developed. In other words, through experiencing the metacognitive mode, the individual begins to shape up and to strengthen an embedded metacognitive program that enables this activity (i.e., procedural knowledge).

Within the metacognitive mode a further type of experience is possible and desirable in metacognitive therapy. This is the experience of *detached mindfulness* (DM; Wells & Matthews, 1994). In this context, "mindfulness" refers to an objective awareness of a thought or belief, while "detachment" refers to two factors: (1) the disengagement of any conceptual or coping-based activity in response to the thought and (2) separating the conscious experience of self from the thought. This latter factor consists of the individual becoming aware of being the perceiver of the thought and separate from the thought itself. Thus, a negative belief or thought can be moved outside the boundary of self, separated from the self-model, at which point it becomes irrelevant for self-regulation. The person no longer defines the self or interprets his or her world with reference to it.

THE METACOGNITIVE MODEL
OF PSYCHOLOGICAL DISORDER

Having introduced some of the important concepts in the metacognitive model of psychological disorder, at this juncture I will describe the model in detail.

The basic model is called the self-regulatory executive function model (S-REF; Wells & Matthews, 1994, 1996; Wells, 2000), so called because it offers an account of the cognitive and metacognitive factors involved in the top-down control or maintenance of emotional disorder. A diagrammatic representation of the model with its meta-level components revealed is given in Figure 1.1.

In the model cognitive processes are spread across three interacting levels involving automatic and reflexive processing (low-level processing), online conscious processing of thoughts and behaviors (labeled cognitive style), and a library of knowledge or beliefs that are metacognitive in nature stored in long-term memory.

In Figure 1.1, the meta-system is differentiated from the rest of the ordinary cognitive system but like other systems is distributed through different levels of processing. The meta-system holds a model or representa-

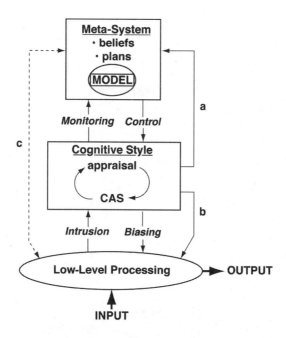

FIGURE 1.1. The S-REF model of psychological disorder with metacognitions revealed. After Wells and Matthews (1994).

tion of current ordinary cognitive processing and guides it toward the goal of an activated plan.

A core principle of MCT is that psychological disorder is linked to the activation of a particular toxic style of thinking called the CAS. For most people periods of emotion and negative appraisal (e.g., sadness, anxiety, anger, worthlessness) are isolated and temporary. However, the CAS has effects that lock people into prolonged or repetitive disturbances of this kind.

The CAS consists of a perseverative thinking style that takes the form of worry or rumination, attentional focusing on threat, and unhelpful coping behaviors that backfire (e.g., thought suppression, avoidance, substance use). This style has a number of consequences that lead to the maintenance of emotions and the strengthening of negative ideas. Generally speaking, the CAS maintains an individual's sense of threat.

An example of the effects of the CAS can be seen in the development of panic disorder. Spontaneous panic attacks are quite common and happen to many people at some point in their lives. However, worrying about subsequent attacks (part of the CAS) prolongs anxiety, and monitoring of bodily sensations (part of the CAS) increases the triggering conditions (intrusion of bodily sensations) for subsequent attacks to occur. Thus, the individual who is prone to activate this cognitive-attentional response pattern is more likely to show a persistence of anxious arousal and to develop repeated panic attacks. Such a pattern will support the growth of beliefs about the uncontrollable and harmful consequences of anxiety.

The CAS arises from knowledge and beliefs, but these are metacognitive in nature and not in the ordinary cognitive domain of beliefs about the self and the world. Two types of beliefs are important: (1) positive beliefs about the need to engage in aspects of the CAS (e.g., "If I worry about my symptoms, I won't miss anything important") and (2) negative beliefs about the uncontrollability, dangerousness, or importance of thoughts and feelings (e.g., "I have no control over my mind; my anxiety could make me go crazy").

At this juncture, before presenting any further detail, I believe that it may be useful to summarize the basic principles of the metacognitive approach:

1. It is proposed that the emotions of anxiety and sadness are basic internal signals of a discrepancy in self-regulation and of threats to well-being.
2. Such emotions are normally of limited duration because the person engages coping strategies to reduce threat and control cognition.
3. Psychological disorder results from the maintenance of emotional responses.

4. They are maintained because of the individual's thinking style and strategies.
5. The unhelpful style, found in all disorders, is called the CAS, consisting of worry/rumination, threat monitoring, unhelpful thought control strategies, and other forms of behavior (e.g., avoidance) that prevent adaptive learning.
6. The CAS is the result of erroneous metacognitive beliefs (knowledge) controlling and interpreting thinking and feeling states.
7. The CAS prolongs and intensifies negative emotional experience through several clearly specified mechanisms/pathways.

THE CAS

The thinking patterns of psychologically disordered individuals have a repetitive and brooding quality focused on self-related topics that is difficult to bring under control. This quality is indicative of the CAS and is marked by heightened self-focused attention.

The CAS consists of excessive conceptual processing in the form of worry and rumination. These are long chains of predominantly verbal thought in which the person attempts to answer "What if . . . ?" questions (worry) or attempts to answer questions about the meaning of events (e.g., "Why do I feel this way?").

In addition to this conceptual component, the CAS is comprised of attentional bias in the form of fixating attention on threat-related stimuli. This is termed "threat monitoring" (Wells & Matthews, 1994). For example, an individual traumatized in a robbery described how he subsequently scanned the environment for potential danger. A patient with low self-esteem reported being sensitive to being ignored by other people; it was discovered that this sensitivity was associated with monitoring for signs that people might not like her.

These conceptual and attentional processes are part of the person's strategy for dealing with threat, self-discrepancies, and the emotion aroused by them. There are additional strategies that constitute the CAS including thought control strategies such as thought suppression and behaviors such as behavioral, cognitive, and emotional avoidance. Some examples of the CAS are evident in the following cases:

A 43-year-old woman described how she had experienced repeated episodes of depression since she was a teenager. The current depression occurred following the birth of her second daughter approximately 14 months earlier. When asked how much of the time she had spent thinking about her feelings and depression in the past week, she explained that she had spent many hours doing so. When asked for an example of this thinking, she described sitting and gazing at a television screen thinking about how abnormal it was to feel this way, why she felt sad, how she did not have the correct feelings for her daughter, why this had happened to her, and what this meant about her suitability as a mother. It was discovered that she was spending a large amount of time ruminating in this way in response to negative thoughts about her daughter. When asked what the goal might be in thinking this way, she explained how she was trying to make her mood worse in an attempt to become angry so that she would be forced to "snap out of depression."

The patient described above responded to her low mood by ruminating and extended focusing on her feelings in an attempt to deal with her sadness. In effect she was trying to "think herself better" by rumination because she held the metacognitive belief that by becoming angry she could escape from her sadness.

One of our male patients was suffering from delayed-onset posttraumatic stress disorder (PTSD) following exposure to a bomb blast. He explained how he had coped well for several years after the event, but recently, as a result of reading about terrorist attacks, he had developed nightmares and had become overanxious when using public transport and visiting the town. He was asked how he was dealing with his unwanted thoughts and nightmares and he explained that he was "trying to get over it." On careful questioning it emerged that he was trying to force himself to think and feel emotion about the trauma because he had read that this was the way to speed up recovery. Furthermore, he believed it was advantageous to worry about terrorist events in the future so that he could be "on his guard" against possible danger.

In this example, the patient's thinking style in response to intrusions was dominated by trying to think (rumination) and feel emotion to speed up recovery. In addition he was worrying about threats in the future as a means of being prepared. These features of the CAS backfired and increased his anxiety and sense of threat.

A 39-year-old female patient described herself as a chronic worrier. Exploration of a recent distressing worry episode established that in response to the negative thought "What if my child is injured?," she had engaged in prolonged worry to try and generate a series of potential ways of coping with such an event. On this occasion she had a panic attack during her worry because she thought she was losing control of her mind. Since then she had been trying to suppress thoughts about her children being involved in accidents, and she was avoiding local newspapers in case they gave her something new she needed to worry about.

In this case, prolonged worry in response to negative thoughts, thought suppression, and avoidance were readily observable components of the CAS. On further questioning the patient described how she believed that worrying was an effective means of avoiding problems in the future, clearly indicating the involvement of positive metacognitive beliefs in the problem as well as negative metacognitive beliefs about losing control.

> A 23-year-old man presented with a problem of anxiety in social situations, in which he feared that he would look anxious and "weird." When asked about his most recent experience of social anxiety, he identified feeling anxious before attending the treatment session. He was asked what he had been thinking and for how long beforehand. The patient described how he had been trying to anticipate what the situation would be like and rehearsing ways of answering any difficult questions. He was also asked if he had been paying attention to himself or to the external environment during the session. The patient answered that he was paying more attention to himself at the beginning of the session and in particular that he had been focusing on how he sounded and might look to the therapist. He was trying to sound and look normal by controlling his behavior.

The feature of the CAS most evident in this case is perseveration in the form of anticipatory worry. It also involves threat monitoring in the form of focusing on an impression of himself, and coping behaviors in the form of trying to sound and appear "normal."

In each of the cases described above it is possible to identify and isolate the CAS. The problem is that components of the CAS lock the person into prolonged emotional experience and produce conflicts in self-regulation that lead to a sense of helplessness and loss of adaptive control over cognition and emotion.

CONSEQUENCES OF THE CAS

What is it that is bad about the CAS? There are several consequences that lead to psychological disturbances. The negative consequences for self-regulation are depicted by the arrows labeled A and B in Figure 1.1. The arrow labeled A depicts the effect that appraisals and coping behaviors have on beliefs. For example, focusing attention on threat reinforces beliefs about the presence of danger, and avoiding experiences such as anxiety prevents the person from discovering the truth about the benign nature of emotion. The arrow labeled B in Figure 1.1 signifies the effect of thinking style and coping on low-level automatic and emotion-level processing. For example, worrying may maintain activation of the anxiety network and divert attention away from processing intrusive images, thereby blocking emotional processing. There are also likely to be direct links between the meta-system's knowledge and the lower level in that certain types of automatic processing may prime the retrieval of knowledge or plans for guiding subsequent processing, as depicted by the arrow labeled C.

Let's now consider in more detail the deleterious effects attributed to the CAS in the model. Worrying and rumination are invariably biased and focus the individual on negative information. This leads to a distorted impression of the self and the world. For instance, worrying focuses on potential danger in the future, but has little relationship with the true probability of dangerous events.

Rumination seeks answers to questions that often do not have a single or identifiable answer, such as "Why me?" Thus, it perpetuates uncertainty and self-discrepancies between what the person knows and what the person desires to know. Furthermore, worry and rumination activate and maintain a sense of threat so that anxiety and depression persist rather than being transient. These processes use up valuable attentional resources and can impair clear and controlled decision making and thinking under pressure. The repeated practice of worry and rumination increases the habit strength of these responses such that the individual has diminished awareness of these activities and allows them to proceed unchecked. Habit strength and lack of awareness contribute to a sense of loss of control of these mental processes. Worry and rumination can interfere with other self-regulatory cognitive processes. For example, worry is predominantly verbal and can interfere with the processing of images that is necessary for emotional processing after trauma. Similarly, ruminating on the past, such as thinking about failures and mistakes, increases the accessibility of this material when making judgments in the future.

The "threat-monitoring" component of the CAS fixates attention on sources of potential threat. This is a problem because (1) it inflates the sense of subjective danger, thereby increasing or maintaining emotional activation; (2) it strengthens a plan or program for guiding cognition that leads the individual to become a skilled and more sensitive threat detector; (3) in cases such as PTSD or trauma, in which cognition needs to retune to the normal threat-free environment, the strategy prevents this process; and (4) threat monitoring may bias fear-processing networks responsible for generating intrusions of stimuli into consciousness. Thus, threat monitoring may increase intrusive mental experiences.

Thought control strategies such as suppression or thinking in special ways are problematic because they interfere with normal emotional processing, such as emotional habituation through repeated exposure to thoughts. Suppression is a problem because it is not consistently effective in stopping unwanted thoughts, and failure can be interpreted as loss of control. In each case persistence in processing of threat occurs. Some regulation strategies have ironic effects because they rely on dissonant processes. For example, a patient might try to think him- or herself out of depression by dwelling on how bad he or she feels and why he or she feels that way. Such dwelling deepens and prolongs the depression because it locks the person onto more negative self-relevant information. Similarly, chronic worriers effectively attempt to worry themselves into a state of feeling that they will be able to cope in the future.

Other coping behaviors such as avoidance and using substances to regulate emotion and cognition are problematic because they deprive the individual of an opportunity to discover that he or she can cope in situations and emotion is not dangerous. A sense of prospective danger is maintained because some coping behaviors prevent reality testing of negative thoughts and beliefs. For example, the nonoccurrence of a catastrophe such as suffering a "mental breakdown" can be attributed to avoiding stress rather than to the fact that the belief about stress causing a breakdown is faulty.

POSITIVE AND NEGATIVE METACOGNITIVE BELIEFS

The CAS is controlled by erroneous beliefs about thinking. Two different content domains of metacognitive belief contribute to this style: (1) positive metacognitive beliefs and (2) negative metacognitive beliefs.

Positive metacognitive beliefs concern the usefulness of worry, rumination, threat monitoring, and other similar strategies. Examples include:

> "If I worry I will be prepared."
> "Focusing on danger will keep me safe."
> "I must remember everything and then I'll know if I'm to blame."
> "If I analyze why I feel this way I'll find answers."
> "I must control my thoughts or I'll do something bad."

On the surface these beliefs may seem reasonable. However, in order to show their erroneous and distorted nature, they are repeated below with some useful questions (printed in *italics*) that the metacognitive therapist uses to reframe them:

> "If I worry I will be prepared."
> *Is it possible to be prepared without worrying?*
> *Is it possible to worry about everything that could happen?*
> *Does worry give a balanced view of the future or a biased one?*

"Focusing on danger will keep me safe."
How do you know which danger to focus on?
Is it the danger you see or the one you don't see that will catch you out?
Could focusing on danger make you less safe because you forget the usual things?

"I must remember everything and then I'll know if I'm to blame."
Is it possible to remember everything?
How will knowing if you're to blame help you feel better and move on?
Can you move on without blaming yourself?

"If I analyze why I feel this way I'll find answers."
How long have you been doing this? How much longer will it take?
What if the answer is stopping your analysis?
What if there is no answer other than changing the way you think?

"I must control my thoughts."
How do you know which ones to control?
Is it possible to control all of your thoughts?
Could controlling your thoughts stop you from finding out the truth about them?

The second domain of metacognitive belief concerns the negative significance and meaning of internal cognitive events such as thoughts and ordinary beliefs. There are two broad subsets of negative meta-beliefs: those that concern the uncontrollability of thoughts and those that concern the danger, importance, and meaning of them. These meta-beliefs lead to a persistence of the CAS because of a failure to attempt control and because they lead to negative and threatening interpretations of mental events. These beliefs can also be extended to emotional experiences or feeling states.
Examples include:

"I have no control over my worrying/rumination."
"Worrying can damage my body."
"Psychological distress can make me lose my mind."
"Bad thoughts have the power to make me do bad things."
"Some thoughts can make bad things happen."
"My thoughts can change me into something I don't want to be."
"Uncontrollable thoughts are a sign of madness."
"If I believe I'm bad then I must be bad."
"Feeling anxious means I must be in danger."
"Thinking something makes it true."

SUMMARY OF THE METACOGNITIVE MODEL

In summary, MCT is based on the principle that psychological disorder persists because of the effects of a state of thinking, the CAS, on emotional experiences and knowledge. The CAS maintains the person's negative sense of self and perception of threat through specific pathways.

The CAS is linked to the activation of negative and positive metacognitive beliefs. The separation of the metacognitive level from the ordinary cognitive level implies that it is possible to experience inner events such as thoughts, beliefs, and emotions in a cognitive or metacognitive mode. This presents a range of possibilities for treatment that focus on removing the CAS, modifying metacognitive beliefs, and developing alternative ways of experiencing and relating to inner events.

A REFORMULATED A-B-C MODEL

One way of understanding the metacognitive model and appreciating how it stands in relation to earlier cognitive-behavioral theories is to examine how it changes the standard A-B-C model that is a basis of cognitive therapies.

In the standard model as depicted in Figure 1.2, an activating event (A) leads to activation of a schema or irrational belief (B), which in turn leads to emotional and behavioral consequences (C).

However, as we have seen, a major unresolved issue in cognitive theories of psychological disorder is the question of what links ordinary negative appraisals or beliefs to persistent negative thoughts and emotions. A further unresolved question concerns what it is that gives rise to difficult-to-control thinking patterns that epitomize psychological suffering.

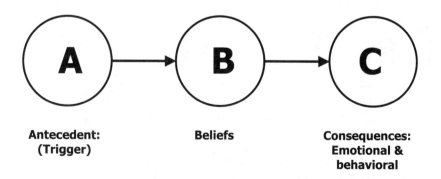

FIGURE 1.2. The A-B-C model.

The MCT reformulates the standard A-B-C model by placing metacognitive beliefs in the center and allowing the activating event to be replaced with an inner experience of a negative thought or ordinary belief. This is depicted as the A-M-C model in Figure 1.3. This is a model that begins downstream of the standard A-B-C model since the antecedent in the reformulated model is an internal cognitive event rather than a situation. In the new model the M component denotes metacognitive beliefs and the CAS. More general negative appraisals or ordinary beliefs (B) are influenced and used by metacognitive processes.

A case example might help to clarify these differences in approach.

A 30-year-old woman had been depressed for a little more than 2 years by the time she presented for MCT. She described feeling depressed and suicidal for much of the time over the past 2 years since leaving her hometown to find a new job. In the week that she was assessed she described that she had been alone and had continuously thought "things won't change," which had led her to feel sadness most of the time and a sense of hopelessness and despair.

An A-B-C formulation of this series of events is presented in Figure 1.4. As evident in this figure, the antecedent was "being alone"

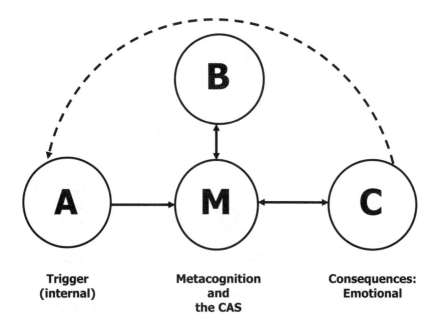

FIGURE 1.3. The reformulated A-M-C model. Adapted from Wells (2000). Copyright 2000 by John Wiley & Sons Limited. Adapted by permission.

which led to the belief "things won't change" and to feelings of sadness and hopelessness.

The metacognitive approach produces a somewhat different analysis by exploring the nature of metacognitions and the CAS. The therapist asked the patient how much of the time she had spent thinking about how she felt and why she felt this way. The patient described how she had spent long periods of time doing this. Her thinking consisted of chains of thought in which she asked herself "Why am I like this, will things ever change, what does this mean, why can't I get things done, why are people happier than me, and will this ever end?" She was asked if there were any advantages in thinking this way and she identified the idea that she needed to think about how bad things are (ruminate) in order to change things, and that by experiencing sadness she could become more motivated. The therapist asked her what she did to try and experience sadness and the patient described that she focused on her thoughts, focused on her feelings, listened to sad music, and reduced her activities to give her more time to think. These metacognitions and the CAS are formulated in Figure 1.5 using the A-M-C model.

By comparing Figures 1.4 and 1.5 it is possible to see the different emphasis of CBT compared to MCT. The former aims to challenge the belief about hopelessness (things won't change), whereas the engine driving persistent and recurrent sadness and hopelessness in the metacognitive formulation are metacognitions and the CAS. MCT therefore focuses on removing the CAS and challenging the metacognitive beliefs that support this response style. Notice also that in the A-M-C analysis the antecedent (A) is specifically identified as an internal trigger, a thought, rather than a situation.

In this example the nature of MCT is evident. It is a treatment that enables patients to recognize the patterns of thinking and coping that lock them into prolonged states of emotional distress, to change those patterns,

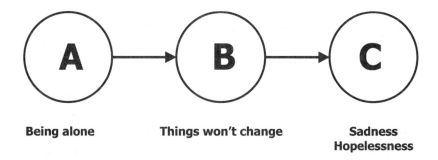

FIGURE 1.4. An example of an A-B-C formulation of a depressed case.

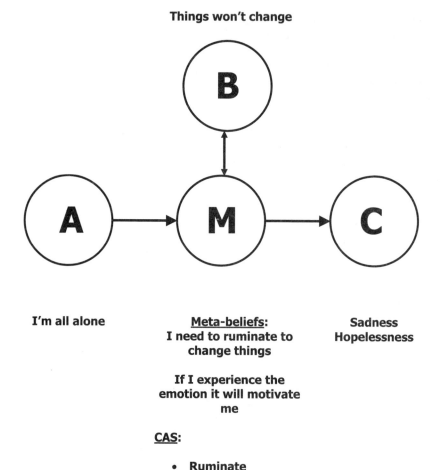

FIGURE 1.5. A metacognitive (A-M-C) formulation of the same depressed case.

and to alter their meta-beliefs about thoughts and feelings. It is not a treatment that focuses primarily on evaluating the reality of ordinary negative beliefs about the self and the world, as would be the case in more traditional forms of CBT. In the depression case we have just examined, the therapist did not reality-test her belief ("Things won't change") by questioning the evidence and reviewing counterevidence. Instead, therapy helped her to develop alternative responses to thoughts about being alone by challenging her metacognitive beliefs and by removing the CAS. The thought or belief about things not changing is seen as persistent and salient because the CAS makes it so.

A NOTE ON PROCESS- VERSUS CONTENT-FOCUSED THERAPIES

Existing CBTs are very much content-focused treatments. Therapists refer mainly to the content of an individual's thoughts and beliefs and challenge that content. MCT is chiefly interested in processes and its focus on content is usually in the metacognitive domain rather than in the social, physical, and world domains of other treatments.

For example, in traditional CBT for depression the therapist focuses on questioning the evidence for negative thoughts and beliefs about the self, the world, and the future. This is exemplified by therapist questions such as "What is the cognitive distortion in your thought?" and "What is your counterevidence?" However, in MCT the therapist aims to reduce the extent of rumination, modifies negative beliefs about the uncontrollability of this process, and challenges positive metacognitive beliefs about the need to engage this process in response to sadness. The metacognitive level of intervention is exemplified by questions such as "Can you postpone your rumination in response to your thought?" and "What are the disadvantages of dwelling on that thought?"

When we refer to the "content of cognition" we are referring to the information-processing system's knowledge, the information that is stored or is current in consciousness. Beliefs can be seen as part of this library of information or knowledge.

When we refer to "processes" we are referring to the actions involved in using that knowledge and in learning new knowledge. To use the library metaphor, processes might be likened to searching for a book, locating it in space, reading the information, and using that information to change what we do, think, or know. Processes link knowledge (beliefs) to emotional and behavioral consequences and processes determine the effect that experiences have on knowledge.

We cannot directly work on knowledge such as the belief "I'm worthless." We can only work on the processes that locate and make use of knowledge. To take this one step further, we might reasonably assume that what we think and consciously believe arises out of the subjective experience of processes. What we know is not content, it is the result of the processes that use content. Patients state that they are "bad," that they are "having a heart attack," and that they are "worthless" because they are repeatedly engaging in processes that generate or sustain this erroneous information.

A central concept in MCT is that it is necessary to alter cognitive processes, namely, the style of thinking, the process of paying attention, and the particular strategies of using internal information to form judgments.

CONCLUSION

In this chapter I have described the theoretical background of MCT and the basic features of the S-REF model on which it is based. The present description leaves aside some aspects of the model less relevant to clinical practice. The reader interested in further issues of cognitive architecture and how the model relates to experimental data on cognitive bias should consult other sources (e.g., Wells & Matthews, 1994, 1996; Wells, 2000; Matthews & Wells, 1999).

The metacognitive model identifies a pattern of thinking called the CAS that causes psychological disorder. This syndrome emerges from the control that metacognitions have over appraisal and coping. Metacognitions represent information about internal thoughts and feelings and also strategies that control the nature of coping and thinking. The metacognitive knowledge base can be thought of as highly proceduralized, representing plans or programs that control cognition.

The implication of the metacognitive model is that treatment can focus on different levels and aspects of the system. This gives rise to a range of new ways of working. The therapist should focus on removing the CAS. Techniques to enable this have been developed. It implies that treatment should focus on modifying erroneous metacognitive beliefs. It also implies that in addition to modifying propositional knowledge or beliefs, it is important to refine the patient's procedural knowledge (implicit metacognitive plans). This means training patients so that they develop new skills for responding to inner events in a flexible and decentered way. It is through the practice of standing back from thoughts and experiencing them in a detached way that the person develops the metacognitive programs necessary to control the effects of unwanted conscious experiences.

In conclusion, three important types of therapeutic change emerge from this analysis: (1) modification of thinking style or strategy (the CAS), (2) modification of declarative metacognitive beliefs, and (3) acquisition of new procedural knowledge or implicit plans for guiding processing and subjective experience. In this book I will describe in detail the implementation of metacognitive therapy that has been systematically developed to produce these effects.

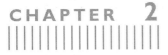

CHAPTER 2

Assessment

In this chapter I describe the methods of assessment used in the treatment of and the research in MCT. This chapter is not concerned with general areas of psychological assessment and diagnosis. If the reader intends to implement MCT, it is important that he or she possesses basic competency in the assessment and diagnosis of psychological disorder.

Despite the fact that MCT is based on a generic theory and could be developed for application in this form (see Chapter 11), it is currently assumed that use of disorder-specific models provides the most effective form of intervention because they capture unique processes and specific metacognitive content in their maintenance. The application of disorder-specific models is aided by accurate diagnosis as a prerequisite to case formulation.

There are four principal goals of assessment: (1) to establish an accurate diagnosis; (2) to obtain information about the severity, history, and development of a disorder; (3) to obtain information necessary for generating a case formulation; and (4) to evaluate treatment progress and overall outcome in relation to target variables. The process of establishing a diagnosis is not covered here. However, diagnostic criteria for each of the disorders covered in this volume is summarized as reference points in the individual disorder chapters. The method of obtaining information for case formulation is dealt with in detail in the individual disorder chapters in the form of case conceptualization interview schedules.

This chapter focuses on the assessment of metacognitive beliefs and the CAS and reviews measurement scales and questionnaires used in treatment and research. Not much detail is given to the psychometric properties of questionnaires, as this information can be obtained elsewhere (e.g., Wells, 2000, and the source articles referenced).

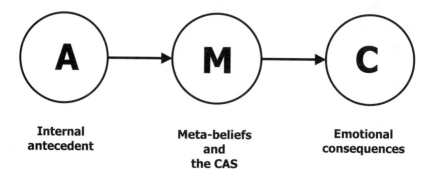

FIGURE 2.1. The central axis of the A-M-C model.

The starting point for the present review of assessment is the central axis of the A-M-C model introduced in the previous chapter and depicted here in Figure 2.1.

OPERATIONALIZING THE **A-M-C** MODEL

Following diagnostic screening, at the assessment phase, the therapist obtains a basic impression of the nature of the CAS, metacognitive beliefs, and symptoms using the A-M-C model as a blueprint. The therapist usually begins this process by exploring emotions and related symptoms (C) in a recent and suitable time frame, say, of the last 2 weeks.

Useful questions for exploring emotions are as follows:

Emotional Consequences (C)

1. "Thinking back over the past 2 weeks, what has your mood/anxiety been like?"
2. "What physical symptoms have you noticed?"
3. "What changes have you noticed in your behavior?"
4. "Have you had any thoughts of harming yourself?" (Consider risk assessment and deterrents if warranted.)

Once the characteristics of emotional and behavioral responses have been clearly determined, it is necessary to assess the base rates of behaviors and emotional symptoms. In particular, the therapist enquires about the frequency and duration of these factors.

Questioning then progresses to exploring the triggering influences on symptoms that are subsumed under activating events (A). Of particular focus in the metacognitive approach are *inner activating* events:

Activating Inner Event (A)

5. "Has anything or any situation made you feel worse?"
6. "What was the initial thought or feeling you had at the time?"
7. "Thinking back to the last time you felt more anxious/depressed, what happened to trigger it? Can you identify an initial thought or feeling that you had?"
8. "Has there been a time when you were more wrapped up in thinking about your problem? What was the thought that started that the last time it happened?"

The therapist searches for an *inner event* that typically takes the form of a negative thought that occurs in an uncued fashion or by situations, sensations, or emotions. Of particular importance is the trigger that precedes a state of sustained thinking about, coping with, or attending to threat. Once the inner event (e.g., the first thought in the worry sequence) is identified, the therapist then proceeds to ask about the nature of the CAS and the metacognitions associated with it.

The CAS and Metacognitions (M)

9. "When you had that experience, what happened to your thinking?"
10. "Did you worry or dwell on things? How long did that last?"
11. "Did you pay more attention to what was troubling you? What was that like?"
12. "Did you do anything to control the way you felt? What did you do?"
13. "Did you do anything to change your thoughts? What did you do?"
14. "Did you try not to think certain things or avoid anything?"
15. "Are there any advantages to worrying or ruminating? What are they?"
16. "Are there any advantages to focusing on thoughts/feelings? What are they?"
17. "How does focusing your attention on threat help?"
18. "What would happen if you didn't control your thoughts/emotions?"
19. "What's the worst that could happen if you continue to feel [or think] like this?"
20. "How much control do you have over your worries or depressive thoughts?"

These questions are usually sufficient to gain a rudimentary impression of the CAS and positive and negative metacognitive beliefs. However, in some cases it is necessary to modulate the patient's level of affect to gain access to the necessary information. This is where behavioral assessment tests can play a role.

Behavioral Assessment Tests in Anxiety

If questions like those cited above fail to identify the broad features of the CAS, the cause may well be limited emotion (e.g., anxiety) during the time frame under question. It may suffice to widen the time frame, but the patient's memory for events can be impaired. It is sometimes the case that the patient has managed to successfully avoid anxiety-provoking situations. In each case the use of behavioral assessment tests (BATs) coupled with the type of questions listed above is recommended.

A BAT involves exposing the patient to a feared situation that resembles the situation that is normally problematic. For example, in social phobia the patient can be asked to role-play a conversation with a confederate or to enter an avoided situation such as standing in line at the bank. A health-anxious patient with cancer concerns can be asked to read a magazine article about cancer detection. The person with generalized anxiety can be asked to identify a situation that would make him or her worry and then seek it out. The patient with obsessions and compulsions can be asked to call up an obsessional thought or to touch a contaminated object. In many cases the mere suggestion of these activities is sufficient to prompt anticipatory worry and unhelpful coping behaviors. The therapist proceeds with a series of modified questions as follows:

Emotional Consequences (C)

1. "Thinking about the situation you have been exposed to, how did you feel emotionally?"
2. "Did you notice physical symptoms [What were they?]?"
3. "Did you notice changes in your behavior?"
4. "Did you notice changes in your thoughts?"

Activating Inner Event (A)

5. "What was the initial thought that started your apprehension?"
6. "Did you get wrapped up in thinking about what could happen? What was the thought that started that?"

The CAS and Metacognitions (M)

7. "When you had that thought, what happened to your thinking?"
8. "Did you worry or dwell on things?"

9. "Did you pay more attention to threat? What was that like?"
10. "Did you do anything to control the way you felt? What did you do?"
11. "Did you do anything to change your thoughts? What did you do?"
12. "Did you try not to think certain thoughts or to avoid anything?"
13. "Are there any advantages to worrying or ruminating?"
14. "Are there any advantages to focusing on thoughts/feelings?"
15. "How does focusing your attention on threat help?"
16. "What would happen if you didn't control your thoughts/emotions?"
17. "What's the worst that could happen if you continue to feel/think this way?"
18. "Do you believe your worries are controllable?"

QUESTIONNAIRE MEASURES

Several questionnaires have been developed to provide a comprehensive assessment of the dimensions of metacognition for research and clinical purposes. All these measures have been psychometrically evaluated. The measures reviewed in this section are the Metacognitions Questionnaires, the Thought Control Questionnaire, the Anxious Thoughts Inventory, the Meta-Worry Questionnaire, and the Thought Fusion Instrument.

Metacognitions Questionnaires (MCQ-65 and MCQ-30)

This instrument is a trait measure of several metacognitive parameters, some of which are central to the metacognitive model of psychological disorder. A large body of empirical evidence supporting metacognitive theory is based on research using the MCQ. The original instrument (MCQ-65; Cartwright-Hatton & Wells, 1997) consisted of 65 items; a more recent 30-item version (MCQ-30; see Appendix 1) with similar psychometric properties is now available (Wells & Cartwright-Hatton, 2004). A copy of the longer and more comprehensive 65-item version can be located in Wells (2000).

The MCQ measures the following domains of metacognition on five separate subscales:

1. Positive beliefs about worry (e.g., "Worrying helps me cope").
2. Negative beliefs about worry concerning uncontrollability and danger (e.g., "When I start worrying I cannot stop").
3. Low cognitive confidence (e.g., "I have a poor memory").

4. Need to control thoughts (e.g., "Not being able to control my thoughts is a sign of weakness").
5. Cognitive self-consciousness (e.g., "I pay close attention to the way my mind works").

The psychometric properties of MCQ-65 are as follows. Internal consistency (Cronbach's alpha) for subscales is .72–.89. Stability as assessed by test–retest coefficients across a 5-week time interval range between .76 and .89 for the individual subscales. The subscales are positively correlated with trait-anxiety, pathological worry, depressive symptoms, and obsessive–compulsive symptoms (Cartwright-Hatton & Wells, 1997; Wells & Papageorgiou, 1998b; Myers & Wells, 2005; Gwilliam, Wells, & Cartwright-Hatton, 2004). There is some specificity in relationships, with the uncontrollability and danger subscale showing the strongest relationships with worry and trait anxiety measures. The uncontrollability and danger subscale discriminated patients with generalized anxiety disorder and obsessive–compulsive disorder from patients with panic disorder or social phobia (Cartwright-Hatton & Wells, 1997). The need for control subscale also appears significantly higher in patients with generalized anxiety disorder when compared to panic and social phobia groups (Wells & Carter, 2001).

In summary, the MCQ-65 shows good reliability and convergent, construct, and discriminative validity. There is evidence that it is responsive to metacognitive treatment (e.g., Papageorgiou & Wells, 2000).

A limitation of the MCQ-65 is its length and the time required to complete it. As a result, a shortened and refined version, the MCQ-30 was developed (Wells & Cartwright-Hatton, 2004).

The MCQ-30 (see Appendix 1) retains the factor structure of the MCQ-65 as verified by confirmatory factor analysis. Cronbach alphas for the individual subscales range from .72 to .93. Retest correlations across an interval of 22–118 days were as follows: total score = .75, positive beliefs = .79, uncontrollability/danger = .59, confidence = .69, need for control = .74, and cognitive self-consciousness = .87 (Wells & Cartwright-Hatton, 2004). In terms of construct validity, positive correlations between the subscales and theoretically appropriate measures have been demonstrated and the factor structure replicated (Spada, Mohiyeddini, & Wells, 2008). The relationships are consistent with those found with the MCQ-65. MCQ-30 subscales are responsive to metacognitive therapy (e.g., Wells et al., 2008).

Thought Control Questionnaire

The Thought Control Questionnaire (TCQ; Wells & Davies, 1994) was developed to assess individual differences in the use of strategies for controlling unpleasant and intrusive thoughts. It is important not to view thought suppression as a unitary construct. Moreover, suppression can be thought of as an objective that can be achieved in different ways. Some strategies in particular may be counterproductive, as suggested by the metacognitive theory.

A factor-analytic approach was used to refine the original conceptually derived pool of items, leading to a reliable five-factor scale (Wells & Davies, 1994). The five-factor solution was subsequently replicated in a sample of patients with depression or posttraumatic stress disorder (PTSD; Reynolds & Wells, 1999).

The five (factors) subscales of the TCQ are:

1. Distraction (e.g., "I do something that I enjoy").
2. Social control (e.g., "I ask my friends if they have similar thoughts").
3. Worry (e.g., "I focus on different negative thoughts").
4. Punishment (e.g., "I punish myself for thinking the thought").
5. Reappraisal (e.g., "I try to reinterpret the thought").

Cronbach alphas for the subscales range from .64 to .79. Test–retest correlations across a 6-week period were as follows: distraction = .72, social control = .79, worry = .71, punishment = .64, and reappraisal = .67 (Wells & Davies, 1994).

As far as construct validity is concerned, the *worry* and *punishment* subscales are positively correlated with a range of different measures of emotional disorder. Relationships between disorder measures and the remaining TCQ subscales tend to be negative and nonsignificant, with the exception of social anxiety, which is significantly negatively correlated with social control. Social control also appears to be significantly and negatively associated with trauma symptoms (e.g., Holeva, Tarrier, & Wells, 2001). However, the use of worry to control thoughts is positively associated with traumatic stress symptoms both cross-sectionally and longitudinally (Holeva et al., 2001; Roussis & Wells, 2006).

The discriminative validity of TCQ is evident in studies that have compared diagnostic and symptom groups. Amir, Cashman, and Foa (1997) showed that individuals with obsessive–compulsive disorder used more punishment, worry, reappraisal, and social control than nonpatients, who in turn used more distraction. The two strongest discriminating strategies were worry and punishment, a finding replicated by Abramowitz, Whiteside, Kalsy, and Tolin (2003). Warda and Bryant (1998) compared people with and without acute stress disorder following road accidents and found that those with stress disorder endorsed greater use of worry and punishment. Subscales also appear to discriminate patients with a diagnosis of schizophrenia from nonpatients, with patients endorsing greater worry and punishment and less distraction (Morrison & Wells, 2000).

Anxious Thoughts Inventory

The Anxious Thoughts Inventory (AnTI) was designed as a multidimensional measure of worry aimed at capturing basic content domains and the distinction between worry and negative appraisal of worry. Worry about noncognitive events (e.g., relationships, bodily symptoms) has been termed Type 1 worry. In contrast, worry about thoughts and worry about worrying has been termed meta-worry or Type 2 worry (Wells, 1994, 1995).

The AnTI (see Wells, 2000) consists of 22 items measuring three categories of worry on separate subscales. The subscales are:

1. Social worry (e.g., "I worry about doing or saying the wrong things when among strangers").
2. Health worry (e.g., "I worry about having a heart attack or cancer").
3. Meta-worry (e.g., "I worry that I cannot control my thoughts as well as I would like to").

Alpha coefficients for the subscales range form .75 to .84, and 6-week test–retest correlations were social worry = .76, health worry = .84, and meta-worry = .77.

The AnTI subscales are positively correlated with another measure of worry, the Penn State Worry Questionnaire (PSWQ; e.g., Wells & Papageorgiou, 1998b), but these associations are modest for the social and health subscales of the AnTI, as might be expected since the PSWQ is a content-free worry measure. Correlations between the AnTI subscales and another measure of meta-worry, the Meta-Worry Questionnaire (see below) showed that the meta-worry subscale had the strongest relationship (0.64) with the Meta-Worry Questionnaire (Wells, 2005a). Relationships between the AnTI subscales and trait anxiety are reported as .63 for social worry, .36 for health worry, and .68 for meta-worry.

The discriminative validity of the AnTI has been established with diagnostic groups (Wells & Carter, 2001). Meta-worry is significantly higher in patients with generalized anxiety disorder (DSM-IV) when compared to groups with panic disorder or social phobia and to nonpatient controls. As would be expected, health worry was highest in the panic group and social worry highest in the social phobia group, but participants with generalized anxiety disorder did not differ significantly from these groups on social and health subscales since they showed high worry across all domains.

Meta-Worry Questionnaire

The AnTI combines items concerning the uncontrollability and danger of worry in its meta-worry subscale. Furthermore, it assesses the frequency rather than the level of belief in meta-worry. The Meta-Worry Questionnaire (MWQ; Wells, 2005a) was conceived as a means of specifically assessing the danger aspect of meta-worry and assessing the frequency of meta-worry and belief level. The instrument was constructed as a means of testing the metacognitive model in the context of DSM-IV generalized anxiety disorder.

The instrument consists of seven items reflecting dangers of worrying. A copy of the scale is reproduced in Appendix 2. Factor analysis of responses in a student sample revealed a single factor for each of the frequency and belief dimensions. The seven items of the scale are listed below:

1. "I am going crazy with worrying."
2. "My worrying will escalate and I'll cease to function."
3. "I'm making myself ill with worrying."
4. "I'm abnormal for worrying."
5. "My mind can't take the worrying."
6. "I'm losing out in life because of worrying."
7. "My body can't take the worrying."

Cronbach coefficients for the frequency scale were .88 and .95 for the belief scale. The MWQ appears to be meaningfully correlated with other measures of metacognition. In particular the MWQ scales show significantly stronger positive correlations with negative beliefs about worry than with positive beliefs about worry measured with the MCQ.

As far as discriminative validity is concerned, the MWQ differentiated nonpatients meeting criteria for DSM-IV generalized anxiety disorder from two groups of individuals classified as having somatic anxiety or no anxiety (Wells, 2005a).

Thought Fusion Instrument

The Thought Fusion Instrument (TFI) was developed originally by Wells, Gwilliam, and Cartwright-Hatton (2001) to assess beliefs about thoughts across "fusion" domains that are considered relevant in the metacognitive formulation and treatment of obsessive–compulsive disorder. Three fusion content domains are captured by this 14-item instrument on a single scale. These domains are Thought Event Fusion (TEF: "My thoughts alone have the power to change the course of events"), Thought Action Fusion (TAF: "If I have thoughts about harming someone, I will act on them"), and Thought Object Fusion (TOF: "My memories/thoughts can be passed into objects").

Factorially a single dimension has emerged in college students. Cronbach's alpha for the scale was .89. Meaningful positive correlations have been found between the TFI, the MCQ, and measures of obsessive–

compulsive symptoms (Gwilliam, Wells, & Cartwright-Hatton, 2004; Myers & Wells, 2005). A copy of the TFI can be found in Appendix 3.

RATING SCALES

While each of the scales reviewed have been subjected to psychometric evaluation and development, several other practice-oriented rating scales are available to assist in the treatment of patients and the weekly monitoring of patient progress. These scales have proven to be valuable tools for clinicians practicing metacognitive therapy although their psychometric properties are not currently known.

The aim of these instruments is to provide useful information for case formulation, to allow monitoring of change in key underlying causal factors, and to bring a particular focus to treatment sessions, thereby reducing therapist drift.

CAS-I

Dimensions of the CAS and metacognitive beliefs can be assessed with disorder-specific rating scales and more generically (though this is not the preferred option) with the CAS-1. These scales provide a means of monitoring changes in worry, threat monitoring, and unhelpful coping behaviors. The scales also contain a measure of metacognitive beliefs that should be the focus of modification. The disorder-specific scales are preferred over CAS-1 when they can be used, as the beliefs and behaviors represented in the former have greater specificity.

CAS-1 (see Appendix 6) contains four sets of items rated on 9-point Likert-style rating scales ranging from 0 to 8. It assesses the proportion of time engaged in worry/rumination, threat monitoring, and coping behaviors. The last item asks for ratings across a range of metacognitive beliefs. These beliefs are divided into negative beliefs and positive beliefs. This instrument is intended for use when diagnosis is uncertain or the patient does not fulfill specific diagnostic criteria that would indicate more appropriate use of the disorder-specific scales.

In the context of a specific diagnosis the disorder-specific rating scales provide a more comprehensive coverage of the types of behaviors and metacognitions that are normally found. Four scales are included in Appendices 7–10 and are recommended for generalized anxiety disorder (GADS-R), posttraumatic stress disorder (PTSD-S), obsessive–compulsive disorder (OCD-S), and major depressive disorder (MDD-S).

These instruments are intended to be administered at assessment and at each treatment session. By necessity they contain a restricted range of items. They are not intended to replace more comprehensive assessment of beliefs by the appropriate questionnaires and inventories reviewed earlier. The scales represent supplementary and frequently used measures that are used for monitoring weekly progress.

Each scale has two conceptually distinct parts: one that assesses the patient's symptoms and responses in the past week, and another that measures the general level of the patient's metacognitive belief. The belief section assesses both negative and positive metacognitions.

Using the Scales to Assess Treatment

The rating scales are administered at the beginning of each treatment session. Then the scores on the items are briefly and collaboratively reviewed with patients. The most important items from the therapist's perspective are those representing the underlying mechanisms thought to maintain the disorder (i.e., items 2 and onwards).

The first item on each scale is a distress/disability index used to assess general treatment effectiveness. Item 2 relates to the extent of perseverative processes, such as worry in generalized anxiety disorder, rituals in obsessive–compulsive disorder, going over events in posttraumatic stress disorder, and ruminations in major depressive disorder. The other items assess unhelpful coping behaviors, many of which are directly aimed at controlling or biasing cognition in a particular way. The final item assesses metacognitive beliefs in the negative and positive content domains.

In each case the aim of treatment is to reduce the distress rating to 0. But this should not be in the context of persistent or increased levels of avoidance. The scales are used by the therapist to focus treatment on underlying causal mechanisms and processes. With this objective the following outcomes should be monitored and achieved:

1. The amount of perseveration (worry, rumination, rituals, etc.) should decrease to levels of 0–1 by the end of treatment.
2. Unhelpful coping behaviors should decrease to 0 as an end-of-treatment target. Residual low-level behaviors are common even when metacognitive beliefs have been eliminated and should be explored (the therapist should question whether untapped idiosyncratic beliefs are causing this).
3. Avoidance should decrease to 0 by the end of treatment. Work on residual avoidance and residual use of coping behaviors may be necessary before termination of regular therapeutic contact.
4. Negative and positive beliefs should be at 0 by the end of treatment. Typically, negative beliefs about uncontrollability are targeted and modified first in treatment. In most circumstances an end point can be achieved in which the majority of beliefs are at 0 by the end of treatment, with at worst a few beliefs having residual ratings of 10.

A SEVEN-STEP ASSESSMENT PLAN

It is useful to have a basic road map for guiding the sequence of assessment and determining how procedures such as assessment of metacognitions fit into the whole assessment session. Below is a seven-step plan that summarizes the typical format of a metacognitive therapy assessment session:

- Step 1: Determine the basic nature of the problem in the past month—for example:
    "How have you been feeling in the past month?"
    "What has your mood/anxiety been like? How much time has it been like that?"
    "What situations trigger anxiety/distress?"
    "What is the effect on behavior, avoidance, etc.?"
- Step 2: Determine a time line—for example:
    "How has the problem developed over time?"
    "Are there multiple problems?"
    "What is the sequence of them? Which came first?"
    "Might they be related?"
- Step 3: Diagnosis (if applicable) and risk assessment.
    Use diagnostic screening methods (e.g., the Structured Clinical Interview for DSM-IV).
    Review medical history and details of medication. Assess level of risk of harm to self and others (act to reduce risk if it is present).
- Step 4: Explore A-M-Cs.
    What are the triggers/situations (A)? (What are the cognitions/beliefs that are internal triggers?).
    What are the metacognitions (M) and the nature of the CAS? What is the effect on emotions?
- Step 5: Select and administer appropriate measures, depending on the diagnosis or the nature of the problem.
    Use general measures of mood and anxiety and disorder-specific measures of cognition and behavior (e.g., Beck Depression Inventory II: Beck, Steer, & Brown, 1996; Beck Anxiety Inventory: Beck, Epstein, Brown, & Steer, 1988; GAD-S, AnTI: Wells, 1994).
- Step 6: Explore and deal with issues of motivation and engagement.
- Step 7: Determine the patient's goals for therapy.

CONCLUSION

In this chapter basic components and tools of assessment were described and the properties of a range of measures were presented. It is beyond the scope of this book to consider issues of reliable and effective assessment in detail. It is assumed that the clinician already possesses the requisite skills for this undertaking. The material contained here is intended to augment existing assessment and diagnostic competencies.

Assessment continues throughout the therapeutic process in the form of monitoring patient progress in terms of symptom levels and the impact of interventions on underlying psychological maintenance processes and mechanisms. To this end questionnaires and specific rating scales should be utilized. The rating scales offer a means of staying "on track" within and across treatment sessions, as the therapist's overall goal of treatment can be operationalized using them. The CAS and metacognitive beliefs are clearly represented in the individual rating scales. CAS-1 provides a generic alternative measure when patients do not satisfy criteria for the disorders covered by the specific scales.

Assessment has been presented in this chapter as a general initial process, but in practice it is extended into the interview that is implemented as a means of generating a case formulation. That process is described in detail later in this book in the individual disorder chapters.

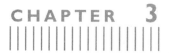

CHAPTER 3

Foundation Metacognitive Therapy Skills

The effective implementation of MCT requires the use of several fundamental skills. There are four particular foundation skills that are important as a keel on which to build treatment. These skills are the focus of the present chapter.

The first skill concerns the therapist's own ability to comprehend the different levels of cognition and to be able to shift between them, that is, to make a distinction between what is metacognition and what is "ordinary" cognition. The second skill is the ability to identify maladaptive cognitive processes that constitute the CAS in their different guises. The third skill is using metacognitive-focused Socratic dialogue. The fourth skill is learning to implement metacognitive-based exposure.

MCT is a skilled undertaking. Practice is the key to efficient and effective use of this approach. Supervision is a powerful ally in maintaining an appropriate focus on metacognitive factors in treatment and in developing greater levels of skill.

IDENTIFYING AND SHIFTING LEVELS

The natural tendency of the patient and the therapist is to conduct therapy at the cognitive level. Cognitive therapists usually engage the patient in reality testing of ideas in order to "encourage a more accurate description and analysis of the way things are" (Beck, Rush, Shaw, & Emery, 1979, p. 152). The focus is on examining the data against which to test the patient's ideas. Reality testing also consists of identifying cognitive distortions in the patient's thoughts and beliefs. It is likely that standard CBT procedures like this accomplish metacognitive changes—for instance, they certainly rely on fostering metacognitive awareness through the daily record of automatic thoughts. But patients are left evaluating thoughts against reality, a conceptual process, rather than simply choosing not to engage with their thoughts (a preferred goal of MCT).

If the therapist chooses the CBT approach, important aspects of MCT are missing because the work conducted is at the object level. The therapist joins with the patient in assuming that the thought or belief might be correct. Therefore great conceptual activity needs to be expended in evaluating the thought. If it is correct, then energy needs to be directed at problem solving. In part this is a form of conceptual processing and goal-directed coping that our patients are already engaged in. For example, a woman recently receiving treatment for generalized anxiety asked, "How do I decide which worries I need to respond to and which ones I can dismiss as distorted?" This person and the therapist were in cognitive mode. Unfortunately, they continued to discuss how it was possible to evaluate how realistic a worry was, and if it was realistic, then how to reasonably deal with it.

Although the therapist and the patient evaluate thoughts in CBT, which involves metacognitive awareness and metacognitive appraisals, treatment clearly operates at the cognitive (object-mode) level since the goal is to reality-test ordinary cognitions rather than to develop or test metacognitions. The metacognitive therapist must shift to a metacognitive level of working instead. For example, in the case of generalized anxiety disorder cited above, the therapist might say, "It seems as if you believe that you need to think about a worry in order to be able to cope. What would happen if you decided to do nothing with your worries?" This approach may elicit metacognitive beliefs about the need to engage in sustained conceptual activity and the possible negative consequences of not doing so, which can be tested. This line of questioning is firmly grounded in the metacognitive level of working and changes the way the patient experiences a worry (i.e., in a detached way) and explores and modifies metacognitive beliefs about worry. There is no attempt to work at the ordinary cognitive level of testing the reality of individual concerns.

The fundamental nature of the metacognitive level of working is that it should enable the patient to become aware of maladaptive thinking styles and processes, and to change the mental model of cognition and ways of experiencing thoughts. This entails more than simply reality testing the content of thoughts and beliefs and requires giving up maladaptive thinking styles (processes) and working at the higher level of testing the validity of beliefs about thinking.

As an example, let's consider the case of a young man who believed that he was "defective." He had suffered a history of abuse. This was his evidence of being defective or "spoiled." A cognitive therapist would be likely to work at the cognitive level and to ask him to consider evidence against this idea, to examine the cognitive distortion in this belief, and to consider alternative conclusions. If the therapist used this approach, it migh well be effective, but it might not provide an alternative way of relating to negative self-beliefs and memories. CBT changes the level of conviction or the content of the belief but it does not help the patient to see that he is more than and separate from his beliefs and his memories. It would be useful to stand back from the belief and see it as an event in the mind rather than an essence of self, as one might with techniques such as detached mindfulness that are used in MCT.

A woman with obsessive–compulsive symptoms believed that she was contaminated with feces. She was concerned that she would become ill and would pass on diseases to her young daughter unless she scrubbed her hands in bleach. In CBT she might be asked to test her predictions that she was contaminated by refraining from washing in bleach and waiting to see if she or her child became ill. This approach would be a reasonable one to take in treatment, similar to exposure and response prevention. But her dysfunctional metacognitions might continue to operate because treatment has worked at the cognitive rather than at the metacognitive level.

   If we were fortunate, this treatment might have enabled her to reality-test the belief that she is contaminated. In essence, we have removed the belief in contamination, just as washing removes that belief, albeit temporarily. In metacognitive therapy we aim to modify metacognitions rather than the lower-level thoughts and beliefs such as those concerned with contamination. Thus, the therapist shifts the focus of discussion in the session away from considering contamination (cognitive level) and explores beliefs about the importance of thoughts about contamination (metacognitive level). The patient does not simply learn that she is not contaminated. Instead she learns that her thoughts concerning feces are unimportant and need not be acted upon in any special way.

A 37-year-old man who had been traumatized in a robbery was continuously troubled by head pain, anxiety attacks, and intrusive memories of the event. When asked about the way he had been coping with these symptoms he said that he had been avoiding going out, using alcohol to "knock himself out," and keeping himself alert to possible danger. He described how he had been going over the event to try and work out if there was anything he could have done differently in the situation. How can the therapist work at the metacognitive level in this case?

   The traditional treatment approach might consist of imaginal reliving of the event and some reality testing of the patient's distorted beliefs about himself and the nature of threat in the world. This would be an example of working at the cognitive level since we are changing the nature of his memory (cognition) and the content of his beliefs about himself and the world (cognition). Alternatively, the therapist could work at the metacognitive level by examining the way in which the patient controls his thinking about the trauma (metacognition), his beliefs about intrusive thoughts (metacognition), and his beliefs about the necessity to cope by going over events using rumination and worry (metacognition).

When the therapist and patient discuss the nature of problems in MCT, the therapist considers the patient's negative thoughts and beliefs about the self and the world as symptoms or triggers of the problem because the true problem rests with how the patient implicitly or explicitly interprets and deals with these cognitive events. Keeping this in mind should allow the metacognitive therapist to make the necessary adjustments to focus therapeutic work at the metacognitive level.

The metacognitive level of working is one in which we ask the patient to step back from the thought or belief and see it as an internal event, as a symptom that does not require a conceptual or analytical response. In order to do that we do not simply appraise its validity but we try to engender a sense or mental model of what it is, an event in the mind, and we modify the metacognitions that give rise to the thinking styles that continuously support it. In contrast, reality testing an ordinary thought or belief to check its validity reinforces the mental model that some thoughts are facts and others are not. This obscures the situation that irrespective of validity, thoughts and beliefs are mental experiences that communicate information. It does not really matter if they are accurate or not, what is important is how we experience them and how we respond to them. The crucial factor is the nature of the metacognitive model that we have of our own cognitions.

DETECTING THE CAS

When starting out practicing MCT, therapists often fail to detect the CAS. Most prominent among these difficulties is the therapist's failure to recognize worry and rumination either in the patient's description of his or her thinking or as a process activated in session. It is essential that the therapist is and eventually the patient should become aware of and able to identify worry, rumination, threat monitoring, and counterproductive coping behaviors.

Periods of patient silence can be an indication that rumination and worry have been activated. Extended justifications of beliefs and repeated reflections on negative emotions are usually indicative of worrying or ruminating. A preoccupation with detail in verbal descriptions of events might be a marker for rumination or avoidant coping. In order to identify the process, the therapist must think beyond the content and validity of what the patient states and be aware of the activation of chains of negative processing. When these are observed they should be pinpointed and labeled to increase patient awareness, and the process interrupted rather than the content reality-tested.

Although these processes frequently play out spontaneously in the therapeutic encounter, a method of detecting them is to ask direct questions about their occurrence. The metacognitive therapist asks questions about dwelling on thoughts, worrying, ruminating, and brooding in response to stresses and emotions. The therapist aims to quantify in terms of frequency and duration the occurrence of these thinking styles. The therapist also asks if the patient has found that his or her attention has become "stuck" on any one thing in particular and what that is. This can be the basis for identifying threat monitoring. The therapist asks if the patient has tried to control thoughts or to cope with emotions or any perceived threat, and what form these responses take and how effective they have been.

The process of threat monitoring may also be observed in session. For example, an obsessional patient could be seen scanning the floor during treatment. This was apparent on the videotape of the session brought to supervision, but the student therapist had not observed this at the time of therapy. At the next session this floor scanning was noted and the therapist asked the patient about it. The patient stated that she was looking to see if there was any evidence that rat poison might have been spilt on the floor. This prompted a very useful discussion about the problem of trying to remain safe through threat-monitoring strategies. In other words, what effect does this strategy have on the frequency of thoughts about contamination and on learning that thoughts about contamination are unimportant?

In another example, a health-anxious patient repeatedly grasped his neck during the assessment interview. When asked about this action, he reported that he had to perform this action to feel his pulse to check whether his heart was beating normally. In this case, the threat-monitoring strategy had been detected by the therapist.

Some maladaptive coping behaviors are covert and readily overlooked by the therapist. The therapist must make a habit of asking about suppression, thought control strategies, emotional control, and avoidance strategies and exploring their idiosyncratic nature. For example, one patient stated that she was trying to stop her thoughts of a traumatic event. The therapist assumed that this meant she was suppressing them and failed to explore this statement in sufficient detail. Later the therapist discovered that the patient was trying to get rid of her thoughts by thinking as much as possible about the trauma because she had read that in order to overcome fear it must be confronted. When the patient was instructed to reduce this excessive thinking, she discovered that her thoughts about the trauma faded.

There are additional strategies for detecting the CAS, such as examining the idiosyncratic rating scales (e.g., CAS-1) and drawing the patient's attention to the occurrence of individual components. The therapist can follow this strategy by instructing patients to record how often they notice themselves dwelling on negative thoughts or trying to suppress ideas that might trigger their concerns.

It should be expected that patients continue to engage in worry and rumination and other aspects of the CAS for some time during the early stages of treatment. It is important for the therapist to repeatedly draw the patient's attention to these processes since they will be manifested in different ways. The demonstration that change in content and focus is not indicative of change in processes is useful in building greater meta-awareness and in arresting perseverative activity.

USING A METACOGNITIVE-FOCUSED SOCRATIC DIALOGUE

MCT uses Socratic dialogue to explore meanings, underlying processes, and beliefs. However, the focus of the dialogue differs from the focus that is typical of CBT. In CBT the therapist uses questioning to explore the content of thoughts and beliefs and to direct treatment to modifying beliefs. In MCT the therapist uses questioning to detect and arrest the CAS. When beliefs or assumptions are a focus, the Socratic dialogue is aimed at detecting and modifying beliefs about thoughts and emotions (metacognitions), rather than thoughts about the self and the world.

The two dialogues presented below first illustrate the traditional CBT approach and then the new MCT approach.

CBT Dialogue

THERAPIST: What led you to feel depressed?

PATIENT: When John didn't want to see me.

THERAPIST: What did that mean to you?

PATIENT: I think no one likes me, I'm just boring.

THERAPIST: So it sounds as if you have negative thoughts when that happens. Do you think everyone gets depressed when this happens?

PATIENT: No, because they don't think it's as important.

THERAPIST: Right, so we need to examine what you think. What does it mean to you when people don't want to meet up?

PATIENT: It means I'm boring, and they're not interested in me.

THERAPIST: How much do you believe it's because you're boring?

PATIENT: I must be, otherwise people would invite me out.

THERAPIST: How does that thought make you feel?

PATIENT: Very sad and lonely.

THERAPIST: So it's the meaning that you give to situations that makes you sad. It's what you believe about them. You think people don't see you because you are boring. What if there are alternative and more likely reasons why people can't see you?

MCT Dialogue

THERAPIST: What led you to feel depressed?

PATIENT: When John didn't want to see me.

THERAPIST: What did that make you think?

PATIENT: I think no one likes me, I'm just boring.

THERAPIST: So it sounds as if you have negative thoughts when that happens. What's the first thought that starts you off?

PATIENT: I think, Why doesn't he want to know me?

THERAPIST: Right. Let's examine how you think in response to that initial thought. What do you go on to think?

PATIENT: I try to work out what's wrong with me. Maybe it's because I'm boring, maybe they don't like me. I try and work out why it's happening to me.

THERAPIST: How much time do you spend doing that?

PATIENT: It can last hours.

THERAPIST: How does that make you feel?

PATIENT: Very sad and lonely.

THERAPIST: So it's the way you respond to the thought "Why doesn't John want to know me?" that makes you sad. You're trying to find an answer by analyzing what is wrong with you. Is that likely to make you feel happy or sad? What if there are better ways of responding to that thought?

The end question of each way of working is very different. In the CBT example the question is "What if there are alternative and more likely reasons why people can't see you?" Compare this with the MCT question: "What if there are better ways of responding to that thought?" The MCT approach focuses on the impact of the rumination process that is triggered by a negative thought and shifts the patient to a metacognitive mode of working. In contrast, the CBT dialogue is operating in object mode in which thoughts are evaluated to determine if they are facts. Furthermore, the patient is encouraged to continue analyzing reasons for not being seen, perpetuating a conceptual process rather than terminating it.

As in the example above, the Socratic dialogue in MCT aims to identify instances of worry/rumination and other features of the CAS. The exploration of different components of the CAS using a metacognitive-focused Socratic dialogue is illustrated further in the following dialogues.

Exploring Worry

THERAPIST: When you had the thought "I could have failed," what did you then go on to think about?

PATIENT: I thought of what I could have done and how I could deal with it next time.

THERAPIST: How long did you think like that?

PATIENT: For the rest of the evening. I couldn't get it out of my mind.

THERAPIST: So you were worrying about the future and how to cope?

PATIENT: Yes, I've got to think about it or I'll never get it out of my mind.

THERAPIST: Can you get it out of your mind so long as you think or worry about it?

Exploring Threat Monitoring

THERAPIST: Have you found that what you pay attention to has changed since you began feeling like this?

PATIENT: Yes, I'm aware of feeling tired and unwell most of the time.

THERAPIST: Is that something you check for?

PATIENT: When I get up in the morning I check to see how I feel, and then I know if it will be a good or a bad day.

THERAPIST: How do you expect to feel if it's a good day?

PATIENT: I should feel relaxed and rested, but usually I feel tired and my mind is hazy.

THERAPIST: How much of the time are you monitoring your mind and feelings?

PATIENT: I'm aware of it most of the time.

THERAPIST: If you are looking for feelings of tiredness are you more or less likely to find them?

Exploring Coping Behaviors (e.g., Thought Suppression, Avoidance)

THERAPIST: When you have the thought "I've got a brain tumor," what do you do to deal with it?

PATIENT: I reduce my activity because I don't want to cause a stroke. I then ask my partner for reassurance. If I'm really worried I make an appointment to see my doctor.

THERAPIST: The ways you cope are to reduce your activities and seek reassurance from your partner or doctor. Has that enabled you to overcome your problem?

PATIENT: No, I still have the symptoms, and I think "What if the tumor is still growing and hasn't been detected yet?"

THERAPIST: So what has happened to your worry since you've been coping like this? Has it stopped?

PATIENT: No, I'm still worried about my health.

THERAPIST: So perhaps we need to explore alternative ways of responding to your thought of a brain tumor. Perhaps you could choose to ban reassurance seeking, postpone your worries, and increase your activities.

Using Socratic Dialogue to Uncover Metacognitive Beliefs

While the examples above illustrate using Socratic dialogue to explore and weaken the CAS, it also serves in searching for metacognitive beliefs. Our patients show a response pattern consisting of the CAS because of the influence of metacognitive beliefs on processing. Uncovering these beliefs and changing them is an important feature of MCT. The following extracts from cases illustrate the use of the Socratic method in detecting metacognitive beliefs (the beliefs are italicized for ease of identification). The questions used typically ask about the advantages and disadvantages of using thinking styles, about the controllability of thoughts, and about the worst consequences of having them.

Detecting Positive Metacognitive Beliefs about Worry

THERAPIST: We identified that you worry about failure and the future. Are there any advantages to worrying?

PATIENT: I'm not sure what you mean by "advantages."

THERAPIST: Does worrying help you in any way?

PATIENT: Yes, it's important to try and anticipate problems so that I can be prepared.

THERAPIST: Do you believe that worrying makes you prepared?

PATIENT: Yes, *if I worry, then I'll be able to deal with problems effectively in the future.*

THERAPIST: How much do you believe that on a scale of 0 to 100%?

PATIENT: Eighty percent. It wouldn't be right not to think about problems.

THERAPIST: So it's either worry or nothing in your mind?

PATIENT: Yes, now that you mention it, but what are the alternatives to worry?

Detecting Positive Metacognitive Beliefs about Threat Monitoring

PATIENT: I've made a complete fool of myself.

THERAPIST: How do you know?

PATIENT: I could see everyone looking at me.

THERAPIST: Do you normally check to see if people are looking at you?

PATIENT: No, it's more like a feeling.

THERAPIST: On this occasion did you check other people or was it a feeling?

PATIENT: Now that you ask, I guess it was more of a feeling.

THERAPIST: What feeling do you use to determine if you've made a fool of yourself?

PATIENT: If I feel awkward and rigid, I'm afraid they can see that.

THERAPIST: So the thing you focus on is whether you feel awkward and rigid?

PATIENT: Yes, I don't want to feel that.

THERAPIST: Are there any advantages to focusing your attention on those feelings?

PATIENT: It stops me from losing control.

THERAPIST: How much do you believe *focusing on your feelings stops you from losing control?*

PATIENT: If I didn't do it things would be worse. I'm sure it helps.

Detecting Negative Metacognitive Beliefs

THERAPIST: It sounds as if you are spending a lot of time analyzing what is wrong and worrying about the future. Does that make you feel better?

PATIENT: Sometimes, but usually it makes me feel more depressed.

THERAPIST: That process of analyzing and excessive thinking is called rumination. Could you stop doing it if it makes you feel worse?

PATIENT: No, I don't think it's controllable.

THERAPIST: How much do you believe *my rumination is uncontrollable*?

PATIENT: One hundred percent.

THERAPIST: Could anything bad happen if you continued to ruminate in this way?

PATIENT: I'm not sure.

THERAPIST: What's the worst that could happen?

PATIENT: I think it's abnormal, it's just further proof that I'm mentally ill, I'll always be a depressive, I can't control the way I think. (*Note:* What is the patient doing right now in this answer? Did you identify the start of a rumination sequence?)

Using Socratic Dialogue to Explore Maintenance Processes in Socialization

The therapist uses Socratic dialogue to communicate the metacognitive formulation and to engage the patient in the treatment process. This "socialization" of the patient to MCT is achieved by exploring maintenance processes as set out in the model. In particular, the therapist aims to show the impact of worry and rumination on anxiety or mood, the ineffectiveness of coping strategies such as thought suppression, and the consequences of threat monitoring on anxiety and appraisals. Some examples of these processes follow.

Threat Monitoring in a Case of Generalized Anxiety Disorder

THERAPIST: What do you think are the consequences of constantly paying attention to how your mind works?

PATIENT: I need to be sure that I'm not losing my mind.

THERAPIST: When you focus on your mind do you notice it is working how you want it to?

PATIENT: No, I usually find that it's not working how I'd expect.

THERAPIST: Could focusing in that way interfere with how well you think it works?

PATIENT: Yes, I suppose it could.

THERAPIST: So you see how one of your coping strategies of monitoring your mind is contributing to your worries. That sounds like it could be a vicious cycle to me.

Thought Suppression in a Case of Obsessive–Compulsive Disorder

THERAPIST: You said you try to control your thoughts. What do you do?

PATIENT: I try not to think about murderers.

THERAPIST: Does that seem to be working?

PATIENT: No, I still get the thoughts.

THERAPIST: Is it possible to forget about something that you are trying not to think about?

PATIENT: No, I suppose you have to remind yourself of what it is.

THERAPIST: That's right. Does pushing the thought away help you discover it is meaningless?

PATIENT: No, I suppose I'm scared of having the thought.

THERAPIST: So the way you deal with it can keep your anxiety going and make the thought more important than it really is.

Coping Behaviors in a Case of Panic Disorder

THERAPIST: How do you stop yourself from suffocating?

PATIENT: I slow down and take deep breaths. I have to get a special deep breath that clicks.

THERAPIST: Do you think there are any problems with doing that each time you think you're suffocating?

PATIENT: Well, sometimes I'm aware that I hyperventilate.

THERAPIST: Yes, that could make your symptoms worse, and that's one maintenance process. Let's explore another one. If you save yourself each time, do you discover that these are simply thoughts about suffocating?

PATIENT: No, I keep thinking it could happen next time.

THERAPIST: That's right. You don't allow yourself to discover that it's only a thought and that you are not going to suffocate. So the thought keeps its importance. (*Note:* The behavior prevents disconfirmation of belief in the thought. It also prevents the patient from relating to the thought as a thought, that is, from shifting from the cognitive level to the metacognitive level and becoming detached from it.)

Worrying in a Case of Hypochondriasis

THERAPIST: You said that worrying and analyzing your symptoms stops you from missing something that could be important and it could save your life. Do you think there are any problems with thinking like that as a way of coping?

PATIENT: Well, I don't suppose it's very positive.

THERAPIST: That's right. So how does thinking that way influence what you believe?

PATIENT: Well, I'm going to end up believing the worst.

THERAPIST: So is your problem a brain tumor or is your problem that you keep thinking the worst?

PATIENT: It might be that I keep thinking the worst.

METACOGNITIVELY FOCUSED VERBAL REATTRIBUTION

The verbal reattribution techniques in MCT are similar to those of CBT, but they differ in focus. They are used to modify negative and positive metacognitive beliefs rather than the content of other thoughts and beliefs. Common types of questions used in both CBT and MCT are as follows:

1. Questioning the evidence for and against the belief
   What is the evidence supporting this belief?
   What is the evidence against this belief?
2. Presenting counterevidence?
   Give information about the benign nature of anxiety.
   Show how worry is different from stress.
3. Identifying the cognitive distortion
   Is this an example of catastrophizing, black-and-white thinking?
4. Questioning the mechanism
   "How can worry or anxiety harm you?"
   "How can worrying keep you safe?"
5. Questioning the advantages and disadvantages of the belief
   "What are the advantages of controlling your thoughts?"
   "What are the disadvantages of controlling your thoughts?"
6. Evaluating the quality of the evidence supporting the belief
   "Would this evidence convince someone else?"
7. Rating and re-rating belief
   "How much do you believe that?"
   "How much do you believe that now that we've reviewed the evidence?"

The following examples illustrate this type of questioning to weaken a range of different metacognitive beliefs.

Negative Belief in Uncontrollability

THERAPIST: How much do you believe that your worry is uncontrollable?

PATIENT: Seventy percent.

THERAPIST: Have you tried to control it?

PATIENT: Yes, but it doesn't work. That's why I know I don't have control.

THERAPIST: How does a worry ever stop if you can't control it?

PATIENT: The problem is no longer there.

THERAPIST: So what happens to your worry if you have to answer the telephone?

PATIENT: Well, then it stops because I have to think about something else.

THERAPIST: So is that some evidence that you can control it?

PATIENT: Yes, a little evidence.

THERAPIST: Let's test your belief in uncontrollability. I'd like to introduce an experiment. . . .

Negative Belief in Danger

PATIENT: I don't want to think these thoughts.

THERAPIST: What's the worst that will happen if you allow yourself to have them?

PATIENT: I might act on them and harm someone.

THERAPIST: How much do you believe having a thought will make you act on it?

PATIENT: Ninety percent.

THERAPIST: What's your evidence?

PATIENT: I don't have any—I'm just worried it could happen.

THERAPIST: Maybe it's just a worry then. Is there any counterevidence?

PATIENT: Well, I've never harmed anyone before.

THERAPIST: That's a good point. How many bad thoughts have you had?

PATIENT: Too many to count.

THERAPIST: So is that evidence that thoughts have the power to make you do something or is it evidence they don't?

PATIENT: Maybe some evidence they don't have power.

THERAPIST: How much do you believe that they have power?

PATIENT: Seventy percent.

Positive Belief about Rumination

THERAPIST: How much do you believe that analyzing the past will help you feel better?

PATIENT: One hundred percent.

THERAPIST: Has it worked yet?

PATIENT: Sometimes I get the answer, so I think it does.

THERAPIST: Have you solved your problem of depression then?

PATIENT: No.

THERAPIST: So where's the evidence that it's working to help you overcome your depression?

PATIENT: Well, I don't really know. But I can't think about nothing.

THERAPIST: Sounds like you have a black-and-white view of your thinking. It's either analyzing the past or nothing as a means of dealing with your low mood. What do you think are the consequences of that?

PATIENT: Well, I guess I'll continue to analyze things.

THERAPIST: How often does that lead you to feel better?

PATIENT: Not always. I can get worse before getting better.

THERAPIST: So perhaps it makes you worse?

PATIENT: Yes, I think it does.

THERAPIST: So how much do you believe it's helping in the long term?

PATIENT: I don't know. Maybe I'm not doing it enough.

THERAPIST: Okay, should we get you to do it more and see if that helps?

PATIENT: No, I don't think it's going to make things better.

THERAPIST: How strong is your belief it helps then?

PATIENT: Less now, probably twenty percent.

METACOGNITIVELY DELIVERED EXPOSURE

Exposure is a component of MCT. However, treatment does not necessitate prolonged and repeated exposures as a means of producing emotional change. The goal of exposure in MCT varies: it is used both to modify beliefs and to strengthen alternative and more adaptive processing. Three types of metacognitively delivered exposure are used to (1) facilitate belief change in general, (2) specifically challenge metacognitive beliefs, and (3) promote adaptive processing of trauma.

General Belief Change

Any behavioral experiment that involves exposure to a feared stimulus with the aim of testing beliefs is an unspecified metacognitive technique since it is evoking the appraisal of cognition. Experiments of this kind can be improved by delivering them in more highly specified metacognitive terms. That is, the way in which a patient processes information during, before, and after exposure can be controlled to maximize belief change. This can be likened to writing a metacognitive script or plan for guiding processing.

> For example, a patient suffering from social phobia typically avoided paying attention to other people's faces during social interactions. She also ruminated about the impression she might have made for hours afterward. Despite the fact that she had been exposed daily to social situations, her belief that "people think I'm stupid" had been present for years. She had received psychological treatment several years earlier in which she had been exposed to social situations while learning to control her anxiety and to use self-assertiveness. This helped at the time, but she felt that her anxiety had continued to be a problem. During MCT she was exposed to social interactions under the instruction to focus attention on other peoples' faces. Specifically she was asked to "try to form a complete impression of what the other person looks like, as if you will need to recognize him or her in a crowd." In addition she was instructed to notice when she began to analyze her performance after the event and to ban this activity and apply *detached mindfulness* to her intrusive thoughts. This procedure of orchestrating her style of processing during and after exposure to situations enabled her to discover that her problem was one of negative thinking and not one of what people might think. For an experimental test of the effects of this type of approach, see Wells and Papageorgiou (1998b).

Challenging Metacognitive Beliefs

In MCT the therapist specifically targets positive and negative beliefs about thinking. Thus, exposure is presented with a rationale that is specifically intended to test metacognitive beliefs.

> For example, a patient with obsessive–compulsive disorder was asked to touch a contaminant and postpone washing to test his belief that "thinking it is contaminated must mean it is contaminated." This is very different from a habituation rationale (e.g., "Do not wash and your anxiety will subside") or a cognitive rationale (e.g., "Do not wash and you will discover that nothing bad will happen"). In the MCT condition the focus is on challenging the belief about the importance of the intrusive thought, not the likelihood of danger actually occurring or responsibility for preventing it. For an experimental test of the effects of this type of approach, see Fisher and Wells (2005).

In another example of MCT in generalized anxiety disorder, the therapist exposed the patient to the worry process as an explicit test of beliefs that worry is harmful (e.g., "Try to worry more to see if you become psychotic"). This differs from standard CBT where exposure involves avoided situations in order to reality-test the content of worry or exposure involves the worry process itself to promote habituation.

Facilitate Adaptive Processing of Trauma

This type of metacognitively delivered exposure aims to remove aspects of maladaptive processing and those coping styles that interfere with self-regulation. It is most often used in MCT for trauma. Here the patient is instructed to respond to spontaneous intrusive thoughts in a particular way that facilitates built-in and automatic self-regulation processes. This is not presented as a test of beliefs but as a way of removing barriers to normal emotional processing. It is not assumed, as is the case in usual CBT practice, that there should be repeated exposure to and elaboration of trauma memories. Instead patients are instructed to acknowledge their intrusions and to refrain from engaging with them in any way such as by analyzing the event, pushing intrusions away, or worrying about future danger. This approach is presented with the rationale that emotional healing is a natural process that occurs spontaneously if it is not disrupted by certain unhelpful responses to thoughts and feelings.

> For example, an individual traumatized by being stabbed in the street reported that he repeatedly had intrusive thoughts about the event and the feeling of heat in his abdomen at the site of the wound. Rather than going over his memory trying to defragment it and promote habituation, as might be practiced in CBT, the MCT therapist explored his typical response to the intrusion. The patient described normally trying to distract himself from the intrusion and analyzing what he could have done to fight off the attacker. The therapist instructed him to abandon these strategies and instead to keep a passive watch over the intrusion without pushing it away, without trying to distract from it, and without analyzing what he could have done. In this way the thought was deprived of its salience and influence and the patient began to notice that it faded on its own.

Using the P-E-T-S Protocol in Exposure

Exposure experiments in CBT have been conceptualized as consisting of four components—preparation, exposure, testing, and summarizing—which have been labeled the P-E-T-S protocol (Wells, 1997). They are normally used to test specific predictions based on the patient's thoughts/beliefs. Each element represents a stage in a sequence. These experiments are used in the treatment of anxiety disorders. Although they incorporate exposure, this is usually brief and is coupled with a specific rationale and a disconfirmatory strategy or test. The P-E-T-S system is depicted diagrammatically in Figure 3.1. This system is also normally used for testing metacognitive beliefs, such as the belief that rumination is uncontrollable, the belief that thoughts can be harmful, and the belief that worry is useful.

The first stage is preparation (P), which consists of focusing on the target metacognition to be challenged. It involves exploring the evidence for that metacognition and the coping behaviors that prevent its disconfirmation. A belief rating is made at this stage. Then a prediction is set up that specifies what should occur if the coping behaviors are modified. In doing so the therapist provides an explicit goal for the experiment as a means of evaluating a thought/belief.

The next phase is exposure (E). This refers to exposing the patient to the internal event that activates the metacognitive belief. For example, this could be exposure to bodily sensations or thoughts in obsessive–compulsive disorder (OCD), or avoided news items that normally lead to a thought that triggers worry in generalized anxiety disorder (GAD).

The third phase consists of the test (T). This is performing a change in behavior that acts as an unambiguous test of a patient's prediction. For

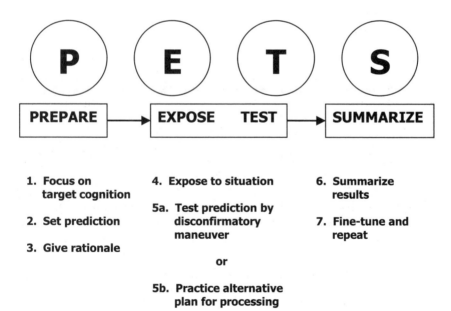

FIGURE 3.1. The P-E-T-S protocol for behavioral experiments. Adapted from Wells (1997). Copyright 1997 by John Wiley & Sons Limited. Adapted by permission.

example, while reading news items about crime a patient with GAD might try to worry intensely to test the prediction that it is possible to lose control of his or her mind. (In the later stages of treatment the test phase is often replaced with a practice phase involving practicing the implementation of alternative plans for processing in order to strengthen alternative response styles.)

The final phase is the summary (S). This involves summarizing the result of the experiment in relation to the original prediction and then rerating belief. The experiment is then refined and repeated in order to further lower the belief level.

An example of implementing an experiment using P-E-T-S can be seen in a patient with OCD who was concerned that he would molest children if he had thoughts of a sexual nature:

THERAPIST: What will happen if you have these thoughts?

PATIENT: Well, nothing will happen if I control them.

THERAPIST: What if you don't control them?

PATIENT: I'm afraid that I could do something.

THERAPIST: So you believe that having the thought has the power to make you act on it?

PATIENT: Yes, and that disgusts me.

THERAPIST: How much do you believe the thought could make you do it?

PATIENT: Sixty percent.

THERAPIST: If I asked you to have those thoughts right now, would that make you act on them?

PATIENT: No, because I'm not in a risky situation.

THERAPIST: What would be a risky situation to expose you to?

PATIENT: If you asked me to drive past a school.

THERAPIST: Okay, so we've identified a belief you have about these thoughts and a situation in which you could have them to test it out. You must challenge your belief about these thoughts in order to overcome your anxiety. What I want you to do for homework is to drive past a school while deliberately repeating these thoughts. In this way you can learn that these are only thoughts and they are not important. Can you think of a school you could try?

PATIENT: Yes, I know where all the local schools are because I try to avoid them.

THERAPIST: At the next session we'll review how the experiment went.

In this example we can identify the elements of P-E-T-S as follows:

P = Find a target metacognition: "The thoughts will make me act on them."

Make a belief rating (60%).

Identify a situation.

Explore the usual coping behaviors as a source of an alternative test strategy by reversing them (e.g., reverse controlling thoughts and avoidance). Set up a prediction ("Let's see if you act on it").

E = Drive past a school to elicit thoughts and activate belief.

T = Ban controlling thoughts and instead deliberately have more of them.

S = In the next session rerate belief and refine experiment as necessary.

Here the summarizing phase is carried over to the next treatment session because this experiment was set for homework. In other situations the whole experiment including the summary phase can be conducted during the treatment session. Some sessions contain several experiments of this kind.

CONCLUSION

In this chapter several foundation skills that are central to practicing MCT were described. Each of these skills represents an example of working at the metacognitive level in treatment, using Socratic dialogue, and implementing specific change strategies. These basic skills will be found reverberating in the material presented in the disorder-specific chapters throughout this book.

The therapist using MCT requires a clear understanding of metacognitive levels of working, and should be able to identify maladaptive processes and metacognitive beliefs. The ability to focus the therapeutic process on this level and away from ordinary cognition is crucial.

The therapist can use the basic techniques of cognitive therapy. However, he or she should implement them in a way that is parsimonious with the metacognitive model. Socratic dialogue should be utilized to explore the CAS, to examine maladaptive metacognitive beliefs, and to socialize to the metacognitive model. It should be used to challenge metacognitive beliefs and coupled with behavioral experiments in this regard.

The optimal use of exposure in MCT considers how exposure can be configured to change metacognitive beliefs or manipulate processing styles that support adaptive learning.

CHAPTER **4**

||||||||||||||||||||

Attention Training Techniques

This chapter introduces metacognitive treatment techniques that directly modify the control of attention. We saw in earlier chapters how patients are conceptualized as "locked into" unhelpful thinking patterns that they find difficult to bring under control. The metacognitive model assumes that the control of attention in psychological disorder becomes inflexible as attention is bound up with perseverative, self-focused, worry-based processing and monitoring for threat. The redirection of attention away from such activity should provide a means of interrupting the CAS and of strengthening metacognitive plans for controlling cognition (improving flexible executive control).

In this chapter I present the treatment manual for one particular strategy called the *attention training technique* (ATT). Later in the chapter I broaden the discussion to briefly consider another strategy called *situational attention refocusing* (SAR). These two techniques have different aims within the metacognitive treatment approach. It is important to note that neither strategy is a means of distraction from internal events or a means of managing or avoiding emotion. The use of distraction in psychotherapy usually entails shifting attention onto neutral or positive stimuli as a means of attenuating attention to painful, emotional, or threatening stimuli and thereby reducing the intensity of reactions to them. The ATT and SAR do not involve shifting attention to neutral or positive stimuli to control or avoid subjective experiences. Instead they involve shifting attention in ways that are specifically designed to strengthen metacognitions that regulate thinking, remove unhelpful thinking styles that impede normal emotional processing, or modify beliefs.

OVERVIEW OF THE ATT

The aim in developing the ATT was to devise a procedure that could impact several dimensions of the CAS and the metacognitions driving it. The first published study reported its effects in the treatment of a panic disorder case (Wells, 1990). In that study the initial objective was to use a technique that could interrupt excessive and inflexible self-focused attention. Self-attention of this kind is a key ingredient in worry/rumination and threat monitoring (e.g., attending to bodily events in panic), which are central components of the CAS.

An important question in the development of the ATT concerned the aspect of attention that should be manipulated as a basis of interrupting the CAS and increasing metacognitive flexibility. Attention is multifaceted and can be divided into aspects of selectivity, switching, parallel processing, and capacity requirements. The ATT was devised with these dimensions in mind and how the technique might interface with the patient's goals.

Several characteristics of the technique were theoretically grounded and specified at the development stage. It was important that it should be attentionally demanding and not become substantially less demanding with practice; otherwise it would not systematically strengthen control processes. It should involve external processing of non-self-relevant material so as to interrupt perseverative self-focused processing. It should not be employed by the patient as a distraction, avoidance, or symptom-management strategy because this could maintain dysfunctional self-focused control and erroneous beliefs about internal events.

Initial attempts to develop an effective technique explored the use of visual attention strategies, but the results were weak. A later attempt involved developing an auditory-based attention procedure that required the spatial allocation of attention. This procedure has remained the basis of the ATT.

The ATT consists of three components: (1) selective attention, (2) rapid attention switching, and (3) divided attention. Each component is practiced in a single seamless exercise. The procedure lasts approximately 12 minutes and is roughly partitioned as follows: 5 minutes for selective attention, 5 minutes for attention switching, and 2 minutes for divided attention.

Selective attention instructions consist of guiding the patient's attention to individual sounds among an array of competing sounds at different spatial locations in the environment, with the instruction to give intense attention to specific individual sounds while resisting distraction by others.

Rapid attention switching consists of instructions to shift attention between individual sounds (and spatial locations) with increasing speed as this phase progresses. At the beginning of this phase approximately 10 seconds is devoted to different individual sounds. Subsequently, the speed of switching is increased to one sound every 5 seconds.

The ATT technique ends with a briefer (1–2 minutes) *divided attention* instruction in which the patient is asked to expand the breadth and depth of attention and attempt to process multiple sounds and locations simultaneously.

The procedure is configured so that it consistently loads attention. To this end multiple simultaneous sounds should be used in a training session. The pace of switching in the switching phase can be modulated. The procedure ends with divided attention so that the technique retains a resource-demanding character.

Between six and nine sounds, combined with spatial locations, are identified or introduced for the exercise depending on the level of demand required. Some but not all of these sounds are "potential sounds" and can be operationalized solely as locations in space. The sounds may not exist during the practice of a particular exercise. For example, the patient is asked to "focus on any sounds in the far distance that might be detected on the right-hand side." In this way attention is allocated to a location in space irrespective of the occurrence of detectable sound events occurring in that space. Thus, the technique utilizes an inner metacognitive map for the spatial allocation, control, and intensity of attention.

Typically a minimum of three actual competing sounds are used at different spatial locations in the consulting room, a further two sounds are identified outside of the consulting room in the near distance, and two more sounds (or locations) are indicated in the far distance (these two "sounds" may consist of "spatial locations"—for example, one to the left and one to the right for focusing attention in the distance). The near distance is usually defined as outside the practice room but within the building and the far distance is defined as outside the building.

Given this range of parameters there is usually enormous scope for varying the precise nature of the technique between sessions, which offsets the effects of practice on task difficulty and provides sufficient flexibility so that the ATT can be implemented in most environments. Recorded versions of sounds have also been used in the implementation of ATT.

Patients are usually asked to focus on a visual fixation point and to maintain their visual focus throughout the exercise. The ATT is practiced when participants are not in a state of anxiety or acute worry. This underscores the point that the technique is not intended as an emotion-management strategy. However, when used in the treatment of depression, the technique inevitably necessitates application during chronic low mood, but even in this case the technique is not intended or used as an immediate alleviation of sadness.

RATIONALE FOR THE ATT

A credible and acceptable rationale is an important component of the ATT. This increases compliance with the procedure and with homework practice. It also frames the technique in an appropriate way that counteracts the effects of some unhelpful processes. More specifically, the rationale emphasizes that the technique is not intended to lead to a "blank mind" free from intrusive inner experiences. Similarly, the rationale counteracts the use of active thought suppression.

Components of the rationale emphasize that inner events that intrude into consciousness should be treated as additional noise and should not be resisted. This facilitates the shift to a metacognitive mode and a state of detached mindfulness.

Unrealistic expectations and assumptions about the technique should be elicited and dealt with before practicing. A common misconception is that the procedure should "block out" unwanted thoughts and feelings. The therapist should emphasize that unwanted intrusive experiences should be regarded as additional noise. The therapist should indicate that it is desirable to be aware of these intrusions and continue to direct attention as instructed even in the presence of this awareness.

Slightly different rationales have been used across disorders that have been tailored to capture the specific nature of the CAS in each case (see Wells, 2000), but they are all based on a generic rationale that can be expressed as follows:

> "Anxiety and depression are unpleasant emotional experiences that signal some kind of threat or loss. They become persistent and a problem when people respond to them by changing their pattern of attention and thinking. Most people don't recognize that their attention has become locked onto dwelling on themselves, their thoughts, and their feelings. This process prolongs and increases negative feelings and negative beliefs about the self. Unfortunately, people are usually unaware of this process and it can be difficult to interrupt. You can see the unhelpful effects of dwelling on your symptoms and thoughts about yourself if you consider what happens when something interrupts this process. If you have to deal with an emergency affecting someone else, what happens to your anxiety/sadness? You will have noticed that you temporarily feel better, but your problem returns when your attention reverts back to your unhelpful pattern of self-focus.
>
> "It is important to become more aware of your focus of attention and to strengthen your control over it. Then it will no longer be habitually locked onto unhelpful patterns of dwelling on yourself and your body. You will learn a technique called attention training that

will make it easier for you to break free of old and unhelpful thinking patterns.

"The aim of the technique is not to distract you from upsetting thoughts or feelings. In fact, these are likely to occur as you practice. You must not try to stop them. The aim is to continue to follow the procedure while allowing these inner experiences to take care of themselves. You can simply think of these experiences as passing inner noises."

CREDIBILITY CHECK

Following presentation of the rationale, the therapist runs a credibility check to determine the extent to which the patient anticipates that the technique will be helpful. The following question should be used:

"How helpful do you think it will be for you to practice this technique? Can you give me a number on a scale from 0, not at all helpful, to 100, representing very helpful?"

Low levels of credibility (i.e., less than 40) should be explored and the rationale for the ATT strengthened. The therapist enhances credibility by reviewing experiences that the patient has had in which he or she has focused more on him- or herself and drawing attention to the impact this has had on thoughts and beliefs. This can be contrasted with the positive effects of being absorbed in externally focused activities to illustrate the role of attention and the importance of strengthening control over it.

SELF-ATTENTION RATING

The self-attention rating is an important index of the effectiveness of the procedure in counteracting the CAS (recall that self-attention is a feature and marker for the CAS). A 7-point rating scale is used to measure level and change in self-attention. This scale is reproduced below and is available to be copied in Appendix 5.

"At this moment in time how much is your attention focused on yourself or on your external environment? Please indicate by giving me a number on the scale":

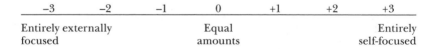

−3	−2	−1	0	+1	+2	+3
Entirely externally focused			Equal amounts			Entirely self-focused

The therapist administers the self-attention rating before the first in-session practice of the ATT and then immediately after practicing. Typically, a reduction of at least 2 points in self-focus is achieved after the first practice session. If this is not the case, the therapist explores the possible reasons for lack of positive change and focuses on dealing with them.

Causes of little change might include a lack of effort due to the low credibility of the rationale or the use of counterproductive strategies during practice, such as thought suppression, daydreaming, and diversion of attention to worry. In these cases the rationale should be reinforced and emphasis given to prioritizing the attention task rather than competing processes. The technique should then be practiced again.

BASIC INSTRUCTIONS FOR THE ATT

A set of instructions for implementing the ATT are given below. In the instructions different sounds are designated as *S1, S2, S3,* etc. While at least three of these sounds are discrete consistent sounds, some designated sounds are often spatial locations in which there is no predetermined consistent sound. These instructions are an updated version of those published earlier in Wells (2000, pp. 145–146):

> "I would like you to focus your gaze on a dot that I have placed on the wall. Throughout the exercise try to keep your eyes fixed on the dot. I'm going to ask you to focus your attention on different sounds inside this room and outside of this room. I will ask you to focus your attention in different ways. It doesn't matter if thoughts and feelings come into your mind. The aim is to practice focusing your attention no matter what you might become aware of.
>
> "To begin with, focus on the sound of my voice (*S1*). Pay close attention to that sound. No other sound matters. Try to give all of your attention to the sound of my voice. Ignore all of the other sounds around you. You may hear them but try to give all of your attention to the sound of my voice. Focus only on the sound of my voice. No other sound matters. Focus on this one sound.
>
> "Now turn your attention to the sound I am making as I tap on the desk (*S2*). Pay close attention to that sound, for no other sound matters (*pause*). Try to give all of your attention to the tapping sound (*pause*). Closely monitor the tapping sound (*pause*). If your attention begins to stray or is captured by another sound, refocus on the tapping sound (*pause*). No other sound matters. Give this one sound all of your attention (*pause*). Continue to monitor this sound and if you are distracted return your attention to it (*pause*).

"Now focus on the sound of (*S3; e.g., the ticking of a wind-up timer*) (*pause*). Pay close attention to that sound, for no other sound matters (*pause*). Try to give all of your attention to the sound of the timer (*pause*). Closely monitor the sound the timer makes (*pause*). If your attention begins to stray or is captured by another sound, refocus on the timer (*pause*). No other sound matters. Give this one sound all of your attention (*pause*). Continue to monitor this sound and if you are distracted return your attention to this sound as soon as you can (*pause*).

"Now focus your attention on sounds that you might hear outside of this room, but nearby. Focus on the space outside and behind you (*S4*). Pay close attention to that space and try to detect sounds that might occur there [if there are specific sounds, the therapist draws attention to them]. Even if there are no sounds keep your attention on that space. Try to give all of your attention to it (*pause*). Closely monitor for sounds there (*pause*). If your attention begins to stray or is captured by a sound elsewhere, refocus on that place. No other sound matters. Give all of your attention to that place and what you might hear there. Continue to monitor and if you are distracted return your attention to it (*pause*)."

The instructions in the above paragraph are repeated for additional sounds (*S5–7*) and/or spaces (e.g., on the left, on the right, and in the far distance).

"Now that you have identified and practiced focusing on individual sounds and locations I am going to ask you to quickly shift your attention between them as I call them out (*pause*). First, focus on the tapping sound (*S2*), no other sound matters (*pause*). Switch your attention and focus on what you might hear behind you in the near distance (*S4*) (*pause*). Pay close attention to (*S4*), no other sound matters. Now turn your attention to (*S7*), no other sound matters (*pause*). Turn your attention again this time to the sound of the timer (*S3*) (*pause*). Now switch and focus on the tapping sound (*S2*) (*pause*). Now focus on (*S6*) (*pause*), now on the sound of (*S5*) (*pause*), (*S4*) . . . (*S2*) . . . (*S3*) . . ., etc.

"Finally, I want you to expand your attention. Make it as broad and deep as possible. Try to absorb all of the sounds and all of the locations that you have identified at the same time. Try to focus on and be aware of all of the sounds both inside and outside of this room at the same time (*pause*). Covertly count the number of sounds that you can hear at the same time (*pause*). Try to hear everything simultaneously. Count the number of sounds you can hear this way.

"This concludes the exercise. How many sounds were you able to hear at the same time?"

PATIENT FEEDBACK

Following implementation of the above procedure the therapist asks the patient to rerate the intensity of self-focus using the bipolar rating scale. Reductions of 2 points are typical in the first sessions. Failure to achieve this level of change is a marker for possible difficulties that must be explored. The ATT should be repeated in these cases with the necessary adjustments made.

Failure to reduce self-focus can be caused by misunderstanding of the rationale for the ATT. In particular, patients might try to control or suppress thoughts, or they might be dividing their attention between continuing with worry/rumination while partially directing attention externally. Some patients are reluctant to relinquish their own mental control strategies which would be necessitated by fully engaging the ATT. In these circumstances fears concerning such a shift in strategy should be examined and challenged.

The therapist also asks about the general experiences that might have occurred as a result of the ATT. The technique can produce perceptual changes such as mild and temporary increased sensitivity to external stimuli and metacognitive experiences that are unusual for patients such as experiences of temporary mental quiescence that should be normalized.

Finally, the therapist should ask about the ease with which the patient could perform the technique. The therapist should state that the technique is intended to be demanding and requires practice. It is most important that the therapist is aware of statements that indicate unhelpful assumptions about the use of the ATT. For example, some patients assume that they were unable to practice effectively because they had intrusive thoughts or feelings during the procedure. Here, the therapist normally reemphasizes that the aim of the technique is not to remove awareness of inner events but to practice controlling attention in a particular way. One strategy is for the therapist to suggest that it is useful to experience intrusive thoughts and feelings during practice as these normally bind attention to them and the aim is to have flexible control even in the presence of these "inner noises."

HOMEWORK

A crucial component of the ATT is consistent practice of the technique for homework. Usually, patients are asked to practice twice a day, but in reality most patients only manage to do this once a day. Practice should be scheduled for approximately 12 minutes and the sequence used in the session should be followed. The ATT Summary Sheet (see Appendix 4) is given as a reminder of how to practice and as a means of monitoring homework.

The ATT Summary Sheet acts as a focus of discussion in which three potential sources of sound can be identified or obtained and noted, thereby increasing compliance. For example, one patient decided to take a radio into a spare room in the house where he would practice, and he tuned this between channels to generate noise. He decided that he would play some music on his stereo that was located in an adjacent room, but he could not think of another type of sound he could use. After some discussion with the therapist he decided to buy a wind-up cooking timer as a further noise-generating device. He built the rest of the procedure around listening for incidental sounds at locations outside. The therapist normally works with the patient in completing the ATT Summary Sheet in the first ATT session.

TROUBLESHOOTING

Occasionally setbacks are encountered in administering the ATT. Some common setbacks and suggested solutions are as follows:

Failure to Practice

Use the ATT Summary Sheet to increase practice rates. Continued failure to practice may be due to poor socialization and lack of understanding of the reasons for using the technique. If this cause is suspected, the therapist should introduce further socialization.

Motivation to Continue the CAS

Some patients do practice ATT but they view it as something that interferes with their preferred strategy of ruminating/worrying. Thus, the motivation to continue the worry component of the CAS remains. There are two ways in which this occurs. First, worry or rumination can continue in parallel with practicing the ATT such that the person has long periods in which he or she has no active mental engagement with sounds because his or her resources are diverted to brooding. Second, the person can view the ATT as a chore that must be done quickly so that he or she can return to focusing on (dwelling on) thinking about problems.

In these circumstances it is necessary to review the disadvantages of worrying and ruminating and help the patient to see how these strategies have not solved problems and are unlikely to do so. The therapist should then introduce worry and rumination postponement strategies (see Chapters 6 and 9) in conjunction with the ATT.

Misuse as Avoidance or Symptom Management

The patient may apply the ATT as a direct means of avoiding emotions and erroneous threat. Some patients have been detected misusing the technique as a form of distraction from emotions, as a means of controlling anxiety or panic, or as a means of suppressing obsessional thoughts. The therapist must detect these instances and reinforce the concept that the technique should not be used as a coping strategy. It is useful in these circumstances to use metaphor to convey the idea that the ATT is a means of general "mental fitness training" and not a form of avoidance.

It is not desirable to use the ATT as a coping strategy because this transforms it into a form of cognitive or emotional avoidance, which is a problem because it may interfere with emotional processing and maintain erroneous negative beliefs about the danger and consequences of thoughts and feelings. Furthermore, the nonoccurrence of catastrophe (e.g., fainting due to anxiety) can be falsely attributed to the use of the ATT and not to the fact that anxiety does not cause catastrophe. By this mechanism false beliefs are more likely to persist. It is helpful for the therapist to explain the counterproductive effects of using the ATT as an active coping strategy.

OUTLINE OF THE FIRST ATT SESSION

The first ATT session should follow the structure and content outlined below:

1. Review the nature of the patient's problem, emphasizing the role of difficult-to-control self-processing in problem maintenance.
2. Present the rationale for the ATT using idiosyncratic material.
3. Socialize by illustrating the role of self-focus in the form of worry and self-monitoring. Use a self-attention socialization experiment if possible.
4. Check the credibility of the rationale. Take steps to increase socialization if necessary.
5. Rate current level of self-focus.
6. Administer the therapist-guided ATT.
7. Rerate the level of self-focus and elicit feedback.

8. Review the ATT Summary Sheet with the patient (see Appendix 4) and complete the list of sounds.
9. Set homework.
10. Elicit feedback and ask the patient to summarize the session.

Subsequent ATT Sessions

Follow-up sessions should begin with a review of homework practice as recorded on the ATT Summary Sheet. Any problems arising should be discussed and resolved. Sessions then proceed with therapist guided practice of the ATT.

The therapist explores competing demands on the ATT effects, such as engaging in checking of the self, worry and rumination, and any attempts to monitor and control inner experiences. The incompatibility of these processes with attention-training effects are highlighted. The patient is asked to ban these processes. For example, the therapist introduces the idea that bodily checking and worry interfere with developing effective levels of mental control and mental agility because they lock attention into familiar and old response patterns that emphasize threat rather than establish control over attention.

CASE EXAMPLE

In hypochondriasis the conceptual component of the CAS can be observed in the form of worry about symptoms and rumination concerning their possible significance and causes. Threat monitoring is evident in the form of mentally scanning the body for signs and symptoms, physically checking parts of the body (e.g., palpating the abdomen), checking bodily processes and mental functioning (e.g., checking memory for names), and searching for information about symptoms. Unhelpful coping behaviors such as excessive resting, avoidance of exercise, taking unnecessary medications that change bodily function, trying to control automatic physiological function (e.g., breathing), and avoidance of medical information can also be readily identified.

A 43-year-old man with hypochondriasis and panic attacks was treated with the ATT. The patient described a range of unexplained symptoms including abdominal pain, chest pain, arrhythmias, dizziness, and feelings of unreality (dissociation). His current main symptom of concern was feeling unreal and chest pain. His medical evaluations had been extensive and were unremarkable, but he was concerned (i.e., worrying) that the tests might have failed to detect a serious medical condition.

The therapist suggested that a technique called attention training be tried to determine if it could reduce his excessive body-focused processing. The therapist explained that the patient had become anxious about his health and preoccupied with his body. The therapist pointed out that this anxiety and preoccupation was an example of altered body awareness that could be adding additional layers of symptoms that needed to be managed before considering further medical testing. The role of these processes was illustrated by asking the patient what happened to his anxiety when he focused on his body ("Do you become more or less aware of your symptoms?"). The therapist also explored what happened to the patient's symptoms when he became intensely worried about his health. This was contrasted with examining what happened to anxiety when the patient was absorbed in a work task. A useful discussion ensued of how the patient would run a mental check of his body when he became aware that he had not been focusing on his symptoms for a while, which was further useful information supporting the role of altered body awareness.

The therapist introduced a socialization experiment to show how alterations in body awareness produced by attention could influence subsequent perception. The patient was asked to focus on sensations in his fingertips to see if there were any feelings there. The patient described a feeling of tingling. The therapist then asked him to be aware of his fingertips but to shut out that feeling. The patient discovered that he was now unable to be aware of his fingertips and to shut out the tingling in them. In this way the therapist helped the patient to understand how turning attention toward the body and dwelling on sensations could lock attention onto them such that it changed his subsequent awareness.

A further socialization technique was also used in which the therapist illustrated the role that assigning personal importance to things has in locking attention onto them. The patient was asked if he had noticed a strange event after buying his most recent car: The fact that many more people now seemed to be driving the same model car. This observation was used as an illustration of how assigning personal significance to events such as cars—or in the patient's case, symptoms—had the power to make someone witness more of them even if little had actually changed. The rationale for the ATT was presented with an emphasis on learning to regain control of attention and reduce worry and the significance given to symptoms so that body awareness could return to a normal state.

The ATT was practiced for eight treatment sessions. In the third session the therapist also introduced worry postponement and instructed the patient to ban his bodily checking at all times. This consisted of asking him to stop checking his pulse and to stop running a mind-check over his body which he was prone to do several times each day.

In later sessions the therapist worked on challenging the patient's positive metacognitive beliefs about the importance of focusing on and worrying about bodily symptoms. In this case the ATT formed a substantive component of metacognitive treatment for hypochondriasis.

SITUATIONAL ATTENTIONAL REFOCUSING

SAR is an attentional modification technique used in metacognitive therapy that differs from the ATT in its aim and nature. Rather than retraining executive control and interrupting perseverative processing, SAR is intended to explicitly enhance the processing of information that is incompatible with the patient's dysfunctional beliefs (e.g., in treating social phobia), or it is used to counteract external threat monitoring in the later stages of MCT for PTSD.

This is a technique that should be applied to stressful or problematic situations as a means of configuring processing in a way that is beneficial for developing adaptive appraisals and beliefs. It is not a coping strategy aimed at preventing emotion or removing threat, but it is applied as a means of disrupting unhelpful attention patterns that maintain an unrealistic sense of threat and as a means of increasing the flow of new information into consciousness to modify beliefs.

The technique has been incorporated in the treatment of social phobia (Clark & Wells, 1995; Wells & Papageorgiou, 1998a) and in the treatment of posttraumatic stress (Wells & Sembi, 2004b). For example, Wells and Papageorgiou (1998a) asked individuals with social phobia to engage in one session of exposure to a feared social situation while focusing attention externally on features of the social environment such as the color of other people's hair and eyes. This condition was compared with one session of exposure alone using a standard habituation rationale. The exposure plus SAR condition was more effective at reducing negative beliefs, reducing anxiety, and changing the image that patients had of themselves afterward.

SAR can be used explicitly to modify beliefs and incorporated as a feature of behavioral experiments. For example, individuals with social phobia often believe that everyone is looking at them. While they claim to be very aware of this attention, their awareness does not stem from looking at other people, but from a sense of self-consciousness. (*Note:* The person's processing configuration is inadequate for discovering the truth and therefore needs to be altered.)

In treatment it is very helpful to ask patients to enter feared social situations and to actively focus on other people to determine how many people are actually looking at them. The patient is further instructed to deliberately make a mistake (e.g., drop something) or to show signs of anxiety while focusing attention on others to determine the truth about the reaction of others even under negative conditions. In these instances showing signs of failed performance coupled with SAR are examples of disconfirmatory maneuvers or "tests" in behavioral experiments as described in Chapter 3 because they actively challenge predictions and beliefs.

In PTSD, patients become hypervigilant for threat and focus their attention on aspects of the environment that could be dangerous as an attempt to minimize danger. Unfortunately, this increases the patient's sense of current danger and vulnerability, thereby maintaining his or her anxiety. SAR consists of asking patients to notice instances of threat monitoring and to ban it during situations that remind them of trauma. Processing is rebalanced and returned to a more normal state by asking individuals to focus on neutral or *safety signals* in the environment instead to counteract bias and retrain an adaptive attentional control plan. For example, one patient scanned for speeding cars whenever she approached a traffic intersection because she feared another collision. She was asked to look out for cars that were slowing down or were stationary instead. She quickly realized that her strategy of looking for danger led her to ignore the actual features of the situation and learned that traffic intersections were generally safe rather than generally dangerous.

CONCLUSION

In this chapter I have described the purpose and nature of direct attentional modification strategies that form a component of metacognitive therapy. While the ATT is generally considered a component of a wider MCT treatment package, evidence suggests that it can be very effective even when used alone (see Chapter 10).

The ATT and SAR have different purposes. While the ATT is designed to increase executive control and to interrupt perseverative self-focused processing, SAR is intended to increase access to disconfirmatory information and to correct attentional strategies that are counterproductive in situations (i.e., it modifies threat-monitoring aspects of the CAS).

Attentional modifications are powerful strategies that impact on metacognition. It is likely that they strengthen plans for controlling and guiding online processing and increase flexibility in cognitive control that is impaired in psychological disorder. The development and investigation of attentional strategies that are grounded in theory linking attention to causative and change mechanisms in psychopathology opens up a wide range of new therapeutic possibilities. As this chapter illustrates, changing attention processes can be developed beyond the use of simple distraction. In MCT it is aimed at modifying central control processes, reversing unhelpful processing styles, and improving the flow of more adaptive information into consciousness that can change the content of what we know. In SAR the manipulation of attention is a basis for implementing metacognitively delivered exposure. The aim is to control cognition in a way that facilitates the acquisition of processing strategies that support access to corrective information.

The metacognitive approach emphasizes the role of control functions in treating psychological disorder. It is proposed that these can be strengthened through the development of attentional technologies such as the ATT. Improved flexible control over attention allows the person to change his or her beliefs and to adaptively process threatening material (e.g., criticism, intrusive thoughts) and modulate emotional processing without triggering the full-blown CAS. (A recorded version of the ATT is available at *www.mct-institute.com*.)

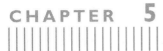

CHAPTER 5

Detached Mindfulness Techniques

The concept of detached mindfulness (DM) was briefly introduced in Chapter 1. In this chapter I examine the concept in greater detail and describe 10 techniques that can be used to train individuals in the rapid and flexible deployment of this metacognitive strategy.

DM was originally described by Wells and Matthews (1994). It concerns the manner in which an individual relates to his or her cognition and the development of flexible control of attention and thinking styles. The ATT reviewed in the previous chapter offers a specific strategy designed to impact on and improve flexible control of attention and to strengthen the ability to disengage from unhelpful ways of relating to inner experiences. DM techniques are focused more on developing meta-awareness in the context of suspending conceptual processing and separating self from cognitive events.

I have previously described DM as

> a state of awareness of internal events, without responding to them with sustained evaluation, attempts to control or suppress them, or respond to them behaviorally. It is exemplified by strategies such as deciding not to worry in response to an intrusive thought, but instead allowing the thought to occupy its own mental space without further action or interpretation in the knowledge that it is merely an event in the mind. (Wells, 2005b, p. 340)

As the name implies, DM has two features: (1) *mindfulness* and (2) *detachment*. DM consists of both features simultaneously. Let's address each of these components in turn, beginning with mindfulness.

We use the term "mindfulness" in DM to refer specifically to being aware of inner cognitive events, namely, thoughts, beliefs, memories, and feelings of knowing. Effectively, the use of the term "mindfulness" is intended to refer to metacognitive awareness of thoughts and beliefs where attention can be flexibly focused on such inner experiences without being locked onto any one of them.

We use the term "detachment" to refer to two further factors. The first and most important dimension of detachment denotes detachment of any reactive engagement with the inner event. That is, the person refrains from further appraisal of or attempts to cope in response to the inner event. The concept of DM contains the antithesis of the CAS. It is about stopping any conceptual or behavioral involvement with inner experiences. It consists of abandoning worry, rumination, suppression, control, threat monitoring, avoidance, or attempts to minimize (nonexistent) threat in response to cognition.

The second component of detachment involves the person experiencing an inner event as an occurrence that is independent of general consciousness of the self (i.e., the individual has a perspective in relation to the event in which consciousness is located separately from it). It is as if the person is aware of the perspective of the self as an observer of the thought or belief. This feature is harder to grasp. Therefore, an example may help to illustrate the construct. This example is based on a male patient with OCD.

THERAPIST: It sounds as if you often have thoughts about contamination.

PATIENT: Yes, every time I see a stain I think, "It must be contaminated" or "I'm contaminated."

THERAPIST: So how aware are you of repeatedly thinking "It must be contaminated"?

PATIENT: I'm always thinking it when I see stains.

THERAPIST: Of course. But how often do you stop and consciously reflect on the fact that you have had that thought again?

PATIENT: I don't, I just act to prevent harm.

THERAPIST: So the first thing you can do is simply to stop and be consciously aware of having the thought. That is called mindfulness.

PATIENT: Yes, but what if it's true?

THERAPIST: Irrespective of whether it is true or not, it is still a thought.

PATIENT: Yes, but I can't ignore it.

THERAPIST: Ignoring the thought isn't the idea. I want you to become aware of it as a thought in your mind that you can observe. I want you to become mindful of it.

PATIENT: How would I know it is just a thought?

THERAPIST: What else could it be?

PATIENT: Well, it could be true.

THERAPIST: Whether it is true or not, it will always be a thought. Whether it is true or not, I would like you to practice detachment from it and see it as a thought separate from yourself.

PATIENT: I'm not sure what you mean.

THERAPIST: Can you have the thought "I'm contaminated" right now?

PATIENT: Yes.

THERAPIST: Look at that stain on the floor. Can you close your eyes right now and have the thought "I'm contaminated"?

PATIENT: Okay.

THERAPIST: Now pay attention to that thought. Don't do anything to change it. Take a step back in your mind and look at the thought and as you do so concentrate on where you are as the observer watching that thought in your head. Concentrate on what it feels like to be detached from that thought. Can you observe that as a thought separate from the sense of yourself?

PATIENT: Yes, I can.

THERAPIST: Can you detach yourself from your thoughts like that in future?

PATIENT: Yes, but I will still need to wash.

THERAPIST: Part of detachment from the thought involves watching it as an observer and postponing doing anything else in response to it. How long could you postpone washing?

PATIENT: I'm not sure.

THERAPIST: What about postponing it for an hour to start with?

In this example the therapist introduces the concept of mindfulness in terms of the patient increasing his subjective awareness of the occurrence of thoughts about contamination. This awareness begins to build the scaffolding to support the shift from the *object mode* in which thoughts are fused with facts to the *metacognitive mode* in which thoughts are events in the mind. In this process the therapist encourages the patient to refrain from evaluating whether or not the thought is a fact by emphasizing that it remains a thought irrespective of its validity. The patient's main task is to be aware of the thought as a mental event and to experience it as such. The dialogue continues with the introduction of detachment in the form of separating the self from the thought and disengaging coping responses (i.e., postponing washing).

Aims of DM

There are several aims in using DM. It can be used to shift patients away from the object mode of experiencing and into the metacognitive mode. It can be used as a means of interrupting perseverative processing in the form of worry and rumination. It can be used to increase executive control over the allocation of attention. It also enables patients to escape the influence of thoughts on self-concept.

The effect of DM is determined by how it is used and the rationale for using it. It is imperative that DM is not used as an emotional or cognitive avoidance technique or as a means of preventing erroneous feared outcomes. For example, a patient may inappropriately use DM as a means of controlling or counteracting the effects of "dangerous thoughts," a misuse that could maintain the mistaken belief that thoughts can cause harm. More specifically, the aim is not to teach DM so that it can become another form of maladaptive thought control strategies. It is not a means of avoiding thoughts. Instead, it is about relating to thoughts and experiencing them in a new way that necessitates overt and covert inaction. It is a "do-nothing" strategy, the antithesis of coping and the CAS. That is why it is a state of "detached awareness." It is also detached awareness because the process of experiencing DM involves disconnection of the sense of self from the contents of consciousness as a more profound and deeper experience. This latter sense can be particularly useful when the thought or "feeling" that intrudes into consciousness is fused with the self-concept.

Elements of DM

I have described how DM is a type of inner awareness that occurs in the absence of effortful conceptually based self-processing. Specifically, it is an awareness of thoughts in which they are experienced as passing events in the mind that are distinct from reality and separate from the self. Since DM is awareness in the absence of conceptual processing, it requires metacognitive control of analytical and perseverative forms of thinking. DM is simply awareness without judgment of the position of the self in relation to a mental event. The psychological elements of DM can be isolated and conceptualized as involving the following:

1. Meta-awareness (i.e., consciousness of thoughts).
2. Cognitive decentering (i.e., comprehension of thoughts as events separate from facts).
3. Attentional detachment and control (i.e., attention remains flexible and not anchored to any one thing).

4. Low conceptual processing (i.e., low levels of meaning-based analysis or inner dialogue).
5. Low goal-directed coping (i.e., behaviors and goals to avoid or remove erroneous threat are not implemented).
6. Altered self-awareness (i.e., experience of a singularity in consciousness of self as an observer separate from thoughts and beliefs).

AN INFORMATION-PROCESSING MODEL OF DM

Progress in the development of useful experiential techniques is most likely to be made by reference to an information-processing analysis of the goals and effects of such techniques. DM is based on such an approach. In earlier work I have described an information-processing model of DM requirements and effects (Wells, 2005b). I briefly summarize that model here (see Figure 5.1).

DM is intended to impact on the CAS and the metacognitive processes and knowledge that drive it. DM can be conceptualized as acting on the interrelated cognitive and metacognitive subsystems. The metacognitive subsystem consists of information about cognition stored as a library of knowledge or beliefs that can be accessed to interpret and control thinking. It also consists of a model of the activities of online processing, which it monitors and controls in pursuit of the goals of processing. The relationship between the metacognitive and the cognitive subsystems can be represented as a flow of information involving monitoring and control, as posited by Nelson and Narens (1990).

The model of the cognitive subsystem held by the metacognitive subsystem is built from the monitoring of events in ordinary cognition (i.e., online processing) and projection of their status into the future in relation to a reference standard. It consists of a current representation of the status of ordinary cognition in relation to a set of goals. The model not only requires real-time feedback from the online level but the accessing of knowledge from long-term memory.

This specification of the components of and the relations between the subsystems leads to hypotheses about the information-processing parameters that have to be met to achieve DM. In this model DM requires the following conditions to be present:

1. Activation of appropriate knowledge (plans) for controlling thinking.
2. A mental model of the mindfulness state.
3. Ongoing monitoring and control of that state.

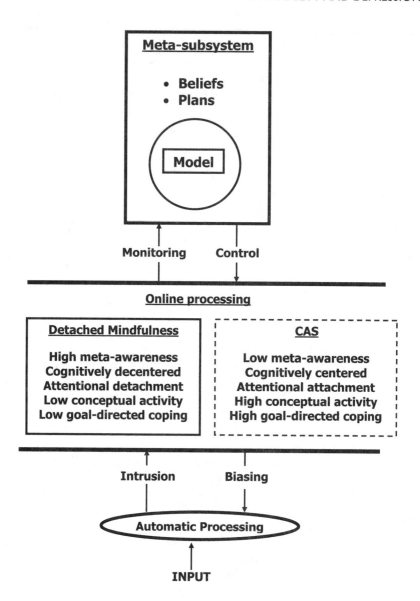

FIGURE 5.1. Metacognitive model of DM grounded in the S-REF framework. From Wells (2005b). Copyright 2006 by Springer Science and Business Media. Reprinted by permission.

4. Sufficient attentional resources and flexibility for executive control to allow accessing and implementation of DM.
5. Development of a model of self that is separate from individual negative cognitions (beliefs and thoughts).

This analysis of the features of DM and its requirements sets the stage for developing specific DM techniques that are grounded in theory. It also means that the effects of different treatment techniques may be formulated in terms of this a priori model. For example, the act of identifying automatic thoughts by using a dysfunctional thoughts record might increase metacognitive monitoring and allow decentering, thereby strengthening metacognitive awareness skills. However, this action might not satisfy the other psychological elements of DM, such as attentional detachment, low conceptual processing, and low goal-directed coping. The process of interrogating thoughts by directing the patient to rationally question them supports the activation of knowledge (plans) that in turn supports a high level of conceptual processing of these thoughts, which is incompatible with DM.

The model (Figure 5.1) and the conditions specified for DM suggest that individuals must be able to activate plans for controlling thinking to accomplish the desired state. In some instances these plans may be disrupted or not highly developed, meaning that initial training to strengthen control plans may be required (e.g., attention training). Most individuals have an intellectual concept of mindfulness but lack the model at the metacognitive level to guide them in experiencing this state. Patients' acquisition of the model can be achieved by encouraging them to experience focal awareness of their cognitive events (e.g., by counting thoughts, engaging in a free-association task—see below). Detachment is facilitated by experiential exercises in which individuals practice (1) suspension of active conceptual processing and control and (2) experiential awareness of self as separate from thoughts. These factors are built into the techniques described later in this chapter.

DM AND OTHER FORMS OF MINDFULNESS

The term "mindfulness" has been used in many different ways in the psychological literature. It has been linked to a state of effortful and conscious controlled processing (Shiffrin & Schneider, 1977), a state that is opposite to "mindlessness." Mindlessness is equated with habitual or automatic processing. This characterization is simply another way of differentiating controlled versus automatic processing. It does not implicate metacognition and conscious awareness of thoughts themselves as does DM.

The heterogenous nature of mindfulness within the psychological and treatment literature is evident in the self-report scales developed to assess this construct. For example, Brown and Ryan (2003) developed the Mindful Attention Awareness Scale (MAAS) to assess the qualities of consciousness associated with well-being. Many of the items appear to assess the tendency not to notice information and to behave as if one is on automatic pilot (e.g., "I could be experiencing some emotions and not be conscious of it until some time later"; "I tend to walk quickly to get where I'm going without paying attention to what I experience along the way"). These items are similar to other psychological concepts such as cognitive failures as measured by the Cognitive Failures Questionnaire (Broadbent, Cooper, Fitzgerald, & Parkes, 1982), a measure of everyday cognitive and performance errors. In these approaches mindfulness is linked either to levels or the efficiency of attentional functioning, but there is limited separation between it and related constructs.

Mindfulness is also fused with concepts such as acceptance (e.g., Hayes, Strosahl, & Wilson, 1999), which means taking thoughts as thoughts and feelings as feelings without the need to avoid them. This is conceptually similar to DM but does not focus specifically on the suspension of worry and rumination and on developing a sense of self as separate from beliefs although it may separate self from thoughts and feelings.

Drawing on previous approaches, Bishop et al. (2004) offer an operational definition of mindfulness that has two components: (1) control of attention so that it is maintained on immediate experience, thereby allowing for increased recognition of mental events in the present; and (2) adopting an orientation of curiosity, openness, and acceptance to one's present experiences. The first component is a feature of DM, and implies greater metacognitive awareness. However, this definition does not include separation of the sense of self from inner events as does DM. The second component takes us further away from DM and introduces the concepts of curiosity and acceptance. It is not clear how such states are implemented, but they are likely to involve active engagement with thoughts, which is not a feature of DM.

Mindfulness has gained prominence as a term equated with Buddhist meditation (e.g., Kabat-Zinn, 1994). DM does have some similarity to the concepts of mindfulness derived from meditation practices, but it is also different from these approaches.

From the meditation perspective, mindfulness has been described as "paying attention in a particular way: on purpose, in the present moment, and nonjudgmentally" (Kabat-Zinn, 1994, p. 4). This is a very broad description that partially covers DM and would also capture some features of attention training (Wells, 1990), but omits some of the unique features of DM.

In the work of Kabat-Zinn (1990, 1994) mindfulness is equated with paying attention. Paying attention to the breath is used as a means of focusing on moment-to-moment experience. Such attention offers a means of directly experiencing the moment without thinking about it. This includes being aware of the thought stream without judging it, cultivating trust in the self, and "letting go," or accepting things as they are. This kind of mindfulness is much more general than the concept of mindfulness in DM, and despite containing reference to awareness without thinking, it is imprecise and somewhat contradictory. In particular, it requires daily practice and focusing on breathing to anchor attention, which suggests some kind of body-focused processing. Furthermore, it is difficult to reconcile cultivating trust in the self and acceptance with the absence of some form of value judgment. The features of mindfulness as practiced in meditation appear to conflict with one another and stand apart from the features of DM that eschew judgment and body focusing.

The conceptual and practical differences between mindfulness in DM and mindfulness used in these other contexts can be summarized as follows:

- DM does not involve meditation.
- DM does not require extensive and continuous practice.
- DM does not require broader features of mindfulness such as increasing present-moment awareness.
- Mindfulness in meditation tends to use body-focus exercises such as focusing on the breath to bring attention back to the present if it is captured by thoughts. DM does not have body-focused anchors for attention.
- DM specifically concerns developing meta-awareness of thoughts rather than present-moment awareness.
- Mindfulness has many meanings with a limited consensus. The definition and features of DM are more tightly specified in advance.
- DM separates meta-awareness from detachment.
- DM is specific about the suspension of conceptual processing.
- DM is specific concerning the suspension of goal-directed coping.
- DM is specific in the concept of separation of sense of self from mental phenomena.

It is likely that the effectiveness of techniques will depend on developing strategies grounded firmly in information-processing models that specify the more or less adaptive means of achieving mindfulness. The principle objective of meditation-derived mindfulness differs from that of DM, whose purpose is to modify well-specified metacognitive structures and processes that cause psychological disorder. The future development of these techniques might be well served by grounding them in a model of their requirements and consequences, as might be offered by the metacognitive approach.

TEN TECHNIQUES

This section presents 10 basic techniques that are used in MCT to promote a state of DM or components of it. This section is based on an earlier paper (Wells, 2005b) describing some of these strategies.

Metacognitive Guidance

"Metacognitive guidance" refers to the use of structured questioning to promote meta-cognitive self-reflection during exposure to problematic situations or stimuli. Useful questions include:

> "Can you look through your thoughts at the outside world?"
> "Can you see your thought and what is going on around you in the situation at the same time?"
> "Are you living by your thoughts or by what your eyes reveal?"

In one case of a patient with washing compulsions the therapist invited the patient to enter a situation that activated his distress and urge to wash, specifically, walking along the street close to a trash can. First, the patient did this without any therapist guidance and was simply told to find a distance from the can that raised some anxiety that was tolerable. Next the therapist asked him to move a little closer to the can and provided metacognitive guidance as follows:

THERAPIST: How distressed are you feeling right now on a scale of 0–100?

PATIENT: Not too bad. I would say 30.

THERAPIST: In a moment I want you to take one step forward and move closer to the trash can. But as you do that I want you to become aware of your inner thoughts. What are you saying to yourself as you step closer? Try that now.

PATIENT: I really don't want to do this.

THERAPIST: What thought did you have that made you feel that way?

PATIENT: I thought it's probably contaminated with bodily fluids.

THERAPIST: Was that a verbal thought or an inner picture?

PATIENT: It was a verbal thought: "What if it has bodily fluids on it?"

THERAPIST: Good. I want you to take that step closer and watch or listen to that verbal thought. See or hear those words in your mind and look through them at the trash can to discover the truth about your thought.

PATIENT: (Takes a step forward.)

THERAPIST: Well done. Could you experience seeing through your thought when you did that?

PATIENT: Yes, sort of.

THERAPIST: Does that tell you anything about your thought?

PATIENT: Well, it's just a thought. Taking that extra step hasn't really changed anything.

THERAPIST: Good. You can learn to relate to your thoughts in a new way without avoiding situations. What about taking another step? This time look through your thought and ask yourself: "Do my eyes reveal to me that I have been contaminated?"

PATIENT: (*Takes a further step.*)

THERAPIST: What do your eyes tell you?

PATIENT: Well, I can't see that I've been contaminated.

THERAPIST: So is it better to live by your thoughts or by what your eyes reveal to you?

PATIENT: Maybe I shouldn't be thinking is it or isn't it contaminated then?

THERAPIST: Could you practice looking through your thoughts instead of washing each time you have a thought?

PATIENT: But when should I wash?

THERAPIST: Only before touching food, after eating, or after visiting the toilet, but certainly not after having the thought.

PATIENT: So you're saying this is just a thought and I don't need to wash?

THERAPIST: That's it. Have you been giving this thought too much importance?

PATIENT: I've been accepting it as true.

THERAPIST: Can you practice relating to this thought in a new way from now on?

Free-Association Task

In this task the therapist asks the patient to sit quietly and watch the "ebb and flow" of thoughts or memories that are triggered spontaneously by verbal stimuli. The aim is not to actively think about items or memories but to watch the spontaneous events or lack of such events in consciousness. The task is introduced in the following way:

"So that you can become familiar with using detached mindfulness, it is helpful to practice in response to spontaneous events in your mind. By doing this you can learn to relate to these events in a new way. In a moment I will say a series of words to you. I would like you to allow your mind to roam freely in response to each word. Do not control or analyze what you think, merely watch how your mind responds. You may find that nothing much happens, but you may find that pictures come into your mind. It doesn't really matter what happens. Your task is to passively watch what happens without trying to influence anything. Try this with your eyes closed. I'm going to say some words now: apple, birthday, seaside, tree, bicycle, summertime, roses.

"What did you notice when you watched your mind?

"The idea is that you should apply this strategy to your negative thoughts and feelings. Just watch what your mind does without getting caught up in any thinking process."

Tiger Task

This is a task that our patients particularly enjoy. In this task participants are asked to passively observe nonvolitional aspects of imagery as a means of experiencing DM. The following instructions are used to implement the procedure:

"So that you can feel what detached mindfulness is like and what you need to do to experience it, I want to introduce you to an exercise. We call this the 'tiger task.' In a moment I'm going to ask you to close your eyes and form an image of a tiger. Let's do that now: close your eyes and conjure up an image of a tiger. Do not attempt to influence or change the image in any way. Just watch the image and the tiger's behavior. The tiger may move, but don't make it move. It may blink, but don't make it blink. The tiger may wag its tail, but don't make it do that. Watch how the tiger has its own behavior. Do nothing, but simply watch the image, see how the tiger is simply a thought in your mind, that it is separate from you and it has a behavior all of its own."

Following practice, the therapist then asks the patient about the movements the tiger made and how the image changed: "Did you make the tiger move or did it happen spontaneously?" When the patient experiences the movements as spontaneous, this is brought to the patient's attention as an experience of DM. The therapist then asks if this process can be applied to spontaneously occurring thoughts of a negative kind.

Suppression–Countersuppression Experiment

When patients are highly invested in controlling and avoiding particular thoughts, and when they erroneously equate the concept of DM with having a blank mind, the suppression–countersuppression experiment is particularly useful. In these cases it is important that the therapist distinguishes between suppression and DM so that patient misunderstanding and misuse of DM is minimized. This technique consists of a brief period of attempting to suppress a target thought contrasted with a subsequent period of thought awareness. An example of this technique is given below:

> "It is important that you learn the difference between detached mindfulness and trying to control or avoid thoughts. Trying to stop thoughts is a form of active engagement with them since you are trying to push them out of your mind. Pushing something is hardly leaving something alone and so this effort backfires and you remain in contact with your thoughts.
>
> "How can you push against a door and not be in contact with it by some means? Let's see this effect in action. For the next 3 minutes I don't want you to think about a blue giraffe. Don't allow yourself to have any thought connected with it, try to push it away. Off you go.
>
> "What did you notice? Did you think of a blue giraffe?
>
> "Let's now try detached mindfulness and see what happens. For the next 3 minutes let your mind roam freely and if you have thoughts of blue giraffes I want you to watch them in a passive way as part of an overall landscape of thoughts. Try that now.
>
> "What did you notice? How important was the thought of the blue giraffe the second time around?"

The therapist should then discuss how suppression gives thoughts extra salience and importance, and how DM can be used to allow thoughts to roam freely as passing events in the mind that do not require an active response. The procedure may then be repeated asking the patient to become aware of being the separate observer of the thought.

Clouds Metaphor

In some versions of this task participants were asked to use imagery to respond to thoughts: thoughts were to be imagined as printed on clouds and allowed to drift across the sky. However, in this form the task involves responding to thoughts and then transforming them. As such it is not a true version of DM. Another version is now preferred in which clouds are simply used as a metaphor to convey the experience of DM. The therapist offers the following account:

> "One way to understand detached mindfulness and what it requires is to consider experiencing your thoughts as you would experience clouds passing you by in the sky. The clouds are part of the Earth's self-regulating weather system, and it would be impossible and unnecessary to try and control them. Try to treat your thoughts and feelings

like you would treat passing clouds and allow them to occupy their own space and time in the knowledge that they will eventually pass you by."

Recalcitrant Child Metaphor

This metaphor helps the patient to understand the different effects of active engagement with thoughts versus detached awareness (mindfulness). The therapist gives the following instruction:

> "You can think of detached mindfulness as similar to the way you might deal with a child. How would you manage a child misbehaving in a store? You could pay a great deal of attention to the child and try to control the child's behavior. But if the child craves attention this response could make things worse. It is better not to actively engage with the child but to keep a passive watch over the child without doing anything.
>
> "Your negative thoughts and beliefs are like that child. If you pay them a great deal of attention, if you control them or use punishment, they misbehave even more. It is better not to try and control or actively engage with them, just keep a watching manner over everything. As you do this, try to be aware of yourself as the observer of these things."

Passenger Train Metaphor

This is an alternative to the clouds metaphor described above. Here the patient is asked to deal with intrusive thoughts and feelings in the same way that he or she would deal with an express train passing through a station:

> "It is helpful to think of yourself as a passenger waiting for a train. Your mind is like a busy station and your thoughts and feelings are the trains passing through. There is no point in trying to stop and climb aboard a train that is passing by. Just be a bystander and watch your thoughts pass through. There is no point in climbing aboard to be whisked away to the wrong place."

Verbal Loop

The repeated presentation of thoughts either by a recording device or through repeated vocalization has the effect of decreasing their attentional salience and diminishing their meaning because they are experienced more as sounds than as inner conveyors of information. This technique is presented with a metacognitive rationale as follows:

"I would like you to listen to a recording of your intrusive thoughts [or repeat quietly to yourself your thought . . .]. As you do so you should relate to them in a special way. Treat the thoughts as a set of sounds and do not engage with them in any other way. They are merely sounds in the outside world. Keep in mind as you listen that you are simply a listener safe in the knowledge that thoughts are not facts, they are simply events in your mind."

Detachment: The Observing Self

We have seen that detachment includes both disengagement of control and conceptual processes and experiencing thoughts or beliefs as an observer with no further divisible sense of consciousness. It is a core, indivisible, felt sense that has no propositional reference and no further point of regression. It is a singular sense of self. In this state the individual is observer of the thought and separate from any thought itself.

This level and experience of DM is accomplished by asking patients questions that direct their attention in a particular way during their monitoring of thoughts. These questions are usually incorporated in the above experiential techniques to intensify the experience of DM once awareness and discontinuation of conceptual processing has been achieved. Specifically the patient is asked during these exercises:

"Are you the thought or the person observing the thought? Try to be aware of your location and what it is like to be the observer. You exist entirely separately from thoughts."

Or:

"Are you the belief or the person observing the belief? Try to be aware of how your consciousness as the observer is separate from your beliefs."

Daydreaming Technique

It is typically the case that our daydreams are experienced in object mode. We become completely immersed in them and live them as momentary reality. The practice of shifting to detached observer during daydreaming can provide a powerful subjective experience of DM.

The therapist asks the patient to engage in a pleasant daydream, such as driving an exotic car or sipping champagne on a Caribbean beach. Then the therapist asks the patient to allow the daydream to continue but to step back and be aware of the self in the present as observer of the daydream as it unfolds.

REINFORCING DM USING SOCRATIC DIALOGUE

On completion of experiential exercises, the therapist reinforces DM during the course of treatment by asking questions when a negative thought or belief is activated. These questions include the following:

> "Are you the belief or the person that observes and uses that belief?"
> "Is that thought important or is it a passing event in your mind?"
> "Can you see yourself as separate from that idea?"
> "What are the advantages of practicing being separate from that thought?"
> "In future, can you separate your sense of self from the mere occurrence of that thought?"

HOMEWORK

The application of DM is a task set for homework. The patient is instructed to notice the triggers for worry/rumination and unhelpful coping behaviors such as avoidance/suppression (the CAS) and to apply DM to the trigger. Typically, DM is combined with other techniques such as the worry/rumination postponement technique (see Chapter 6), which facilitates detachment of continued processing from initial intrusions.

The therapist reviews the range of thoughts to which DM is applied in the first few sessions, with a view to increasing this application and enhancing the patient's awareness of triggers for the CAS. The therapist makes careful note that DM is not being inappropriately applied as a coping strategy aimed at preventing erroneous threats.

In order to determine an effective frequency of the technique, the therapist asks about the proportion of triggers to which DM has been applied. As a rough rule of thumb, the therapist aims to achieve a 75% application rate during treatment. The effective use of DM can also be gauged by examining scores on the CAS-1 rating scale. In particular, items 1 and 3 (worry and coping) are indicative of the level of maladaptive engagement with internal triggers (i.e., the antithesis of DM).

APPLICATION OF DM IN MCT

MCT is not a treatment based on individual techniques. It is quite possible to effectively implement MCT without specifically training patients in DM. It is important that the therapist does not see this technique or any other technique as the mainstay of treatment. However, DM is a component of MCT that can act as a catalyst for meta-level change.

Application of DM early in therapy is recommended in conjunction with postponement of worry and rumination (see Chapter 6). Usually the technique is introduced in the first or second session but is not intensively practiced thereafter. In the treatment of depression we prefer the regular practice of the ATT at each session as a more structured and intensive means of achieving executive control and with the aim of accomplishing important features of DM.

Throughout its usage the therapist normally tracks the patient's goals in using the technique and monitors examples to ensure that it is used appropriately. The therapist should be aware of misuse of DM as a distraction technique, a means of avoiding anticipated threat, and as a means of anxiety control.

> A 26-year-old woman undergoing MCT for depression described how she had inconsistent results applying DM, stating that "I'm not always successful in making my thoughts go away." A very useful discussion followed in which the therapist discovered that she had been inappropriately trying to stop negative automatic thoughts (e.g., "I'm worthless") rather than applying DM to them and interrupting further conceptual analysis of her failings and weaknesses.

Later in treatment it may be necessary to ban the use of DM as a prelude to or in conjunction with experiments designed to challenge negative beliefs about loss of control and the danger of thoughts and symptoms. The continued use of DM can prevent some patients from discovering that they cannot lose mental control since they attribute the nonoccurrence of the catastrophe to use of the technique.

CONCLUSION

DM is a state of relating to inner thoughts and beliefs in a particular way. It is intended to increase flexible control over thinking styles and promote the development of a new model of the significance and importance of thoughts and beliefs.

There are several differences and some similarities between DM and other mindfulness practices. DM is intended to impact on the CAS and enable the development of new metacognitive knowledge. The features and information-processing requirements of DM can be specified in the context of the metacognitive model.

Ten strategies for achieving DM as part of MCT were described. In MCT the therapist uses these techniques most often as part of the early sessions of treatment. They form only a component of the treatment process. They should not be considered as intensive training exercises or as procedures that determine the success of the intervention, but instead as useful tools that can be used to facilitate metacognitive change and the transition between cognitive and metacognitive levels (or modes) of working.

|||||||||||||||||||||

CHAPTER 6

Generalized Anxiety Disorder

Generalized anxiety disorder (GAD) is the most prevalent anxiety disorder and its core processes represent the elementary processes in all anxiety disorders (e.g., Barlow, 2002).

GAD is characterized by excessive and difficult-to-control worry combined with several anxiety symptoms. To meet criteria for GAD the individual must exhibit a minimum of two different worry content domains, such as health, social, family, or financial worries. The DSM-IV-TR (American Psychiatric Association, 2000) diagnostic criteria for this disorder are summarized in Table 6.1.

Individuals presenting with GAD often state that they have been worriers much of their lives. Worry and anxiety can interfere very significantly with their social and/or occupational functioning. The focus of the person's predominant worry changes over short to long time intervals, but the focus is not confined to nor can it be better explained by another Axis I disorder. For instance, the worry is not confined to speaking in front of a group (as in social phobia), physical illness (as in hypochondriasis), or having a panic attack (as in panic disorder). Domain-specific worries like these may be better accounted for by another diagnosis.

Since worry is the key cognitive feature of the disorder, the therapist must be able to identify this activity and differentiate it from other types of similar mental activity, namely, rumination or obsessional thinking.

Worry has been defined as a chain of negative thoughts that are predominantly verbal and aimed at problem solving (Borkovec, Robinson, Pruzinsky, & DePree, 1983). The chain-like verbal nature of the worry process can be clearly seen in the example given below taken from a patient entering our MCT treatment program:

TABLE 6.1. Diagnostic Criteria for GAD

Criterion A

Presence of excessive anxiety and worry occurring more days than
not for at least 6 months. At least two worry topics.

Criterion B

The person finds it difficult to control the worry.

Criterion C

Anxiety and worry are associated with at least three of the
following symptoms: restlessness, easily fatigued, concentration or
memory difficulties, irritability, muscle tension, sleep disturbance.

Criterion D

The focus of worry is not confined to another Axis I disorder.

Criterion E

Anxiety, worry, or physical symptoms cause significant impairment.

Criterion F

Anxiety is not due to substances or a medical condition.

Note. Summarized from American Psychiatric Association (2000).

"I was worrying before I even got to work. I thought what if my car
breaks down, I would be late for the meeting, I would have to make an
excuse, my supervisor could be angry at me, what if she asks my opin-
ion and I'm not prepared. I was worrying constantly, thinking have I
done the right thing, have I made a mistake in the report? What if it
isn't good enough? They would think I was incompetent. What if they
regret taking me on? What should I say, what if they ask me something
I don't know? It was all too much. I was worrying before and throughout the meeting and when I got back to my office I just couldn't take it
anymore. I just lost it and burst into tears."

Worry involves catastrophizing and is subjectively difficult to control.
The process has been viewed as a coping mechanism but the process itself
can become the focus of worry (Wells, 1995). Such worry about worry is a
key concept in the metacognitive approach to treating GAD.

Worry can be described as ego-syntonic, meaning that it is usually
perceived as characteristic of the self and does not violate the person's
self-view. In contrast, other types of persistent negative thinking such as
obsessional intrusions are ego-dystonic, meaning that they are viewed by
the person as inappropriate, abhorrent, and disgusting. An example would
be a religious person having blasphemous thoughts.

In a comparison of normal obsessions and worry several differences emerged (Wells & Morrison, 1994). Obsessional thoughts were of shorter duration and involved more imagery, while worry was more verbal, more realistic, and more voluntary. Another distinction between obsessional intrusions and worry is that the former can consist of urges and impulses that are not characteristic of worry. Depressive rumination is also ego-syntonic in the sense that the person often sees it as a means of understanding feelings and working out problems. Although there are many similarities between anxious and depressive thoughts (Papageorgiou & Wells, 1999b), there also appear to be some differences. Worry is more future-oriented while depressive rumination focuses more on the past. Worry and anxious thoughts involve themes of danger while rumination is concerned more with loss, failure, and personal inadequacy.

THE UBIQUITY OF WORRY

The metacognitive model of psychological disorder assumes that worry is a central component of the CAS thought to contribute to all types of pathology. GAD might be considered as the archetypal manifestation of the CAS. The application of MCT in this disorder provides a platform for understanding how to conceptualize and treat uncontrollable worry processes across a spectrum of disorders.

Many of the strategies presented in this chapter will find a place in the treatment of other disorders, although their precise usage and implementation will need to be adjusted to meet the specification of causal factors in disorder-specific case formulations.

It might be logical to assume that there is something special or unique about GAD worry that makes it such a problem for individuals suffering from this disorder. The research evidence appears to show that this is not the case. The content and nature of GAD worry is very similar to normal worry (e.g., Ruscio & Borkovec, 2004). There is, however, one way in which GAD worry appears to be markedly different as predicted by the metacognitive model. Worry in GAD is associated with more negative thoughts and beliefs about worry (Wells & Carter, 2001; Ruscio & Borkovec, 2004).

IS WORRY CONTROLLABLE?

Worry is often experienced as difficult to control. This does not mean that it cannot be controlled easily. The patient and the MCT therapist need to understand the essence of possible and impossible control and effective and ineffective strategies.

Worry is a slow conceptual process involving the contemplation of relatively novel future events and ways of coping with them. It is readily modified by feedback from internal or external sources. The conscious strategic nature of worry should mean that it is amenable to high levels of volitional control even if awareness of such control is low or nonexistent. However, it is important to distinguish between intrusive thoughts that might be more automatic and involuntary and act as triggers for worry and the sustained conceptual nature of worrying itself, which represents a response to such intrusions. An aim in MCT is to lessen or stop sustained conceptual-based (worry-based) thinking in response to intrusions. This is the type of control that the therapist and the patient aim for and not control or suppression of the intrusive thoughts that trigger worrying. Furthermore, the control of sustained thinking or worry in MCT is used as a means of challenging metacognitive beliefs.

THE METACOGNITIVE MODEL OF GAD

The metacognitive model of GAD (Wells, 1995, 1997) is presented diagrammatically in Figure 6.1. It proposes that people with GAD tend to use worrying as their predominant means of anticipating future problems and generating ways of coping. Worrying is usually triggered as a coping strategy in response to an intrusive negative thought (e.g., "What if I'm involved in an accident?"). This is not necessarily a problem because it is theoretically possible to be a "happy worrier" so long as the person believes that his or her work of worry is effective and prevents danger. General worry about external events and about social and physical health concerns in response to triggers is called "Type 1 worry." The use of worry as a means of coping is linked to positive metacognitive beliefs that most people hold to some extent. These include beliefs such as "Worrying helps me avoid problems in the future"; "Worry means I'll be prepared"; and "Worrying helps me cope." However, it is the activation of negative metacognitive beliefs that is most important in the transition to GAD.

GAD develops when the person activates negative beliefs about worrying. Two types of negative belief are important: negative beliefs about the uncontrollability of worry and negative beliefs about its harmful or dangerous consequences. The latter category contains beliefs that worry can lead to physical (e.g., heart attack), psychological (e.g., mental breakdown), or social (e.g., rejection by others) catastrophe. Examples of metacognitive beliefs are presented in Table 6.2.

Once negative metacognitive beliefs are activated, the individual negatively appraises worrying, that is, he or she worries about worry, leading to increased anxiety and feelings of being unable to cope. Worry about worry

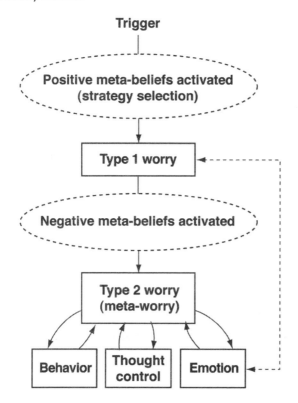

FIGURE 6.1. The metacognitive model of GAD. From Wells (1997, p. 204). Copyright 1997 by John Wiley & Sons Limited. Reprinted by permission.

is an example of a metacognitive appraisal (an interpretation of a thought process). It has been called "meta-worry" or "Type 2 worry" (Wells, 1994) to signify that it is the negative appraisal of worry and associated symptoms. Examples of meta-worry are "I'm losing control," "I'm going crazy," and "I'm harming my body." Anxiety symptoms are often misinterpreted as a sign of the dangerous and damaging effects of worrying that leads to a strengthening of negative beliefs and a spiral of immediately intensified anxiety. Panic attacks can occur when such interpretations concern an immediate impending catastrophe such as a heart attack or loss of mental control.

Type 2 worry (meta-worry) leads to two further factors that contribute to problem maintenance. These are separated out in the model as *behavioral responses* and *thought control strategies*. The main reason for this is to simplify socialization, as we shall see later. In particular, an interesting dynamic in the thought control responses used by the patient rewards closer scrutiny.

**TABLE 6.2. Examples of Metacognitive Beliefs
about Worry in GAD**

Positive metacognitive beliefs

- "Worrying helps me cope."
- "If I worry I'll be prepared."
- "Worrying keeps me in control."
- "If I worry I can anticipate and avoid problems."

Negative metacognitive beliefs—Uncontrollability

- "I have no control over worry."
- "My worries have taken control of me."
- "I have lost control of my thoughts."
- "My worries are uncontrollable."

Negative metacognitive beliefs—Danger

- "I could lose my mind with worrying."
- "Worrying will damage my body."
- "I could go crazy with worry."
- "I'm going to have a mental breakdown because of worry."

Coping behaviors consist of reassurance seeking, avoidance (though this is often subtle), information search (e.g., surfing the Internet), distraction, use of alcohol, and so on. These behaviors maintain negative appraisals and beliefs about worry because they subvert the process of self-control by handing control over to external factors. For example, one patient asked her husband to telephone her at set times each day to confirm that he was safe. Otherwise she would not be able to contain her worry. This process prevented her from discovering that she could control her own worries, and it therefore maintained her belief in uncontrollability. It also provided a greater range of opportunities for uncertainty when her husband was unable to telephone on time, which acted to intensify her triggers for worry. Some patients attempt to control or avoid worry by searching for information by "surfing the Internet." One patient described how he had recently worried about the appearance of a dark patch of skin on his upper arm. As a means of trying to control his worry he had explored information on the Internet about the nature and causes of skin discoloration. He had hoped that he would find information that would lead him to worry less, but in fact he had discovered dangerous possibilities that he had not even thought of, which became the triggers of sustained worry. Thus, some strategies backfire and act as further triggers for worrying. Even when they do stop worry they prevent the person from discovering that the worry process can be suspended by internal means. They also prevent the person discovering that even if worry continued it would not lead to negative consequences such as a heart attack or a mental breakdown.

Another process in the model refers to the patient's use of thought control strategies. There is often an unhelpful use of strategies involving suppression of worry triggers and a failure to disengage from the worry process once it is activated. Suppression involves trying not to think thoughts that might trigger worrying. So, for example, a person currently concerned about his or her performance at work will try to suppress all thoughts about work when away from that environment. Unfortunately, suppression is not entirely effective and its failure can reinforce beliefs about loss of control and/or lead to an increase in the salience of triggering thoughts. The second important process is the individual's failure to disengage the worry process once it is activated. This is made manifest as continuing to think through the worry in order to cope, or trying to reassure the self with self-talk. It is a continuation of conceptual activity in which the patient fails to interrupt the perseverative coping process. Several factors can contribute to this failure. For instance, the person often believes that not worrying would be equivalent to not attempting to cope (as worry is a main coping strategy) or the person lacks awareness of the control he or she has, assuming, for instance, that the problem is intractable (e.g., worrying is part of my personality). Often the individual has had few personal experiences of self-control of the worry process that would challenge his or her beliefs about its uncontrollability.

THE MODEL IN ACTION

A walk-through of the model as it operates in a worry episode will serve to illustrate the operation of each of its components.

A distressing worry episode is triggered by an initial intrusive thought, usually in the form of a "What if . . . ?" question (e.g., "What if my partner is involved in an accident?"), but sometimes in the form of a negative image. This trigger activates tacit positive metacognitive beliefs about the need for sustained catastrophic thinking (Type 1 worry) as a means of anticipating and coping with problems. This Type 1 worry immediately leads to increases in emotional symptoms, but may subsequently lead to reductions in negative emotions if the person satisfies his or her goal of worrying. The goal is often the feeling that one will be able to cope or an appraisal that most dangerous possibilities have been covered.

During the worry sequence in GAD, negative beliefs about the uncontrollability and dangerous nature of worry are activated. This leads to negative interpretation of worry (i.e., Type 2 worry) and increased anxiety. At this point the person finds it harder to achieve a goal that signals it is safe to stop worrying and may begin to see the self as less able to cope.

Now behaviors and thought control strategies aimed at avoiding worry and preventing its negative effects are initiated. Many of these strategies

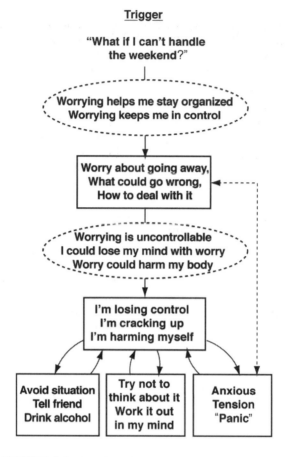

FIGURE 6.2. An idiosyncratic GAD case formulation.

are unhelpful or backfire, leading to a preoccupation with and a strengthening of negative beliefs about uncontrollability and danger, so that these beliefs are more likely to figure predominantly in future worry episodes. An example of this model drawn out for a recent worry episode reported by a patient is presented in Figure 6.2.

STRUCTURE OF TREATMENT

Treatment can be usefully conceptualized as movement through a sequence of stages. The number of sessions required to meet each stage varies depending on patient and therapist factors. Patient factors are level of insight, motivation, and engagement with homework. Therapist factors include level of skill and experience in implementing MCT. The sequence of stages is as follows:

1. Case conceptualization
2. Socialization
3. Inducing the metacognitive mode
4. Challenging metacognitive beliefs about uncontrollability
5. Challenging metacognitive beliefs about the danger of worry
6. Challenging positive metacognitive beliefs about worry
7. Reinforcing new plans for processing worry
8. Relapse prevention

Treatment typically ranges from five to ten sessions, with the modal number of sessions being eight when delivered by therapists with some experience of MCT. In the remainder of this chapter the implementation of each of these stages is described in detail.

CASE CONCEPTUALIZATION

Measures

Tools required during this stage are:

1. Generalized Anxiety Disorder Scale—Revised (GADS-R)
2. GAD Case Formulation Interview
3. Session checklists

The therapist begins by administering the GADS-R and examines the negative and positive metacognitive beliefs endorsed in order to obtain a preliminary impression of the types of beliefs that should be amenable during formulation. The GADS-R can be found in Appendix 7. This scale also provides an impression of the types of behaviors used to avoid worry and danger, which can be subtle in GAD. Other measures normally considered that are completed before the session are the Beck Anxiety Inventory (BAI; Beck et al., 1988) and the Beck Depression Inventory II (BDI-II; Beck et al., 1996).

Agenda of the First Session

The treatment session begins with setting an agenda:

"In today's session I would like to explore a recent episode of worry in which you became distressed by the worry. In doing this we can explore the factors that are keeping your worry problem going and begin to examine ways that you can overcome your anxiety. I would also like to explain a little more about MCT and what you might expect from treatment. Is there anything you would like to put on the agenda and talk about today?"

Generating a Case Conceptualization

The next step is to proceed with generating an idiosyncratic version of the metacognitive model that represents the events in a recent distressing worry episode. It is important that the therapist focuses on an actual recent episode rather than trying to conceptualize processes more generally, which can be a major source of in-session drift.

A straightforward means of generating the case conceptualization is to follow a particular sequence of questions. This sequence is depicted by the numbering 1–8 in the GAD Case Formulation Interview presented in Appendix 11. Each number links a particular interview question to eliciting the material required for each part of the model.

An example dialogue using these questions is presented below. The case conceptualization resulting from these questions is presented in Figure 6.3.

THERAPIST: When was the last time you were worried and distressed by your worry?

PATIENT: It was about 2 weeks ago.

THERAPIST: Was that a typical worry episode?

PATIENT: Yes, but I didn't panic on that occasion.

THERAPIST: Fine. Let's look at that worry. Briefly, where were you?

PATIENT: I was at home and saw a police car drive by, and then I started worrying that one day they could be coming to give me bad news and how I couldn't cope with that.

THERAPIST: Okay, I need to slow things down. What was the first thought that went through your mind when you saw the police car? Was it a "What if . . . ?" question or an image of something bad happening?

PATIENT: I think it was more like: "What if my husband has been killed?"

THERAPIST: So that was the trigger, an initial "what if" thought about your husband.

PATIENT: Yes, and I thought how bad it would be.

THERAPIST: So it sounds as if you were into the worry now. What did you then go on to worry about?

PATIENT: I thought what if I couldn't manage the children on my own, how

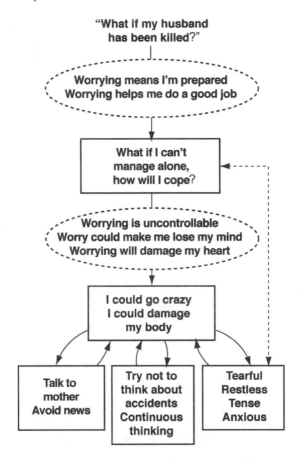

FIGURE 6.3. GAD case formulation arising from the dialogue.

would I cope with the finances, what if I ended up alone, how could I deal with those things?

THERAPIST: So it sounds as if you were deeply into worry. What happened to your emotions when you were worrying like that?

PATIENT: I felt terrible, I was tearful, restless, tense, I felt anxious.

THERAPIST: When you were feeling anxious and you were worried, did you think anything bad could happen because of the way you were thinking and feeling?

PATIENT: I'm not sure.

THERAPIST: What was the worst that could happen if you continued to feel and think like that?

PATIENT: That's terrible, I don't want to get into that. When you get into that you think you're going to lose your mind and that's when panic sets in.

THERAPIST: When you're really worried do you think you could go crazy?

PATIENT: Yes.

THERAPIST: Do you have any other negative thoughts about your worries and anxiety?

PATIENT: I think I could damage my body, especially my heart, if I go on like this.

THERAPIST: Why don't you stop yourself worrying if it's so harmful?

PATIENT: I can't, I have no control.

THERAPIST: So it sounds like you have some beliefs about worry. That it is uncontrollable, that it can make you lose your mind, and that it can damage your heart, is that right?

PATIENT: Yes.

THERAPIST: How much do you believe it is uncontrollable on a scale from 0 to 100%?

PATIENT: Ninety percent.

THERAPIST: How much do you believe it can make you lose your mind?

PATIENT: Seventy percent.

THERAPIST: How much do you believe worry can damage your heart?

PATIENT: Seventy percent.

THERAPIST: These sound like negative beliefs about worry. Can I ask you, do you have any positive beliefs about worry? That is, do you think worry is helpful in any way?

PATIENT: It means I can be prepared, it helps me be aware of problems, and it helps me do a good job.

THERAPIST: How much do you believe that?

PATIENT: I believe all of those things about 70 percent.

THERAPIST: When you were worrying on this occasion did you do anything to stop yourself worrying?

PATIENT: I talked to my mother about it to get some reassurance. She is good, as she gets me to look at it logically.

THERAPIST: Anything else, such as avoiding things, or searching for evidence to put your mind at rest?

PATIENT: I avoid watching the news and reading newspapers as there's always something to worry about.

THERAPIST: I want to ask you about two other things in response to worrying thoughts. Do you try not to think certain thoughts in case they trigger a worry?

PATIENT: Yes, I try not to think about illness and accidents.

THERAPIST: Okay. Have you ever decided not to respond by worrying when you have a negative thought like that?

PATIENT: No, I feel I'm right to worry about it, that it wouldn't be good otherwise. I have to think about these things, otherwise I won't be able to deal with them.

THERAPIST: Okay, I'll put that in the model too. Let's call it "continuous thinking."

A Note on Eliciting Metacognitions

Metacognitive beliefs concerning uncontrollability and danger are at center stage in the case conceptualization and treatment. It is crucial that these can be effectively elicited. Novice MCT therapists sometimes find it difficult to elicit negative metacognitive beliefs, often because they are implicit in the patient's description. While negative beliefs about danger are *typically* present, negative beliefs about uncontrollability are *always* present. For example, a patient stated that he had no negative beliefs about worrying, just that worrying made him feel bad. The therapist asked him why he didn't reduce his worrying if it made him feel so bad, to which the patient replied that he couldn't because he had no control. As this example shows, uncontrollability beliefs are an implicit part of this patient's problem.

A strategy for eliciting negative metacognitions consists of asking about the disadvantages of worrying. The disadvantages correspond to negative beliefs. Asking about the advantages of worrying can provide a means of eliciting positive beliefs about the activity.

The therapist might also find it useful to ask about the "worst consequences scenario" to determine negative beliefs about worry. An example of a worst consequences question combined with an exploration of meanings follows:

THERAPIST: How do you feel when you're worried?

PATIENT: I feel stressed and anxious.

THERAPIST: What's the worst that could happen if you continued to worry like that?

PATIENT: I'd really lose it.

THERAPIST: What do you mean by "really lose it"?

PATIENT: I don't know really, it would be taken out of my hands.

THERAPIST: What's the worst way of losing it?

PATIENT: I'd crack up or something.

THERAPIST: What would that look like?

PATIENT: I'd have a breakdown and be paralyzed with worry.

THERAPIST: Do you believe that worry can cause a breakdown?

PATIENT: Yes, if I go on like this.

SOCIALIZATION

The process of socialization has effectively begun while the therapist systematically traces out the components of the case conceptualization. However, the next step is more explicit in explaining the mechanisms in the model. The therapist proceeds by sharing the diagrammatic case formulation (or, better still, this has been mapped out already in real time on a marker board). The following steps are usually followed:

Step 1: Sharing the Conceptualization

The therapist explains briefly how the model works:

"Looking at the diagram we have mapped out, it is possible to see some important factors that help us understand the causes of your worry problem. On this occasion your worry was triggered by an initial intrusive thought [state patient example], and went on to worry about what this would be like and how to deal with the situation if it happened [point to Type 1 worry]. This was associated with feeling anxious [trace link between Type 1 worry and anxiety]. But that wasn't the end of things because you then began to worry about what you were thinking and feeling. We call this 'worry about worry' or Type 2 worry [point to Type 2 worry]. On this occasion you thought [state patient's Type 2 worry]. What effect did thinking that have on your anxiety?

"So you see that part of your problem is worry about worry and the negative beliefs you have about worrying. This is directly increasing your anxiety. You have also developed some other coping behaviors that may not actually help [point to behaviors box in the case formulation]. For example, have these things worked yet, have you been able to overcome your worry problem? It these things don't work, what does that lead you to believe about the controllability of worry?

"There are also some interesting thought control strategies that you use. You try not to think thoughts that might trigger worrying. You also don't seem to interrupt the worry process consistently when it is activated. If you allow yourself to engage in continued thinking, does that give you the sense that you can control it?

"Apart from your negative beliefs you also have some positive beliefs about worry. We will deal with these later. But let me ask you now, Do you think that having positive beliefs about worry might contribute to a persistence of worrying?

"So you see how your problem is maintained by what you believe about worry and the strategies you use to control it. We need to change these things in treatment so that you can recover."

Step 2: Hypothetical Questions

Hypothetical questions are then used as a means of illustrating the contribution of metacognitive beliefs to the problem:

"I can illustrate the role of beliefs about worry by asking you a question. If you believed that worry was only a good thing to do, how much of a problem would worry be?"

"If you suddenly discovered that you could control worry, how much of a problem would remain?"

"If you discovered that worry could not harm your mind or body, would worry be so distressing?"

Step 3: Dissonance (Two-Minds Strategy)

A further means of conveying the message that beliefs about worry are central to the problem is by illustrating how metacognitive beliefs place the patient in a no-win situation that can only lead to the process of difficult-to-control worry:

"It appears that you are in two minds about worry. On the one hand you believe it is a beneficial thing to do, but on the other hand you believe it is uncontrollable and harmful. How easy is it for you to stop worrying so long as you are in two minds about it?"

Or:

"As we have seen you are in two minds about worry. Are two minds better than one in this instance? What problems do two minds create?"

Step 4: Question the Effects of Behaviors

By questioning the effects of behavior the therapist can help patients discover that their self-regulatory behaviors have not been effective. This act of discovery allows the therapist to pose an important question that leads neatly into the first therapy exercise of applying DM and worry postponement. Questions to use are as follows:

"How effective have your behaviors been in getting rid of worry in the long term?"

"What have your behaviors enabled you to discover about the controllability of worry?"

"Your inability to control worry could mean it is uncontrollable, but could it also mean you have been using the wrong strategies to control it? Have you thought about it like that before?"

Step 5: Suppression Experiment

Next, a suppression experiment is used to illustrate how some thought control strategies are counterproductive or ineffective and do not provide useful information about worry. Here the patient is asked to suppress a neutral thought. The experiment is normally introduced with very little rational in the following way:

"Let's see how some of your strategies might not be helpful. We can try with a neutral thought. Let's assume that you worry about blue rabbits. For the next 3 minutes I want you to stop yourself from having any thoughts of blue rabbits. What ever you do you must not think of a blue rabbit in any shape or form. Off you go.

"Okay, you can stop now. What happened when you tried to suppress that thought?"

Typically, the patient reports that the suppressed thought occurred. This result can then be used to illustrate how trying to suppress worry triggers is not very effective. The therapist can ask, "If it is not effective, what does this lead you to believe about the controllability of worry?"

In some instances the patient is able to suppress the target thought. In such cases the therapist should simply ask, "It seems that you could suppress the thought. Is that something you can do with all of your worry triggers?" The answer to this question can be used to show how the strategy is not consistently effective.

BRIDGING FROM SOCIALIZATION TO METACOGNITIVE MODIFICATION

As the process of initial socialization draws to an end the patient should be asked to summarize what he or she has learned about the cause of worry. The therapist gives a brief description of the nature of MCT as follows:

"Treatment will focus on examining more effective ways of responding to your thoughts that trigger worry so that you can discover that worry is not uncontrollable. We will then try to deal with the negative beliefs that you hold about the danger of worry. These beliefs give rise to high levels of anxiety so we should deal with them soon. Later in treatment we will look at the positive beliefs you have about worry and a range of alternative ways of responding to negative thoughts."

QUESTIONING UNCONTROLLABILITY BELIEFS

The next stage is the use of verbal reattribution to explore and weaken beliefs about the uncontrollability of worry. Discussion of modulating influences on worry is used to provide evidence that worry is subject to control and can be readily displaced by alternative processing demands. For example, the therapist asks:

> "What happens if you are worrying and the telephone rings and you answer the phone? What happens to your worry?"
> "If worry truly is uncontrollable, how does it ever stop?"

The latter question can elicit some intriguing answers. As the following dialogue illustrates, the therapist should attempt to carefully explore the patient's concept of control and distinguish control of worry from suppression of thoughts:

THERAPIST: How much do you believe worry is uncontrollable?

PATIENT: Eighty percent.

THERAPIST: If worry truly is uncontrollable, how does it ever stop?

PATIENT: It doesn't, unless the thing I was worried about is no longer there.

THERAPIST: So what happens to your worry when you sleep?

PATIENT: It's there even when I'm asleep. I wake up feeling tired.

THERAPIST: Is feeling tired the same as worry?

PATIENT: No, no, it's different, I suppose.

THERAPIST: So if worry is uncontrollable, how do you ever sleep?

PATIENT: Well, sometimes sleep is difficult, but I suppose it does stop.

THERAPIST: Yes, that's right. What happens to your worry if you have to do something important like answer the telephone? Does it stay the same?

PATIENT: No, it's very much switched on and off.

THERAPIST: That's right. So does that suggest worry is uncontrollable?

PATIENT: No, I do have some control. But maybe not over big worries.

THERAPIST: Well, we need to examine what we mean by "control." You can't always control initial thoughts that trigger worry, but you can choose not to engage in the extended worry process that follows. And that's what I'd like us to look at next.

DETACHED MINDFULNESS AND WORRY POSTPONEMENT

Socialization should have begun to shift the patient to a metacognitive perspective (level) of viewing the problem. At this stage of treatment it is useful to check that the patient understands that the problem is one of beliefs about worry and unhelpful strategies for regulating thoughts.

The next step is building on the suppression experiment and developing the skills of DM. In Chapter 5, we saw a range of techniques for inducing DM. The strategy used in the treatment of GAD is identifying the trigger, applying DM to it, and postponing the worry process that normally follows the trigger.

This can be thought of as a means of decoupling intrusions from the control of subsequent processing so that the patient develops greater metacognitive flexibility. Furthermore, this is used as part of a subsequent behavioral experiment to test negative metacognitive beliefs about the uncontrollability of worry.

Detached Mindfulness

With reference to the suppression experiment and/or the ineffectiveness of coping strategies, the therapist should remind the patient how trying to control initial triggers for worrying has not been effective in overcoming the problem. What is required is a new approach that can enable the patient to discover the truth about the uncontrollability of worry. The following questions are used to introduce this stage:

> "Have you ever decided not to worry in response to a triggering thought?"
> "Have you ever tried to hold in mind a trigger and just leave it alone?"
> "Have you ever seen your negative thoughts as merely events passing through your mind?"

After setting the scene in this way, the therapist instructs the patient about applying DM to thoughts. This is typically practiced with neutral thoughts and then followed by DM's application to two or three typical worry triggers. The therapist introduces the exercise in the following way:

> "We have seen how trying to control triggering thoughts doesn't provide a long-term solution to worry. It's time to try something new, something called detached mindfulness. This will enable you to develop a new relationship with your thoughts and discover the truth about worry. In a minute I will ask you to have a thought about a tiger and allow the thought to exist in its own space in your mind. I'd like you to just watch the thought and do nothing to control it or influence it in any way.
>
> "Okay, can you have the thought now? Just watch the tiger. You may notice that it is moving, but don't make it move. You may notice the thought fades, but don't make it fade. You may notice other thoughts but they should not be of your deliberate making. Just watch the thought in a detached way."

After approximately 2 minutes the therapist should determine if the task was successfully implemented. If there were difficulties, these difficulties should be explored and corrected. For instance, some patients report that they were unable to "hold onto" the thought. This problem should be discussed as an indication that the person was trying to do something with the thought, which is not the objective of the exercise. It is helpful to gently remind the patient that the objective is to watch the thought in a detached way no matter what happens. The task should be repeated or an alternative DM strategy such as free association (see Chapter 5) should be implemented until the patient has the necessary experience.

The next step is application of the technique to a recent worry trigger. First the therapist identifies a recent trigger in the following way: "Think about your most recent worry. What was the triggering thought?" At this point a negative image or What if . . . ? thought is pinpointed. The therapist proceeds to repeat the DM procedure for this trigger:

> "I'd like you to bring to mind that worry trigger. Allow the trigger to be in your mind but do nothing with it. Don't push it away, and don't try to reason with it and work it out. It's only a thought."

Worry Postponement Experiment

After the experience of applying DM, the idea of postponing the worry process that is normally connected with triggering thoughts is introduced as a means of enhancing DM but also as a means of challenging the belief that worry is uncontrollable. In doing so it is crucial that the therapist makes a clear distinction between *thought suppression* (which is undesirable) and *worry postponement*. The following explanation is normally given:

> "For homework I would like you to apply detached mindfulness to each of your triggering thoughts. Then follow this with postponement of any worry or thinking-through process. Perhaps you can say to yourself: 'There's a worry thought, I don't need to dwell on this and activate my worry now, I'll wait and do that later.' Then later in the day I'd like you to set aside a time when you can take time to worry through that thought. That time should be restricted to 10 minutes, and not be just before bedtime. The worry time is not compulsory—most people forget to do it—so I'm not suggesting that you must try to use that time. By using worry postponement you can test out how uncontrollable worry really is. Have you ever used a strategy like this before?
>
> "It is important that you know the difference between thought suppression and postponing your worry. I'm not asking you to not think a thought. The thought that acts as a trigger can still be in your mind, but you choose not to engage your thinking and reasoning process. For example, you may have a trigger about work, something like 'What if I can't cope?' I don't want you to try and suppress thoughts like that. Say to yourself, 'There goes a worry trigger. I'm going to leave it alone and not deal with it now. I'll deal with it later.' The thought can remain and you choose not to deal with it with your usual worry response. Can you see what I'm asking you to try? This is an experiment to see how uncontrollable worry truly is."

The therapist then takes a belief rating in uncontrollability and does so again after a week of implementing the experiment for homework. Note that an index of belief change in the uncontrollability domain can also be obtained from the sessional administration of the GADS-R.

CHALLENGING UNCONTROLLABILITY BELIEFS

Verbal Methods

Further challenging of belief about uncontrollability is achieved by reviewing counterevidence. For instance, the therapist asks what happens to the patient's worry if he or she is distracted by the doorbell or needs to answer the door? Or if his or her child requires urgent attention? The therapist aims to show how worry is displaced by these competing demands and therefore must be responsive to the patient's responses and priorities. The therapist also asks what happens to worry when the person sleeps, which is further evidence that it is subject to control. (*Note:* sleep disturbance caused by worry is not evidence that worry cannot be controlled. It is simply the case that the patient has not used *appropriate* control.)

Loss-of-Control Experiments

Refinements of the worry postponement experiment are required to fully modify beliefs about uncontrollability. In the next stage, treatment progresses to "pushing worry" in two contexts: during a postponed worry period and during a worry episode. The aim is to provide unambiguous evidence that worry cannot become uncontrollable even when the patient tries to lose control.

The loss-of-control experiment is best introduced and first practiced during a treatment session. This reduces patient fear associated with implementing the procedure for homework, thereby facilitating compliance.

In the session, the therapist asks the patient to think of a recent or current worry, and then to begin worrying about it with the aim of worrying as intensely as possible to test if it is possible to lose control of the activity. The procedure is introduced as follows:

> "You've discovered that worry isn't uncontrollable by using worry postponement. But what would happen if a really big worry came along? How much do you believe you could lose control?
>
> "It is important to be sure that you cannot actually lose control of worry. One way to do this is to deliberately push your worrying. Can you think of a current or recent worry?
>
> "I'd like you to dwell on that worry and to engage your worry process, worry as much as you can, really catastrophize and try to lose control of the activity. Off you go, try that now."

It is then suggested that the loss-of-control experiment be practiced for homework during a postponed worry period and then again at the actual time that a worry trigger is experienced. Some patients feel confident enough to go straight into pushing worry during a worry episode and so pushing worry in a postponed period can be omitted. As with all behavioral experiments, the therapist monitors belief change throughout this procedure by using verbal ratings of belief in uncontrollability and/or the self-report index relevant to this provided by the GADS-R.

Some patients question the usefulness of pushing worry in the treatment session or discount the experience as "artificial" and not capable of providing evidence about real worry. This is only natural because the situation is contrived and is simply used to reinforce the need to practice the procedure for homework in order to test beliefs in real situations. The therapist should be aware of the possibility that resistance of this kind may be a sign of avoidance and that the procedure should be implemented anyway.

CHALLENGING DANGER METACOGNITIONS

Once beliefs concerning the uncontrollability of worry have been effectively challenged, as indicated by scores of zero or as close to zero as possible on the GADS-R, it is appropriate to move on to challenging danger-related metacognitions.

Verbal and behavioral reattribution methods are used to weaken and modify danger-related metacognitions. Several verbal strategies are used before introducing behavioral experiments. These verbal methods involve (1) strengthening dissonance, (2) questioning the evidence, (3) exploring counterevidence, (4) questioning the mechanism, and (5) providing new information.

Strengthening Dissonance

When positive beliefs about the usefulness of worry are evident from the outset of treatment, they provide an opportunity to emphasize the conflict that exists between such beliefs and metacognitions concerning danger. Dissonance induction has the potential to change any side of the equation: it may lead to a weakening of positive or negative beliefs. The following questions are useful for this purpose:

> "You seem to believe that worrying has advantages but also that it is harmful. How can both be true?"
> "Is it true that worry is good and bad in equal measure?"
> "If worrying is harmful, how can you also believe that it helps you cope?"
> "Have you ever thought that worry might not be useful or harmful, and that it is irrelevant?"

Questioning the Evidence

The therapist questions the evidence that the patient has to support negative danger-related metacognitive beliefs. Worry is often equated with the concept of stress. Because the patient believes that stress is harmful, he or she also believes that worry is harmful. When this is the case we have found it helpful to discuss how stress and worry are different entities. One way to do this is to show how worry is a coping strategy in response to stress and negative thoughts. Therefore it is not *equivalent* to stress but is instead a *response* to stress.

Further discussion should focus on the fact that there is limited evidence that psychological stress is directly damaging. The relationship appears to be subtle and mediated by appraisals of control and aspects of personality. The stress response can be seen as part of a wider anxiety response that represents a survival mechanism for dealing with threat. If stress was harmful, natural selection would have selected out vulnerable individuals. Some specific questions that therapists can use during this phase of treatment are:

"How do you know that worry is harmful?"
"How long have you been worrying? Have you come to harm yet?"
"How many people on your street do you estimate worry, and how many have become mentally or physically ill as a result?"
"Would your belief that worry is dangerous stand up in a court of law given the state of evidence?"

We have found the book *The Truth about Stress* (Patmore, 2006) to be a useful resource for those who wish to explore the stress myth further with their patients.

Generating Counterevidence

We saw above how the therapist might draw the patient's attention to counterevidence by questioning how long the patient has been a worrier, and whether or not psychological or physical catastrophes have occurred as a consequence. This maneuver can backfire insomuch that the patient may have health issues that he or she mistakenly attributes to worry. In these circumstances it is necessary to show how worry and the health issues might be correlated, but that this does not mean worry causes health problems (i.e., that the patient worries about his or her health because of health symptoms: poor health leads to worry, but this does not mean that worry is the cause of poor health).

Observations that contradict predictions based on danger-related beliefs should be explored. One strategy is to ask the patient if he or she knows anyone else who is a worrier, and to ask if that person has suffered significant physical and mental health problems as a consequence.

We have seen how worry is often equated with stress. The belief that stress or worry is harmful can be challenged by asking the patient to think of people who are exposed to intense stress, for example, race car drivers or soldiers in combat training. These situations are likely to activate high levels of anxiety and worry, and yet these people do not show physical or psychological breakdown as would be predicted if the patient's beliefs were accurate. Direct counterevidence can be cited such as the finding that the incidence of civilian psychological disorder decreases in wartime.

Questioning the Mechanism
and Searching for Counterevidence

One way to challenge beliefs about the harmful consequences of worry is to question the mechanism that links worry to negative outcomes. Often, this will be the first time that the patient has explored such issues. This process alone, when it yields insight into the absence of an explanation, can weaken negative beliefs. The therapist aims to challenge the existence or validity of any mechanism. Useful basic questions include:

> "What's the mechanism by which worry causes [insert idiosyncratic danger outcome]?"
> "How does worry cause harm to the body?"
> "How does worry cause harm to the mind?"

Typically, these questions are answered with reports of symptoms.

For example, a 53-year-old woman undergoing MCT for GAD was asked by her therapist, "How does worry harm the body?" She answered, "It increases blood pressure, and I know that high blood pressure is associated with heart problems." The therapist went on to make a distinction between chronically elevated blood pressure that poses a cardiac risk and the transient increases in blood pressure associated with worry and exercise. By drawing parallels between the effects of worry and exercise, the therapist was able to show how transient increases might actually improve cardiac resilience.

When there are fears concerning the negative effects of worry/anxiety on the body involving cardiovascular events, it is useful to explore the mechanism by which anxiety influences physiology as a means of eliciting disconfirmatory evidence. For instance, a patient was concerned that worry would lead to heart damage. His fear was based on the observation that whenever he was worried and anxious he noticed changes in his heart rhythm. The therapist explored the effect of anxiety on the production of adrenaline and using guided discovery helped the patient to see how adrenaline could be used to save life in the event of a heart attack as follows:

THERAPIST: Do you know why your heartbeat changes when you're anxious?

PATIENT: Because I'm scared.

THERAPIST: That's right, and when you're scared what substance does your body produce that makes your heart beat faster?

PATIENT: Is it adrenaline?

THERAPIST: That's it, you produce adrenaline, which acts on your body so that you can survive danger. Have you seen those medical dramas where they have to start someone's heart following a heart attack?

PATIENT: Yes.

THERAPIST: What do they do to restart someone's heart?

PATIENT: They give electric shocks.

THERAPIST: That's right. And what do they inject directly into the heart?

PATIENT: Adrenaline.

THERAPIST: That's right. So do you think they would do that if adrenaline could damage the heart?

PATIENT: No.

THERAPIST: So you can see that adrenaline can save your life. Even if you have had a heart attack and your heart is probably weaker as a result, adrenaline can save your life. Do you think doctors would use adrenaline if it was going to make matters worse?

PATIENT: No, I see what you mean. So adrenaline is not going to harm me then?

THERAPIST: What do you think now that we have examined some of the counterevidence?

PATIENT: No, it probably won't, it could even be a good thing.

THERAPIST: Can you think of anything else that increases your heart rate.

PATIENT: Like exercise, you mean?

THERAPIST: Yes, good example. Would you say that exercise is bad for your heart?

PATIENT: No, it's recommended as something that can protect against heart disease.

THERAPIST: That's right. So can you see how an increase in heart rate is not good evidence that your heart will be damaged by worry.

The evolutionary perspective can be a valuable tool in counteracting negative beliefs about worry and anxiety/stress. The therapist uses guided discovery to help the patient explore how evolution would have extinguished a tendency in which worry or stress disadvantaged the organism through adversely affecting psychological or biological well-being. The following transcript illustrates the use of this technique:

THERAPIST: Think about the evolution of humans. Do you think early environments were stressful for our ancestors?

PATIENT: Yes, they must have been.

THERAPIST: In what way do you think they were stressful?

PATIENT: I guess there was a lot that people didn't know back then. So many things that we don't worry about today would be the source of stress.

THERAPIST: I'm sure you're right. Do you think that there was a lot to worry about?

PATIENT: Yes, much more than there is today.

THERAPIST: So if worry and stress caused mental illness, do you think humans would have evolved and still be around as a species today?

PATIENT: No, probably not.

THERAPIST: So, looking at some of the counterevidence, how much do you believe that worry is harmful to your mental health?

The evolutionary strategy can be usefully coupled with the survival mechanism explanation, in which the therapist presents information that the anxiety response is part of the person's built-in survival mechanism. Such a mechanism would not be effective if it caused dangerous outcomes such as mental or bodily breakdown. The following transcript illustrates this approach:

THERAPIST: Do you think there could be advantages to anxiety?

PATIENT: No, I just don't want to have it. If I could worry without the anxiety that would be one solution because the anxiety is damaging me.

THERAPIST: Have you heard of the fight-or-flight response?

PATIENT: I think so, but I'm not sure.

THERAPIST: It's part of a person's built-in survival mechanism and anxiety plays a central role. When a person is exposed to danger, his or her anxiety is activated. This leads to changes in thinking and in bodily arousal that prepare the person to take emergency action. For instance, the heart beats faster and blood is redirected away from the gut and to the muscles to supply them with more oxygen. You may have noticed that your thinking speeds up and so on. This is to help the person fight or to run away from the situation. So you can see anxiety is there to help you survive danger. Do you think it would have served humans so well as a survival response if it harmed them in some way?

PATIENT: No, I don't suppose so. I hadn't thought that anxiety could be helpful.

THERAPIST: Can you think of any other ways that anxiety could be helpful?

PATIENT: What, you mean for survival?

THERAPIST: I was thinking more about whether some anxiety could improve performance.

PATIENT: Well, I've heard that athletes try not to be too relaxed before competing.

THERAPIST: That's right, being anxious or psyched-up can actually improve performance. So maybe that's some further evidence that anxiety is not bad for you.

BEHAVIORAL EXPERIMENTS

The preceding section examined some of the common verbal reattribution techniques used to weaken negative beliefs concerning the danger of worry. Dealing with these techniques should be followed by the use of behavioral experiments that consolidate what the patient has learned and test his or her specific predictions. The therapist should not assume that verbal strategies alone are sufficient to produce the complete and stable changes in a patient's negative metacognitive beliefs that are required in treatment.

Behavioral experiments should be a consistent and mandatory component of treatment. Five examples of the behavioral experiments commonly used in MCT to challenge negative beliefs are given in the examples that follow.

Minisurveys

A 51-year-old patient was very concerned that his worry was abnormal and a sign that his mind was weak and vulnerable. He believed that his worry was a warning that he was "losing his ability to think." The therapist discussed with him possible ways to test his belief that his worry was abnormal and a sign that he must be losing his ability.

It was decided that a useful way for the patient to find out would be to interview four people and ask them questions about worry. It was reasoned that if the patient's worry was abnormal then other people would report worrying little and having no difficulty controlling their worries. Three questions were generated: (1) "Do you ever worry?," (2) "Do you ever have difficulty controlling worry?," and (3) "How often do you worry?" The patient was asked to interview some people whom he thought hardly ever worried and some whom he thought might worry a lot. The therapist also agreed to ask three people the same questions. When asked what responses he predicted, the patient stated that he thought most people would say they did not worry and if they did it would not be frequent and not associated with difficulties in control.

The results of the survey were a great surprise to him. He had asked his wife about worry and was shocked to discover that she worried more than he did. Indeed, she found her worry uncontrollable at times, but she did not have GAD. The results changed his belief that he was abnormal and losing his ability to think. He concluded that this was further evidence that he simply worried too much about worry.

Going-Crazy Experiment

In a treatment session with a 27-year-old woman the therapist asked, "What is the worst that will happen if you worry more?" The patient replied that she would "have a mental breakdown." The therapist asked what the symptoms of a mental breakdown would be like and discovered that the patient had a particular fear of schizophrenia. The therapist explored how the patient might know that she had schizophrenia, to which the patient explained that she would develop visual hallucinations.

An experiment was run in which the patient was asked to worry about a recent concern during the therapy session and to increase her worry to its maximum degree to test if she could induce hallucinations. She found that hallucinations did not occur, a finding that reduced her belief level from 65% to 30%. The therapist asked what was keeping the remaining belief going. The patient replied that she had not experienced any physical symptoms like she would if she was anxious. Further exploration revealed that the patient's main physical symptoms were racing thoughts and tightness in her arms. The therapist refined the experiment and asked the patient to worry intensively while exercising and tensing her arm muscles to determine if this caused hallucinations. After trying this experiment her belief fell to 20%. The remaining belief was tackled by asking the patient to conduct homework in which she deliberately pushed her worry higher the next time she felt anxious.

Damaging the Body with Worry

A 31-year-old patient believed that he could damage his body with worry. He believed that he could induce a heart attack. After establishing that the patient was in good physical health and there was no risk for him to perform vigorous exercise, the therapist asked him to worry while jogging around the outside of the clinic. The patient predicted that this would lead to physical collapse or even to a heart attack.

After this experiment the patient's belief in worry damaging his body dropped by 30%.

Evaluating Effects of Worry on the Body

When patients believe that worrying can have damaging effects on the body the therapist first weakens this belief by reviewing the evidence and counterevidence. Next the therapist runs a behavioral experiment to evaluate the effects of worry on bodily reactions.

A patient was concerned that worry could harm her body. Her evidence for this belief was that worry could increase her heart rate. The therapist took her pulse under three conditions of (1) light exercise, (2) sitting in a chair having neutral thoughts, and (3) sitting having worrying thoughts. The results showed that exercise led to an increase in heart rate but there was little difference in her heart rate between worrying and having positive thoughts. This result was used as evidence against the idea that worrying had a marked effect on her body.

The therapist refined the experiment by asking the patient what would happen to her heart rate if she worried while exercising compared to exercising without worry. The patient predicted that her heart rate should be much higher, at least 20 beats per minute higher when she worried. The therapist asked the patient to do 10 step-ups while worrying, then 10 while not worrying, and compared the patient's pulse rate in the two conditions. The patient discovered that there was little difference in rate between the two conditions. This discovery was successful in challenging her belief.

CHALLENGING POSITIVE METACOGNITIVE BELIEFS

The model specifies that positive metacognitive beliefs about worry are normal and not specific to pathology. However, the problem in GAD is that patients lack the flexibility of selection and implementation of a range of strategies for dealing with intrusive thoughts and emotion. That is, positive beliefs in GAD monopolize the style of processing in response to negative thoughts and emotions. In turning the spotlight on positive metacognitive beliefs, the therapist is normally entering the final third of treatment. Positive beliefs become the focus only after negative beliefs about uncontrollability and danger have been effectively challenged.

The modification of positive beliefs is considered important as a means of freeing up the patient's capacity to use alternative means of responding to internal events, and to increase motivation to break the habit of responding with extensive conceptual activity. Strong positive beliefs may serve as a vulnerability following treatment as they underlie a continuation or reinstatement of worry responses.

Several strategies have been developed in MCT to weaken positive beliefs. These include standard verbal reattribution techniques, the specific mismatch strategy, and worry modulation experiments.

Verbal Reattribution

The therapist usually begins this part of treatment by questioning the evidence supporting the advantages of worrying. This step is introduced in the following way:

> "We have examined your negative beliefs about worry, and you've been able to discover that worrying is controllable and harmless. We should now turn our attention to the positive beliefs you hold about the usefulness of worry. Such beliefs support the continued overuse of worry as a coping strategy. We should now look toward expanding and maintaining the new ways you have learned of relating to your thoughts."

The therapist challenges the patient's beliefs by questioning the evidence supporting them and reviewing counterevidence. Some examples of typical questions are as follows:

> "Do you have any evidence that worrying is helpful?"
> "What is the mechanism that leads worry to be helpful?"
> "Have you ever done something and not been able to worry? What was the outcome?"
> "What happens to your concentration when you worry?" ("How does that fit with worry being helpful?")
> "What happens to your mood when you worry? So how helpful is worrying?"
> "If worrying is effective for avoiding problems, it must mean that people who worry often must have fewer problems in their life. Is that right?"
> "How often do situations turn out the way your worry depicted them? So if worry exaggerates reality, how useful can it really be?"
> "Does worry let you look at things from all angles, including the positive? If it is biased, how useful is it in helping you?"

An example of using these questions during treatment with an older patient with GAD is represented in the following dialogue:

THERAPIST: What do you think is the main benefit of worrying?

PATIENT: It means I won't make major mistakes. I can avoid them.

THERAPIST: Do you have any evidence that worrying stops you from making mistakes?

PATIENT: Well, I've been a worrier most of my life and I suppose I haven't made any really big mistakes.

THERAPIST: Have you been able to worry about everything in your life?

PATIENT: No, I don't suppose it's everything.

THERAPIST: So, have the things you haven't worried about been a mistake?

PATIENT: No. Sometimes you can be pleasantly surprised by the things you don't anticipate.

THERAPIST: So what's your evidence that worry is necessary to stop you from making mistakes?

PATIENT: I suppose there isn't any. But it might help sometimes.

THERAPIST: What's the mechanism that makes worry help sometimes?

PATIENT: Well, I might be correct in anticipating a problem.

THERAPIST: How often do situations turn out exactly like you anticipated?

PATIENT: Sometimes they do.

THERAPIST: So they are exactly how you anticipated them, is that right?

PATIENT: No, maybe not, because worry is so negative.

THERAPIST: That's right. Does worry paint an accurate picture or is it biased in some way?

PATIENT: It's pessimistic, so it's not really realistic.

THERAPIST: That's right. So how much do you believe worry is helpful in preventing mistakes?

PATIENT: It probably isn't very useful.

Worry-Mismatch Strategy

The worry-mismatch strategy is designed to illustrate how the content of worry does not fit closely with the nature of reality. This strategy is not principally a means of challenging the content of worry (although it may have that effect), but instead a means of challenging the validity of beliefs about the usefulness of worry (metacognitions).

There are two types of mismatch strategy, the *retrospective* mismatch and the *prospective* mismatch. Both strategies involve obtaining a detailed patient description of the content of steps in his or her worry process, and then comparing these steps with a description of the events as they actually occurred in a situation. This strategy can be implemented for a past event (retrospective mismatch) or for a forthcoming event (prospective mismatch).

In the retrospective version, the therapist first identifies a recent situation that the patient was exposed to and had worried about beforehand. The therapist elicits a detailed description of the content of the steps involved in the worry episode and writes them out in one column of a two-column table. This column is headed "Worry Script." The steps in the worry sequence are elicited by the therapist repeatedly asking, "And then what did you think or worry about?" Alternatively, the therapist repeats "What if that happens?" at each step until no new information is generated.

In the next column, headed "Reality Script," the therapist writes a description of the true sequence of events in the worry situation. The therapist repeatedly asks, "And what actually happened in the situation?" The therapist then directs the patient to assess the level of agreement or "fit" between the two scripts, emphasizing the discrepancy that exists. The technique is rounded off by the therapist asking, "If worry does not closely match reality, how useful can it really be?" An example of a completed mismatch script can be seen in Table 6.3.

The therapist uses the prospective mismatch when a patient is intending to engage in a future activity but is currently worrying about it. It is also useful when the patient avoids situations because the thought of entering them causes him or her prolonged worry. In these circumstances the worry script is written out in a treatment session and then for homework the patient is asked to enter the avoided or worried-about situation and later to write out the reality script and bring it along to the next session. At that session the therapist and the patient retrieve the worry script from the file and write out a more detailed reality script based on the patient's notes for comparison with the worry script.

Worry Modulation Experiments

If positive beliefs about worry are accurate and worry is helpful, then it logically follows that increases and decreases of worry in the patient's life should have an observable effect on outcomes. Since the patient has

TABLE 6.3. A Completed Mismatch Script

Worry script	Reality script
Situation: *Visiting friends for a few days*	
Trigger: *"What if I arrive late?"*	
"I'll miss the train."	"I arrived early."
"I will arrive last of all."	"Not many people were there."
"Everyone will be drunk."	"I had some great food and wine."
"I won't be able to join in."	"I met a couple of really nice guys."
"I'll get anxious."	"I'm looking forward to visiting my
"I'll have to leave."	friends again next month."
"I'll end up on the streets."	
"I'll be lost."	
"Someone will attack me."	
"I could die."	

already experienced decreasing the extent of worry earlier in treatment, the effect of this decrease on outcomes can be questioned by the therapist to weaken positive beliefs:

> "We might already have some evidence that can address the issue of whether worrying is helpful. Can you think back to earlier in treatment when you postponed your worry? Did you find that unhelpful? Did you find that you coped less well or things didn't work out when you worried less?"

This questioning can be followed by an experiment in which worry is increased and decreased with the specific aim of assessing its impact on daily outcomes such as work performance, coping, and daily events. In order to facilitate the experiment, the therapist should operationalize with the patient observable signs of worrying being helpful and not worrying being unhelpful. The aim is to test the prediction that not worrying will result in poorer outcomes than worrying.

> For example, a patient who believed "Worrying means I'll perform better" was asked to worry more on the first day at work after the treatment session, and then to ban worry on the next day to see if there was a difference in her performance. At the following treatment session the therapist asked the patient if she had noticed any difference in performance on the two days in question. The patient reported that there was no difference. She had realized that she was a cautious person in any case and that worrying did not improve her performance.

NEW PLANS FOR PROCESSING

Once negative and positive metacognitive beliefs have been effectively modified, the final step of treatment, which contributes to relapse prevention, is consolidation and strengthening alternative metacognitive plans (proceduralized—"experiential"—knowledge) that can control responses to intrusive thoughts/stress.

Proceduralization of replacement plans requires repeated practice of new processing strategies. That the patient maintains awareness of the perseverative process is particularly important, since changes in content can mask the fact that the process is still intact.

> For example, a patient reported that she no longer worried like she used to. However, she wanted to talk with the therapist about something that was bothering her. She went on to disclose that she had seen a movie about someone undergoing therapy who recovered memories of childhood abuse. After seeing this movie the patient was

analyzing her own experiences to try and work out if the source of her GAD could be that she had been abused but had repressed memories of the abuse.

The therapist helped her to see that this analysis of whether she might have been abused was just another manifestation of worry/ rumination: the reason she felt the way she did was because she was still engaging in the worry process. This patient continued to hold on to persistent positive beliefs about the usefulness of worry and analytical thinking as a strategy for finding solutions to negative feelings. She needed further strengthening of skills for recognizing and detecting the worry process (irrespective of content) as part of her alternative plan for processing. The alternative plan for processing would become detecting of the worry process, applying detached mindfulness to the triggering thought, and allowing emotions to ebb and flow without trying to understand them.

A range of alternative plans for processing can be built up. Some examples of strategies commonly used as components of new plans are given in Table 6.4. It is important to note that this part of treatment is only implemented after successful modification of negative beliefs about danger because alternative plans should not inadvertently become sources of avoidance.

TABLE 6.4. Examples of Components Used in New Plans

Old plan	New plan
1. "If I have a negative thought, then worry about what could happen and how to avoid it."	"If I have a thought, then leave it alone and wait and see what happens."
2. "If I have a negative thought, then cover all possibilities so I'm not taken by surprise."	"If I have a negative thought, then imagine one thing positive rather than covering all possibilities."
3. "If I'm worried, then focus on evidence supporting or counteracting my worries."	"If I'm worried, then don't search for any evidence; simply stop the thought process."
4. "If I need to do something new, then try to stop thoughts of danger."	"If I need to do something new, then allow thoughts to ebb and flow like tides."
5. "If I'm worried, then use alcohol to help me cope."	"If I'm worried, then avoid alcohol (push worry if I need to prove it's harmless)."
6. "If I'm worrying, then ask my partner for reassurance."	"If I'm worrying, then ban asking for reassurance."
7. "If I do anything novel, then try to anticipate problems before doing it."	"Do more novel things; break my routine without giving much thought first."

RELAPSE PREVENTION

Relapse prevention consists of reviewing residual scores on metacognitive variables that are hypothesized as constituting continued vulnerability. In GAD negative beliefs about uncontrollability and danger concerning thoughts are a proximal cause of GAD. The therapist should check that these beliefs are at 0% or as close as possible to this level. More extensive evaluation of such metacognition is therefore recommended in the last two treatment sessions by close scrutiny of the GADS-R and administration of further tools such as the Meta-Worry Questionnaire and the MCQ-30. If residual beliefs in these domains persist, then further modification should be attempted by returning to and refining the strategies used earlier in treatment.

A further cause of subsequent problems is the continued use of worry or rumination as a coping strategy. It is important that the therapist checks for other subtle forms of ongoing patient worry that are activated in situations and emphasizes awareness and abandonment of this process. The presence of remaining positive beliefs about worry should be explored in this context. If necessary, further work should be undertaken to modify them.

Avoidance of situations and other behaviors such as reassurance seeking or information search are markers for residual beliefs about the uncontrollability and threat imposed by emotions such as anxiety. These responses should be identified and reversed before termination of treatment.

Finally, the therapist and the patient work on writing out a therapy blueprint, which contains a summary of information about GAD and worry, an example of the case formulation, the results of behavioral experiments to test negative and positive metacognitions, and the new plan for dealing with stress/intrusions.

Booster treatment sessions can be scheduled for 3 and 6 months after treatment as an opportunity to monitor patient gains and reinforce the knowledge and strategies he or she has acquired.

GAD TREATMENT PLAN

An overall 10-session treatment plan for implementing MCT in GAD is presented in Appendix 15. This is intended as a guide to treatment structure and content and should be applied flexibly as individual circumstances require. The plan should be implemented with direct reference to the strategies described in this chapter.

||||||||||||||||||||||

CHAPTER 7

Posttraumatic Stress Disorder

When symptoms of stress persist for more than 1 month after a traumatic event an individual may fulfill criteria for a diagnosis of posttraumatic stress disorder (PTSD). It is not advised that treatment is offered before this time, during the acute-stress phase, as most cases of traumatic stress remit spontaneously. We currently do not know if the implementation of MCT during the acute-stress phase can potentiate recovery in those individuals prone to the development of PTSD. Caution is advised because interventions during this phase might run the risk of increasing the likelihood of disorder. For instance, evidence suggests that critical incident debriefing given in the immediate aftermath of trauma can make people worse (e.g., Bisson, Jenkins, Alexander, & Bannister, 1997).

The metacognitive model of PTSD (Wells, 2000) is grounded on the principle that most people have a built-in capacity to adapt following trauma and do not go on to develop prolonged problems. However, the activation of the CAS in the aftermath of stress increases the likelihood of persistent symptoms. It might be the case that some interventions delivered soon after exposure to traumatic events increase conceptual processing and inadvertently potentiate CAS-like processes, increasing the likelihood of abnormal stress responses in some individuals.

The treatment described in this chapter has been successfully applied to both short-term (1–3 months) and chronic (greater than 3 months) cases of PTSD. Our evaluations of treatment effects have included a wide range of traumas including physical and sexual assault, road traffic accidents, terrorist attacks, threats to life, and exposure to other crimes. To date, this treatment has not been evaluated specifically in combat stress or in treating intrusive memories of childhood abuse.

TABLE 7.1. Diagnostic Criteria for PTSD

Criterion A

Exposure to a traumatic event involving actual or threatened death or serious injury with a response involving a sense of intense fear, helplessness, or horror.

Criterion B

At least one of the following re-experiencing symptoms: recurrent and distressing recollections, images, thoughts, or perceptions / distressing dreams / reliving / intense distress on exposure to reminders / physiological reactivity when exposed to reminders.

Criterion C

At least three of the following avoidance symptoms: efforts to avoid thoughts, feelings, conversations linked with the trauma / activities, places, or people that cause recollections / inability to recall important aspects of trauma / diminished interest or participation in activities / feeling detached or estranged from others / restricted emotions / sense of a shortened future.

Criterion D

At least two of the following increased arousal symptoms: difficulty falling or staying asleep / irritability or anger / difficulty concentrating / hypervigilance / exaggerated startle response.

Criterion E

Duration of symptoms at least 1 month.

Criterion F

The disturbance causes significant distress or impairment of functioning.

Note. Summarized from American Psychiatric Association (2000).

A diagnosis of PTSD requires that the individual has been exposed to events that involve actual or threatened death or serious injury, and that his or her response consists of intense fear, helplessness, or horror (DSM-IV-TR; American Psychiatric Association, 2000). The symptom clusters of PTSD are (1) re-experiencing the traumatic event, (2) persistent avoidance, and (3) persistent symptoms of increased arousal. The DSM-IV-TR criteria are summarized in Table 7.1.

CAS in PTSD

Before describing the metacognitive model of PTSD, it will be useful to examine the nature of perseveration, threat monitoring, and maladaptive self-regulatory behaviors as they constitute the CAS in this disorder.

Perseveration: Rumination, Worry, and "Gap Filling"

In the previous chapter we saw how perseveration in GAD is dominated by the process of worry, a future-oriented conceptual activity aiming to answer questions such as "What if . . . ?" and concerned with anticipating and dealing with danger. Another type of perseverative conceptual activity is rumination, which is predominantly past-focused and asks questions such as "Why?" and "What does it mean?" Rumination also includes wishful thinking characterized by thoughts such as "If only. . . ." Both worry and rumination are important in PTSD. But there is an additional form of dwelling that occurs in this disorder that I will call "gap filling." Gap filling refers to going over events in memory and trying to fill in specific gaps. Gap filling is typically supported by the belief that success in doing so will lead to knowledge concerning blame and responsibility for negative events or to the belief that it will facilitate avoidance of threat in the future. For example, a woman who had been sexually assaulted by a stranger repeatedly traced her memory for a social situation to try and remember what her assailant looked like so that she might recognize him and avoid him in the future. She became more anxious as she repeated this process because all she could recall was that he had dark-brown hair and an accent, which meant he could be one of many people.

It is normal to have incomplete memories of events irrespective of whether events are traumatic. The metacognitive approach is not based on the idea that absence of memory or fragmentary memory is central in the genesis of PTSD. However, meta-memory processes consisting of preoccupation with gap filling and the negative interpretation of memory phenomena can be important factors in individual cases.

In summary, perseverative conceptual activity constituting the CAS in PTSD involves worry, rumination, and repeated attempts to review or complete memories.

Threat Monitoring

The threat-monitoring component of the CAS takes the form of increased attention to potential danger with a view to reducing risk. In some cases this occurs in the form of scanning the environment for stimuli that resemble those associated with the index event, but monitoring often extends beyond this narrow focus to looking for a wide range of potential dangers.

For example, a patient who had been knocked down by a car and sustained serious leg and head injuries reported that he was constantly scanning the street for speeding vehicles. However, further exploration of his attentional strategy revealed that he scanned for a wide range of dangers that included holes in the road, rickety scaffolding, wobbly ceiling fans, and uneven pavement slabs.

Threat monitoring is expressed in different ways by our patients. Some describe being "more aware" of dangers, others state that they "keep a lookout" for danger, while still others say that they maintain a state of "readiness" or scan for threat. In some cases threat monitoring takes the form of repeated checking. For example, a patient who had been burgled while asleep subsequently tried to be aware of noises and would listen closely for them before going to sleep. On hearing something, he would get out of bed and check for intruders. This was happening several times a night, significantly impacting his sleep pattern.

Behaviors

There are other unhelpful coping behaviors in addition to the responses described above. These include avoidance of situations in which the trauma occurred and avoidance of reminders of the trauma (e.g., television medical dramas). Behaviors also include attempts to suppress intrusive thoughts or memories of trauma and the use of alcohol or drugs to self-medicate symptoms and emotions. Behaviors can be quite idiosyncratic, as in a recent case of a patient who checked her pulse regularly in response to feelings of dissociation as a means of proving to herself that she was "still alive."

METACOGNITIVE BELIEFS

What is the content of metacognitive beliefs in PTSD? Positive beliefs concern the use of worry, rumination, threat monitoring, gap filling, and the control of trauma-related intrusive thoughts. Negative metacognitive beliefs concern the meaning and danger of symptoms such as intrusive thoughts, dreams, and anxiety.

Beliefs about worry focus on it as a means of avoiding potential future threats and of planning ways of coping (e.g., "Worrying about being attacked in the future will help me avoid it happening again").

Beliefs about rumination focus on using it as a means of determining blame, responsibility, and causes of events. In so doing the person typically believes that he or she can develop better ways of coping or can prevent problems in the future by developing a better understanding of what happened in the past (e.g., "I must analyze what happened in order to cope better next time").

The process of gap filling is similar to rumination and is supported by beliefs such as "I must remember everything I did just before the accident to determine if it was my fault."

Threat-monitoring strategies are supported by positive beliefs concerning the need to focus attention or to channel awareness in a particular way. Examples of these beliefs include the following:

"If I maintain a state of readiness, I'll be prepared."
"I must look out for signs of danger wherever I go."
"Paying attention to suspicious people means I won't be taken by surprise."
"If I try to be alert, I can detect danger before it's too late."
"Listening for people behind me means I'll be ready to act."
"If I check the street, I know it will be safe."

Positive beliefs often also concern the need to control thoughts. Both positive and negative beliefs about thought control are implied by the following types of patient statements:

"I must not think about the trauma or I'll never get over it."
"If I don't think about it, then I won't get upset."
"Some aspects I won't think about because it's too much to take."

Negative metacognitive beliefs focus on the meaning and significance of thoughts and symptoms. These include beliefs that intrusive thoughts or flashbacks are a sign of serious mental instability, that they could cause "mental breakdown," or that they are a sign that the person is being punished or is to blame for the traumatic event. For instance, patients have believed that (1) intrusions are a sign of "brain damage," (2) repeated thoughts of a sexual assault "must mean I wanted it to happen," and (3) arousal symptoms are "abnormal" and a sign of "mental weakness."

In the next section I describe the way in which the CAS and metacognitions operate in explaining the persistence of traumatic stress symptoms.

THE METACOGNITIVE MODEL OF PTSD

The model (Wells, 2000; Wells & Sembi, 2004a) is depicted diagrammatically in Figure 7.1. It is based on the assumption that following a traumatic event an individual's internal survival objective is the formation of a metacognitive plan that can guide his or her cognition and action in future encounters with potential threats. The formation of such a plan is influenced by the experience of symptoms such as orienting reactions, exaggerated startle reactions, arousal responses, and the running of mental simulations of acting in different ways.

This process, termed the reflexive adaptation process (RAP), normally proceeds unhindered. It is automatically initiated by intrusions and when it is effectively completed symptoms subside. However, this normal process can be disrupted by the thinking styles and coping strategies adopted by the individual.

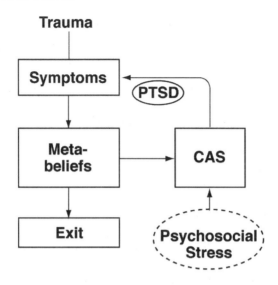

FIGURE 7.1. The metacognitive model of PTSD.

Specifically, the CAS interferes with the RAP and the return of cognition to processing a normal threat-free environment. Metacognitive beliefs underlie the activation of the CAS and lead to negative interpretations of symptoms, thinking, and attentional styles that enhance the processing of danger, and to coping behaviors that prevent cognition returning to a normal state of threat-free processing.

The CAS causes sustained threat-related processing termed "trauma-lock" (Wells & Sembi, 2004b) because the person's cognition is locked onto dwelling on the trauma, worrying about future threats, attending to danger, and negatively interpreting symptoms. By engaging these processes the individual is inadvertently strengthening his or her metacognitive plans for detecting and processing danger and is thereby becoming an increasingly sensitive and skilled threat detector, leading to an array of situations activating an anxiety response.

The CAS stems from positive and negative metacognitive beliefs. Take, for example, the positive belief that one must worry in order to be prepared and the negative belief that intrusive thoughts are a sign of intractable psychological damage. In combination or alone, these metacognitions configure the individual's processing style and interpretations such that they give rise to an erroneous sense of danger, thereby maintaining anxiety and its associated symptoms.

In the model (Figure 7.1) traumatic events produce a stress response and its associated symptoms. This normal stress response includes intrusive thoughts, hyperarousal, exaggerated startle reactions, and attentional orienting responses. These act on cognition as biasing agents and lead to selection and strengthening of metacognitions for controlling thinking and coping. It is probably adaptive for such reactions to persist for a period of days or weeks after stress since it is advantageous for the organism to be in a state of preparedness to deal with danger.

Intrusions in the form of images provide the impetus for the individual to imagine dealing with the trauma in different ways. This is a process of *mental simulation* that couples behavior with information in a dynamic way across time to form a script or plan for guiding action. Such mental simulations probably have survival value since they facilitate the laying down of the rudiments of motor programs that can be called up by threats in the future. It is safer to simulate dealing with danger than to be actually exposed to it as a means of learning new responses.

Anxiety symptoms are part of the RAP and naturally subside over time. However, when metacognitive beliefs specify the use of rumination, worry and/or gap filling, threat monitoring, thought suppression, and avoidance, and/or they lead to threatening interpretations of symptoms, threat perception persists and anxiety is maintained.

What are the mechanisms linking components of the CAS to a perpetuation of symptoms? To begin with, worry and rumination are predominantly verbal processing activities that deplete attention that could be used for imaginal simulations. Thus, mental simulation can be impaired by depletion of resources. Worry and rumination are negative in content and so they maintain anxiety or negative affect, increasing the likelihood of emotion-related intrusive thoughts.

Gap filling causes the person to be preoccupied with replaying specific aspects of the trauma rather than allowing trauma-related material to decay in processing. Threat monitoring focuses the person on processing potential threats in the environment and consequently heightens his or her sense of present danger. Suppression of thoughts and memories increases the salience of this material and is difficult to consistently achieve, which contributes to an individual's sense of loss of control. Negative interpretations of symptoms lead to anxiety and contribute to the sense of danger arising from emotion itself. Other coping strategies such as avoidance and dissociation interfere with processing of the true environment so that the person continues to overestimate danger.

THE MODEL IN ACTION

This section examines a sequential analysis of how the model operates in a typical case.

The RAP is triggered by intrusive symptoms, which are typically thoughts in the form of images or memories depicting aspects of the trauma. In some instances the trigger is a bodily sensation that reminds the person of an injury or emotion occurring at the time of trauma such as a feeling of pain or sudden arousal.

The trigger activates metacognitive beliefs that guide the way the individual responds to it. In PTSD the metacognitions are maladaptive because they lead the individual to ruminate/worry or gap-fill, to pay attention to threat, and to avoid or suppress thoughts of trauma. These strategies (the CAS) keep symptoms going by blocking emotional processing (the RAP) and maintain anxiety by perpetuating the processing of threat-related stimuli.

In addition to activating positive metacognitions that guide coping responses, the person typically holds negative metacognitive beliefs about the meaning of symptoms that lead to threatening interpretations of symptoms and to further anxiety.

Psychosocial stressors can also contribute to the process of worry/rumination and threat monitoring. These stressors include threats that are difficult to bring under personal control, ongoing threats or intimidation, lack of social support, and blame.

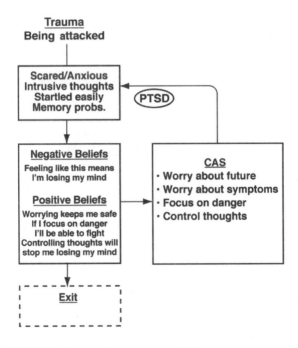

FIGURE 7.2. An idiosyncratic PTSD case formulation.

The conceptualization in Figure 7.2 is based on the experiences of a patient who was attacked with a weapon during a robbery at work. His predominant symptoms were repeatedly feeling anxious and scared, enduring intrusive thoughts, being easily startled, and experiencing difficulties with memory and concentration. He misinterpreted these symptoms as signs that he was losing his mind. This misinterpretation in turn led to worry about his symptoms, which maintained his sense of anxiety. The worry also further impaired his concentration and memory. The patient believed that he should worry about future threats in order to be prepared for them and therefore safer. This worry about potential threats in the future maintained his sense of danger and anxiety. He believed that he must focus on danger so that he could put up a better fight in the future. This attentional strategy increased his sense of living in a threatening environment.

In this case the patient believed that he must control his thoughts about the trauma, which led to suppression attempts, which backfired and increased the frequency and duration of his intrusive thoughts. Thought control attempts and worry collectively impaired his memory and concentration. Thus, clear feedback loops involving the CAS were responsible for maintaining his symptoms and anxiety, giving rise to PTSD.

STRUCTURE OF TREATMENT

MCT sessions are usually held on a weekly basis. Treatment is often brief. Initial sessions are typically 45–60 minutes in duration. Once patients effectively implement detached mindfulness and control over their worry/rumination, sessions may be reduced to 30–40 minutes.

In evaluations of the effectiveness of treatment, 8–11 sessions were required to achieve PTSD-free status. As usual in MCT, treatment progresses through a series of stages. The sequence of treatment in PTSD is as follows:

1. Case conceptualization
2. Socialization
3. Training detached mindfulness
4. Worry/rumination postponement; banning gap filling
6. Challenging metacognitive beliefs
7. Attention modification
8. Reinforcing new plans for processing
9. Relapse prevention

Treatment does not involve imaginal exposure or reliving or challenging thoughts about the trauma. Apart from a description of the trauma during assessment, treatment does not normally go into a detailed discussion of the traumatic event.

CASE CONCEPTUALIZATION

Measures

Tools required during this stage are:

1. Posttraumatic Stress Disorder Scale (PTSD-S)
2. PTSD Case Formulation Interview
3. Session checklists

The therapist begins by administering the PTSD-S and examines the negative and positive metacognitive beliefs endorsed by the patient in order to obtain a preliminary impression of the types of beliefs and behaviors that should be explored and incorporated in the case formulation. The PTSD-S is reproduced in Appendix 8. This scale provides an impression of the types of responses made to intrusive thoughts and memories of the trauma. Other measures that the therapist might consider that can be completed before treatment are the Beck Anxiety Inventory (Beck et al., 1988), the Beck Depression Inventory II (Beck et al., 1996), and a specific PTSD measure such as the Impact of Events Scale (Horowitz, Wilner, & Alvarez, 1979), the Post-traumatic Stress Diagnostic Scale (Foa, 1995), the Penn Inventory (Hammarberg, 1992), or the Davidson Trauma Scale (Davidson, 1996).

Agenda of the First Session

The agenda should reflect the goals of each session. For the first session the goals are the mapping out of a case formulation, increasing patient awareness of the factors maintaining disorder, and implementing specific initial strategies of MCT. The first change strategy introduced is DM and rumination/worry postponement. The first session is introduced in the following way:

> "In today's session I want to explore a recent episode when you had intrusive thoughts about the trauma. In doing so we can find the factors that are keeping your stress symptoms going and begin to examine ways that you can overcome your problem. I would also like to explain a little more about metacognitive therapy and what you might expect from treatment. I would also like to introduce you to some new ways that you can respond to your symptoms. Is there anything you would like to put on the agenda and talk about today?"

Generating a Case Conceptualization

The next step is to proceed with generating an idiosyncratic version of the metacognitive model that represents the events activated in response to an intrusive thought, memory, or feeling associated with the trauma. Because intrusions or emotions such as fear are readily detected, there is usually little difficulty in identifying a trigger for mapping the case formulation.

Furthermore, the process of case conceptualization does not necessitate detailed recounting of the details of the trauma. This can be an advantage because it circumvents cognitive-affective avoidance.

The therapist usually begins by identifying a recent experience of symptoms that includes emotional shifts (i.e., affect shifts) or intrusive thoughts as a starting point for case conceptualization. The affect shift is often fear/anxiety, but it can also be sadness or anger:

> "Can you think back to the most recent time when you noticed a change in your emotions related to thoughts about the trauma? When was that? What was the internal event that triggered your initial emotion? Was it a thought, a memory, or a feeling?"

An effective sequence for obtaining information for the case conceptualization is to ask about symptoms/affect first, and then to ask about the strategies used to manage or avoid symptoms. The therapist next asks about attentional monitoring for threat and about worry/rumination. Questions are then directed at eliciting beliefs about symptoms, worry/rumination, and threat monitoring. The sequence and nature of case conceptualization questions is presented in the PTSD Case Forumulation Interview in Appendix 12.

An example dialogue using these questions is presented below; the resulting case conceptualization is presented in Figure 7.2.

THERAPIST: What are the symptoms that have been troubling you in the past month?

PATIENT: I've changed. I'm not like I used to be.

THERAPIST: In what way have you changed?

PATIENT: I'm just jumpy all the time, and people really annoy me.

THERAPIST: You said jumpy. Does that mean you are easily startled or anxious all the time?

PATIENT: Yes. Sudden noises make me jump, and I feel scared and anxious much of the time.

THERAPIST: Have you had any other symptoms such as intrusive thoughts about the trauma?

PATIENT: Oh yes, all the time. I keep thinking of being on the ground and thinking that I could die, and I can feel the blood running from my head.

THERAPIST: Does that thought occur often?

PATIENT: Yes, it keeps coming back.

THERAPIST: When was the most recent time that you were distressed by such thoughts?

PATIENT: This morning I had the thought. It's whenever I have to leave the house.

THERAPIST: Do you do anything to try and cope or to manage your symptoms?

PATIENT: I'm not sure.

THERAPIST: Are you trying to avoid or control thoughts about what happened?

PATIENT: I try not to think about it, I tell myself that once I'm home I'm not going to think about what happened.

THERAPIST: How do you stop your thoughts?

PATIENT: I tell myself not to think about it, and if I get a thought I try to control it.

THERAPIST: Are you paying attention to things differently now?

PATIENT: What do you mean?

THERAPIST: Have you found that what you pay attention to has changed since the event?

PATIENT: Yes, I pay more attention to certain types of people in the street and I'm always monitoring for sounds behind me. Like the sound of footsteps. I check out what people are wearing to see if they could be carrying a weapon.

THERAPIST: Let's call that "Focus on danger" for short. Are you spending time dwelling on or going over what happened?

PATIENT: I try not to think about it.

THERAPIST: Are you going over things and asking yourself questions such as "What happened?", "Why me?", "What does it mean?", "If only . . . ", and thoughts like that?

PATIENT: Yes, I'm thinking like that quite a lot.

THERAPIST: How much time each day are you thinking like that?

PATIENT: Now that you mention it, I think it's a lot of the time.

THERAPIST: Are you worrying about bad things that could happen in the future?

PATIENT: Yes, much more than I used to. It's like many things now seem dangerous.

THERAPIST: What sorts of things are you worrying about in this way?

PATIENT: I think about being involved in accidents, or being attacked, and recently I've been worrying about being involved in a terrorist attack. Like, what if I'm blown up like those people recently?

THERAPIST: What are you trying to achieve by worrying about the future?

PATIENT: I'm trying to be prepared so that I can avoid dangerous situations.

THERAPIST: What are your concerns about your symptoms?

PATIENT: I think I'm abnormal for feeling like this.

THERAPIST: What do you mean by that?

PATIENT: I think I'm heading for a nervous breakdown. Do you think I could be?

THERAPIST: It depends what you mean.

PATIENT: Maybe it means I'm losing my mind.

THERAPIST: What's the worst that could happen if you continue to feel like this?

PATIENT: It might mean I'm going to lose my mind.

THERAPIST: Are there any advantages to going over what happened?

PATIENT: I don't think so.

THERAPIST: Are there any advantages to worrying about what could happen in the future?

PATIENT: Yes, it means I can avoid getting into danger, it will keep me safe.

THERAPIST: Are there any advantages to paying attention to danger?

PATIENT: Yes, it means I can be prepared, and I'll be able to fight.

THERAPIST: How does controlling your thoughts help?

PATIENT: It will stop me losing my mind.

SOCIALIZATION

Socialization proceeds by presenting the case formulation. The therapist emphasizes the theme that PTSD symptoms are a normal part of adaptation to traumatic experiences. The therapist also emphasizes that under usual circumstances the symptoms subside over time as this natural psychological healing process occurs. The therapist notes, however, that this process is disrupted when the individual engages in particular types of thinking and behavior. The factors that block adaptation include:

1. Worrying or ruminating about the trauma or one's responses to it.
2. Worrying about danger in the future.
3. Going over memories of what happened.
4. Paying too much attention to threat and danger after the event.
5. Trying to avoid or excessively control thoughts about the event.
6. Negative beliefs about the meaning or consequences of symptoms.
7. Avoidance of situations.

In the next step the therapist draws attention to the prevalence and role of worry/rumination. For example, the therapist says:

"Looking at your case formulation we can see that you are spending time dwelling on what happened in the past and what could happen in the future. We call this rumination and worry. How much of the time each day are you doing this? Does thinking in this way help you to become less anxious or does it keep your sense of threat and anxiety going?"

Next, the therapist questions the consequences of thinking strategies to help the patient see how they contribute to a perpetuation of anxiety by maintaining a sense of danger and threat:

"Do you think there are any problems with going over what happened?"
"Has going over things helped you move on from the event?"
"What is the consequence of worrying? Does worrying help you feel less anxious? Does it make you feel safe? What happens to your sense of danger when you worry?"
"Are there any disadvantages to paying attention to threat? Does it increase your sense of safety or increase your sense of vulnerability?"
"How effective have your attempts to stop thinking about the trauma been?"

PRESENTING THE TREATMENT RATIONALE

Patients are introduced to the idea that their intrusive thoughts, arousal responses, flashbacks, nightmares, and startle responses are normal and necessary after trauma.

The symptoms are described as a sign that the person's cognitive system is attempting to process the trauma and adjust to the event in a way that enhances future coping. However, the patient's present coping strategies and thinking style have the effect of preventing this process from reaching completion. The therapist emphasizes the point that it is important not to avoid symptoms because they are part of the recovery process. The "healing metaphor" is used as a means of illustrating that spontaneous recovery does not require excessive use of present strategies.

Presenting the "Healing Metaphor" and the Goals of MCT

The therapist uses the following explanation:

> "Overcoming a psychological injury caused by trauma is very much like overcoming a physical injury such as a cut to the skin. If you think of a physical injury the body has its own way of healing itself over time. But what would happen if you tried to make the injury heal, say by picking at the scar and repeatedly cleaning the wound? How quickly would it heal?
>
> "Trauma symptoms are like this. Over time the mind can heal itself and this often occurs. However, just like a flesh wound, if you interfere with the healing process it can take longer and symptoms can persist. You are interfering with the healing process by engaging in worry/rumination, by avoiding thoughts, and by keeping attention focused on threat. The goal of treatment is to remove these unhelpful responses so that normal healing can be resumed. If you look at the case formulation we will be emptying the box (in Figure 7.2) labeled maladaptive strategies (or CAS), and getting you to do some new things instead so that you exit the PTSD cycle."

The case formulation provides a vehicle for illustrating the course of treatment. In Figure 7.2 the adaptive processing or "Exit" box is empty. The therapist describes to the patient how treatment will consist of emptying the unhelpful processing box: "CAS" and practicing new strategies in treatment that will fill the adaptive "Exit" box as a means of promoting the healing process and exiting the PTSD cycle.

DETACHED MINDFULNESS AND RUMINATION/WORRY POSTPONEMENT

The aim of the next stage in treatment is to increase awareness of the nature and occurrence of worry/rumination (and where necessary, gap filling) as a prerequisite to developing alternative responses to intrusive symptoms. The patient is asked to think about the frequency and duration of time spent thinking about trauma or worrying about future calamities over the past week. The therapist looks for circular negative thinking based on ""What if . . . ", "If only . . . ", "Why . . . ", and "Why me" questions.

After identifying this thinking pattern, particularly in response to intrusive thoughts about the trauma, the therapist then focuses on introducing alternative responses. The aim is to (1) increase patient awareness of the disadvantages of worry, rumination, and gap filling, (2) to introduce DM, and (3) to implement worry/rumination postponement (and banning gap filling). Let us now examine these in turn.

Advantages–Disadvantages Analysis

The therapist works to help the patient see that engaging in worry/rumination serves little purpose and contributes to locking him or her into merely replaying negative aspects of the trauma or thinking about future threat. In order to do this and to weaken positive beliefs about the need to engage in this type of persistent thinking, the therapist guides the patient through an advantages and disadvantages analysis of worry/rumination. The aim is to weaken the advantages and strengthen the disadvantages to facilitate implementation of worry and rumination postponement. The following dialogue illustrates this process:

THERAPIST: I would like us to explore the advantages and disadvantages of rumination and worry. Let's start with rumination, which refers to thinking back and dwelling on what happened and analyzing it. We will list the advantages of doing that first and then list the disadvantages. What do you think are the advantages of repeatedly going over the event?

PATIENT: It helps me get clear in my mind what happened.

THERAPIST: Okay, I'll write that down. Does rumination help in other ways?

PATIENT: It means I can work it out if I'm to blame.

THERAPIST: I'll add that to the list. Any other advantages?

PATIENT: I can't think of any.

THERAPIST: Could it help you prevent similar situations in the future?

PATIENT: Yes, if I can understand why it happened I might be more cautious next time.

THERAPIST: Okay. Anything else?

PATIENT: No, I don't think so.

THERAPIST: Let's look at the disadvantages of rumination. What do you think the problems are?

PATIENT: Well, you've started me thinking that it keeps my anxiety going.

THERAPIST: That's a good one. I'll add that to the disadvantages list. Any other problems with it?

PATIENT: It doesn't let me forget about what happened.

THERAPIST: Good. It keeps your mind focused on threat. Anything else?

PATIENT: I can't think of anything.

THERAPIST: Does ruminating make you feel happy and positive?

PATIENT: No, quite the opposite, it makes me feel angry and sad.

THERAPIST: Okay, so let's write that down too.

In the next stage the therapist revisits the advantages of rumination and challenges them as follows:

THERAPIST: Let's return to the advantages listed. Have you been able to get a clear impression of what happened since you've been ruminating?

PATIENT: Well, no, I don't think it was my fault, but I can't remember everything.

THERAPIST: How much rumination would be needed to remember everything?

PATIENT: I don't think any amount will make it better than it is already.

THERAPIST: So has rumination really helped you sort things out?

PATIENT: Maybe, a little, but not really.

THERAPIST: Does rumination make you more cautious?

PATIENT: Yes, I'm sure it does.

THERAPIST: At what price? Look at the disadvantages.

PATIENT: Yes, I can see it has problems.

THERAPIST: Do you think it is possible to be cautious without ruminating about the past?

PATIENT: Yes, I suppose it is possible. I hadn't thought of that.

THERAPIST: So, when you look at it in detail, are there any strong advantages to ruminating?

PATIENT: No, it doesn't look as if there is. But I'm not sure I can stop it that easily.

THERAPIST: As a matter of fact, stopping it is not such a problem. We'll move onto that in a minute.

The advantages and disadvantages analysis as illustrated above should be undertaken in examining the motivations (i.e., beliefs) about other unhelpful coping behaviors. Specifically, worry, thought suppression, and (later in treatment) alcohol or drug use and avoidance as appropriate.

When avoidance of thoughts or thought suppression is a feature of the formulation, the advantages–disadvantages analysis is usually supplemented with an in-session suppression experiment to illustrate how attempts to avoid thoughts can be a problem. Here the therapist normally asks the patient to try not to think a target thought (e.g., "Try not to think about a blue tiger for the next few minutes"). Then after the patient spends a couple of minutes engaging in the task, the therapist asks what happened. Typically, the patient reports experiencing the thought. This result is used as evidence to illustrate how thought control is not particularly effective and might even increase preoccupation with intrusions.

Detached Mindfulness

The next step is introduction of the concept of responding to initial negative thoughts or intrusions related to the trauma with DM rather than with rumination and worry.

As described in Chapter 5 DM refers to establishing a new perspective in relation to intrusive thoughts in which they are observed in a detached way, without interpreting, analyzing, or controlling them. Patients are instructed to respond to negative thoughts, intrusive thoughts, flashbacks, and nightmares as follows:

> "When you have an intrusive thought [flashback, etc.] it is important that you do the following. First acknowledge to yourself the presence of the thought, then remind yourself that this is part of the healing process and that it is unhelpful to engage with it. Try saying to yourself: 'This is just a thought. I don't need to do anything with it. I'm just going to leave it alone to occupy its own place.'"

Analogies can be used to aid comprehension of the concept of DM. The recalcitrant child (Chapter 5) or "pushing clouds" metaphors are particularly useful. For example, the therapist says:

> "You can interact with intrusive symptoms in the same way that you would treat clouds in the sky. Clouds are part of the environment's self-regulating weather system. They come and go and there is nothing we can do to influence them. Trying to push them away or worry about them is not necessary or helpful. Even if you could influence them it would disturb the balance necessary for rainfall and the cli-

mate. The best thing to do is to let clouds occupy their own space and passively watch their behavior over time. This is an approach you can use with your intrusive thoughts and symptoms. Treat them as if they were clouds passing by and merely watch them passively from a distance."

This explanation is followed by practice in DM to neutral thoughts so that the patient can gain experiential awareness of this state. For example, the free-association or tiger task can be used (see Chapter 5). In the free-association task the therapist asks the patient to sit quietly and let his or her thoughts roam freely during free association. The instructions for this task follow a format like this:

"One way to experience a sense of detached mindfulness is to apply it to general thoughts and feelings. In a minute I will say a series of words and I would like you to sit and passively watch the movement of thoughts in your mind. You may have many thoughts or you may have none. That doesn't matter. The aim is to be aware of what happens without influencing it in any way. Do not try to deliberately form thoughts or to activate feelings or memories. Simply watch your spontaneous inner experiences without influencing them. Let's start (*pause*). Apple (*pause*), ocean (*pause*), tree (*pause*), birthday (*pause*), bicycle (*pause*), home (*pause*), chocolate (*pause*), holiday (*pause*). Were you able to stand back and watch your thoughts and experiences happen spontaneously without influencing them?"

Rumination/Worry Postponement

Once the patient understands the concept of DM and completes in-session practice, the therapist introduces the rumination/worry postponement strategy. The therapist instructs the patient that whenever he or she experiences an intrusive thought or symptom (e.g., sudden increase in arousal), he or she should acknowledge that the symptom has occurred, and then tell the self not to ruminate, worry, or analyze the trauma or symptom now, to just let the symptom fade in its own time, and to actively think about it later.

Patients are asked to allocate a 15-minute thinking time each evening. This should take place at least 2 hours before going to bed. During this time the individual can analyze and think about the trauma and symptoms as much as he or she feels necessary. However, the therapist emphasizes that this thinking or worry time is not compulsory. Indeed, most patients decide not to use it. Patients are instructed to stop worrying at the end of their 15-minute worry period, and to deal with any further worry by applying DM and carrying thoughts over to the next day's worry period if necessary.

APPLICATION OF DM
AND RUMINATION/WORRY POSTPONEMENT

The therapist asks the client to apply DM and worry/rumination postponement in response to all intrusive thoughts about the trauma. It is important that the therapist closely monitors the practice of these strategies. This is enabled by careful discussion of how the technique is implemented for homework.

Early in the use of these strategies most patients state that they are using them. However, the therapist's careful analysis typically shows that they are not being applied consistently to all intrusions or that they are being applied inappropriately. An example is given below to illustrate how it is necessary for the therapist to closely examine and "debug" or improve the implementation of DM and worry postponement.

THERAPIST: Have you been practicing detached mindfulness and worry postponement?

PATIENT: Yes, I've been using it.

THERAPIST: How often have you used it?

PATIENT: Every day, whenever I get a thought, like you said.

THERAPIST: So how much of the time have you been thinking about the trauma?

PATIENT: Well, I still think about it.

THERAPIST: When was the last time you thought about it?

PATIENT: Today, on the way to the session.

THERAPIST: What thoughts did you have?

PATIENT: I was thinking about why I hadn't worked out the problem for myself.

THERAPIST: It sounds like you were analyzing things. How long did that last?

PATIENT: I'm not sure, probably on and off while I was driving here.

THERAPIST: What was the thought that triggered it?

PATIENT: It was the thought of coming to treatment. Not everyone needs treatment just because they've had an accident.

THERAPIST: So the thought was something like "What's wrong with me?"

PATIENT: Yes, something like that.

THERAPIST: It sounds as if that was an example of a rumination. What do you think?

PATIENT: Yes, I suppose it was. I wouldn't have seen that unless you'd pointed it out.

THERAPIST: How many times have you let ruminations like that occur in the last week?

PATIENT: Quite a few. I need to be more aware of it happening.

THERAPIST: Good, so you need to be aware of prolonged thinking about the trauma and postpone it. If you have a thought such as "What's wrong with me?" apply detached mindfulness and disengage any prolonged thinking about it. You don't need to answer those questions.

It is important that the therapist assesses the effective and optimum use of DM. This is achieved by following some basic guidelines:

1. The therapist asks patients to estimate the percentage of time they have been able to apply the technique to intrusive thoughts. It is important that the therapist and the patient do not confuse this as a rating of distress. The aim is not to rate the percentage of time the patient has been able to experience intrusions without distress. The therapist should emphasize that the aim of the technique is not primarily to reduce distress, but to allow natural processing to occur without excessive thinking. As a rule of thumb, the aim is that DM should be applied to at least 75% of intrusions, and occurrences of worry/rumination should not exceed 1–2 minutes each. It usually requires several sessions and refinements to practice to achieve these targets.

2. The patient is asked if there has been any decrease in the usage of the technique over time, and if so what the cause of decrease is. If this is due to a reduction in distress associated with the intrusion, the therapist emphasizes that the technique should be applied to most intrusions irrespective of distress levels.

3. A reduction in usage of DM due to a reduction in the frequency of intrusions is acceptable, but the aim of the technique is not to actively stop intrusions. The therapist asks if the patient has tried to stop intrusions or whether they have decreased spontaneously.

4. The therapist asks about the breadth of application of DM. It is important that it is applied to all types of intrusions relating to the trauma and its consequences. Some patients report specific recurrent intrusions that predominate. Having applied DM to this major intrusion they notice other intrusions but do not apply DM to these events as they should.

5. The patient is questioned about any nonusage of the technique. Reduced usage is to be expected if worrying has decreased. However, early in treatment a decreased usage of DM in response to particular intrusions should be a signal for its application to other broader worry domains where appropriate (see "Generalization Training" below). Failure to implement

the technique may be linked to strong positive metacognitive beliefs about the need to actively analyze the trauma or worry about future threat in order to cope or avoid danger. In these circumstances Socratic challenging of positive metacognitive beliefs about worry is recommended to facilitate implementation.

GENERALIZATION TRAINING

The therapist proceeds to the next stage of MCT by introducing the idea that worry/rumination postponement should be applied to all types of worry and persistent negative thinking, irrespective of whether or not worry/rumination is related to the trauma. At this stage it is useful to generate a list of current concerns to increase awareness of the pervasiveness of negative recyclic thinking. All types of dwelling, worry, and rumination are then targeted for the application of postponed worry for homework.

The therapist then examines the application of DM to the after-effect of nightmares. Trauma-related dreams/nightmares are often followed by preoccupation with thoughts and feelings elicited by them. The therapist introduces the idea that negative feelings and thoughts are natural in the aftermath of dreams/nightmares, but it is important to acknowledge these thoughts and feelings without actively analyzing or trying to suppress them. The patient is instructed to apply DM to any such after-effects when they occur.

ELIMINATING OTHER MALADAPTIVE COPING STRATEGIES

The next stage is examining the presence of other maladaptive coping strategies that are counterproductive for adaptation. The therapist carefully reviews the usage of other strategies for controlling symptoms, minimizing threats, controlling thoughts, and reducing anxiety.

Typical strategies to identify include use of alcohol or other drugs, thought suppression, avoidance of reminders of the trauma (e.g., TV programs), avoidance of people or places, avoidance of activities (e.g., driving), and checking (e.g., checking the street, checking one's body or memory).

Having identified these behaviors, the therapist helps the patient to see how they are a problem. For example, some of these strategies can be seen as a form of avoidance of thoughts and memories. This leads to a discussion of the problems caused by cognitive avoidance. Once the unhelpful consequences of each of the patient's strategies is identified, the therapist asks the patient to ban using them. Table 7.2 can be used by the therapist as a guide to thinking about the problems associated with using some of these coping strategies.

**TABLE 7.2. A Guide to Thinking about Consequences
of Unhelpful Coping Strategies**

Coping strategy	Therapist questions	Unhelpful consequences
1. Avoiding situations	"Can you forget about the trauma so long as you avoid reminders of it?"	"In order to avoid, I have to constantly think about what I'm doing and the danger involved."
	"How does avoidance help you to return to the way you used to be?"	"It means I've changed as a person and I'm keeping it going."
	"If you avoid situations, what is your sense of danger based on?"	"It's based on an absence of information. Time has moved on—it means I'm afraid of a memory."
2. Using alcohol	"What are the disadvantages of using alcohol to cope?"	"It means I'm not dealing with it myself. I'm trying to shut it out and interfering with natural recovery."
	"How long will you need to use alcohol before it works in the long term?"	"It won't work, it's just a quick fix. It stops me discovering the long-term solution."
3. Checking	"If checking helps you feel better, why do you need to continue checking?"	"It helps me feel safer at the time but it doesn't last."
	"If you continue checking, can you return your sense of danger to how it used to be?"	"It keeps my sense of danger going. I didn't always think this way."
4. Thought suppression	"How effective have you been in stopping your thoughts?"	"Sometimes I stop them, but they keep coming back."
	"What are the disadvantages of continuing with a strategy that doesn't work?"	"I keep failing and think I have no control."

ATTENTION MODIFICATION

The attention modification component of treatment is introduced when patients have successfully implemented DM and worry/rumination postponement for at least 1 week as operationalized by DM applied to at least 75% of intrusions, and worry/rumination periods lasting no longer than 1–2 minutes.

In this phase of treatment the focus turns to hypervigilance and threat-monitoring strategies that maintain perceptions of danger and associated anxiety. Two types of attention-monitoring strategy are relevant: (1) attention to internal sources of threat (e.g., sensations, bodily events, emotions, thoughts) and (2) attention to external threats in the form of scanning the environment for sources of danger. These patterns of attention may coexist, exist alone, or oscillate depending on the situation. Reversal of threat monitoring is important because it shifts patients out of threat modes of processing that repeatedly generate information concerning danger in environments that previously were processed in a nonthreatening way. Rather than persisting in a loop of processing danger that increases sensitivity to unlikely threats, the patient is encouraged to develop a new plan for controlling attention that allows threat-related processing to decay.

The attentional modification component of treatment is implemented in four stages:

Stage 1: Explanation and Rationale

The therapist introduces the topic by describing how attention maintains PTSD. It is helpful to link this insight with the information the patient has already discovered about the unhelpful role of worry in order to form a bridge from the early part of treatment. The following introduction is used as a basis for the rationale:

> "You have seen how worry/rumination and attempts to control symptoms can maintain your problem. You have been successful in reducing those unhelpful responses. It is now time to consider another type of unhelpful response that can keep a sense of danger and threat going. Has your sense of danger changed since the event?

> "It is quite normal following trauma to become overly aware of potential dangers. This is a type of focusing of attention that maintains a sense of danger and stops you returning to a more balanced view of the world."

The rationale is illustrated by asking questions about the consequences of threat-monitoring strategies. It is best if these questions are directed at exploring the patient's own specific strategies. For example, the therapist might ask:

> "Are there any problems with constantly scanning the environment for signs of threat?"
> "Is scanning for threat likely to increase or decrease your anxiety?"
> "Does paying attention to threat give you a balanced impression of how safe a situation really is?"
> "What effect does paying attention to threat have on your anxiety?"
> "Does paying attention to threat mean that you will always cope better?"

In this way the therapist aims to build a conceptualization of hypervigilance or threat monitoring as another form of preoccupation or coping behavior that is similar to worry/rumination in being unhelpful. The following interchange illustrates the use of these questions:

THERAPIST: Has your focus of attention changed since you were robbed?

PATIENT: What do you mean?

THERAPIST: For instance, when you are walking in the street do you notice things that you didn't before?

PATIENT: Yes, I'm looking for people on bikes and people wearing their hoods up. I just look for anyone who might be acting suspiciously.

THERAPIST: Anything else you pay more attention to?

PATIENT: I'm more sensitive to the things I read in the newspaper. I'm checking to see if the crimes reported have happened near to anywhere I visit.

THERAPIST: Are there any problems with scanning for things in this way?

PATIENT: No, it means I'll stand a better chance of avoiding problems in the future.

THERAPIST: Does paying attention to threat mean you will always cope better?

PATIENT: No, I suppose you can't pay attention to everything.

THERAPIST: If you had paid more attention to your surroundings before the trauma, would it have prevented what happened to you?

PATIENT: No, because they approached me from behind. I suppose I would need to be looking backward all the time.

THERAPIST: What effect does paying attention to threat in this way have on your anxiety?

PATIENT: It makes me feel scared, and I'm more aware of how much crime there is.

THERAPIST: So is it that crime has increased since you were robbed, or has something else changed?

PATIENT: No, it's just that I'm noticing it more.

THERAPIST: Does noticing it more mean that you're safer?

PATIENT: It could.

THERAPIST: What about the things you don't notice?

PATIENT: Well, those are the really dangerous things.

THERAPIST: So I guess you need to notice everything even if it hasn't happened yet.

PATIENT: Yes, I try to think about what could go wrong.

THERAPIST: That sounds like your worry process again. Can you see the similarity?

PATIENT: Yes, if you describe it like that.

THERAPIST: What will be the long-term effect on your anxiety?

PATIENT: I'll just keep on feeling anxious.

THERAPIST: That's right. So we need to reduce your threat monitoring so that you can return to a more balanced view of the world.

Stage 2: Weakening Positive Metacognitive Beliefs about Monitoring

Before the patient is willing to give up threat monitoring, he or she often needs therapist guidance to weaken the positive beliefs that support its usage. Some examples of positive beliefs include the following:

> "If I pay attention to threats, I'll be able to protect myself."
> "Being alert to danger means I can avoid problems before it's too late."
> "I must keep a state of readiness in order to be prepared."
> "Staying on edge means I won't be taken by surprise."

To challenge these beliefs the therapist asks whether maintaining attention on threat would have actually averted the traumatic event. In particular, how would the patient have known precisely which danger to look out for before the event happened?

Reinforcing the disadvantages and negative consequences of engaging in threat monitoring also provides a means of weakening positive beliefs. The therapist helps the patient see how attention to threat creates a greater sense of danger. An experiment can be run to reinforce this message in which the patient is asked to change his or her attentional strategy and look out for accidents "that are waiting to happen," such as cars speeding and driving too close together. In this way the therapist can pose the question "Does attention to threat give you an accurate impression of danger or an inflated sense of danger? Because it is inflated it is necessary to return to a balanced sense that will involve reducing threat monitoring."

Stage 3: Awareness and Abandonment

Once the patient understands his or her problem with threat monitoring, the therapist asks the patient to consciously acknowledge the focus of attention the next time anxiety is experienced in a situation. Next, the patient should be helped to stop threat monitoring by shifting attention to neutral stimuli such as counting the number of blue-colored objects that can be seen. In order to apply this strategy the patient is encouraged to return to a normal pretrauma routine, and if possible to the situation in which the trauma occurred.

Subsequent sessions at this stage should assess the extent to which the patient is returning to his or her normal pretrauma routine. If avoidance of low-risk situations is an issue, the patient should be encouraged to enter specific situations for homework while practicing the abandonment of threat monitoring.

Stage 4: Attention Refocusing—Safety Signals

After abandonment of threat monitoring the next stage is active attentional refocusing. This consists of asking the patient to deliberately refocus attention away from him- or herself and away from threat onto safety signals in the environment when in situations that remind him or her of the trauma. The therapist introduces this concept in the following way:

> "In order to allow thinking to retune to the normal environment it is helpful to practice focusing attention in a benign way. This means looking for signs of safety instead of signs of low probability threat."

This goal is implemented by practicing refocusing strategies in the treatment session. First, the patient is asked to sit in the waiting room and then focus on aspects of the environment that make it a safe place to be. Next, the patient might be asked to walk along the street with the therapist and practice focusing on safety signals.

For example, a patient who had been knocked down by a speeding motorist described how he was nervous crossing the road and was constantly looking out for speeding vehicles (i.e., threat monitoring). The therapist asked him if this was the best thing to focus on when planning to cross a road, and what might be better information. After some discussion the therapist suggested that it might be better to focus on large gaps in the traffic as a means of judging if it was safe to cross the road. The patient agreed that this was better than focusing on speeding vehicles as a means of determining that it was safe to cross. On practicing the alternative attentional strategy the patient reported that he began to feel more comfortable in the situation. If necessary, "metacognitive guidance" (Chapter 5) can be applied in these situations.

RESIDUAL AVOIDANCE

At this stage of treatment the therapist identifies any remaining avoidance of situations and aims to reverse this strategy. Some patients continue to avoid the scene of the trauma. In these circumstances they are asked to visit the scene while applying *external* monitoring of the *current* safe environment. There may be a tendency to process the image or memory of the trauma activated in the situation but the patient is encouraged to apply DM to the intrusion and to "look through it" at the external present safe environment.

NEW PLANS FOR PROCESSING

Once maladaptive strategies have been removed and the positive meta-cognitive beliefs supporting them have been modified, the final step of treatment, which contributes to relapse prevention, is consolidation and strengthening of alternative metacognitive plans that can be used to control responses to trauma-related intrusions in the future.

Of particular importance is that the patient maintains awareness of worry/rumination and threat monitoring and avoidance. The new plan for processing should reflect responses that are incompatible with these responses. To facilitate this, a "plan summary" (see Appendix 19) can be completed representing the maladaptive old plan and summarizing the new responses to be repeatedly practiced in response to idiosyncratic triggers.

Implementation of this strategy has three important components. First, a comprehensive range of triggers for symptoms must be elicited so that awareness can be enhanced. Second, a detailed set of statements written in the first person should be scripted on the summary that capture the old plan and the new plan to be practiced. Third, the patient must be encouraged to repeatedly implement the new plan as an alternative to the old plan. Let us take a closer look at each component:

"My Triggers" contains a list of typical internal events that activate old styles of processing and coping. Typical examples include:

1. Intrusive thoughts (e.g., a flashback or memory fragment).
2. Negative thoughts (e.g., before leaving the house the patient thinks "Is it safe?").
3. Arousal symptoms (e.g., being startled or feeling anxious).
4. Cognitive symptoms (e.g., difficulty concentrating).
5. Physical symptoms (e.g., aches and pains).
6. External events (e.g., hearing an unexpected noise).

"Thinking style" consists of a description of the old ruminative and negative brooding thought process. For example, "I try to work out why this has happened to me, why I feel this way, what this means about me as a person, what if it had been different." The new plan should capture an instruction that encapsulates alternative responses learned in treatment: "I must interrupt any dwelling on the issue and postpone analyzing it. If negative thoughts occur, I will apply detached mindfulness, and continue with what I am doing."

"Behaviors" should be completed with a statement about avoidance and maladaptive coping such as alcohol use. For instance: "I must avoid dangerous places, I must try to sleep more, if I have a drink I can numb the thoughts." The new plan can then be "I must continue with my original lifestyle, I must interrupt my worries and apply detached mindfulness to my thoughts."

"Attention focus" refers to the old tendency to monitor for signs of threat which should be replaced with a new attention plan. We have seen how threat in PTSD often consists of monitoring symptoms or external sources of danger. For instance, a patient explained how he would check the street for gangs of youths before leaving the house and before going to bed. He would also check his memory for the traumatic event to see if he could remember the face of his assailant. The old plan was written as: "I must check for groups of youths in order to feel safe. I must recover my memory so that I can be safe in the future." The new plan that was developed was written as: "I must ban checking for danger. I must leave my memory alone. I must focus on different signals in the environment such as the presence of safety."

RELAPSE PREVENTION

During relapse prevention the therapist reviews residual scores on the PTSD-S, paying particular attention to the frequency and duration of worry/rumination, positive beliefs about strategies, and attentional threat monitoring and avoidance. Residual elevated scores on these dimensions should be explored and modified because they are potential contributors to relapse.

The therapist checks for other subtle forms of rumination or similar perseverative processes that may have developed more recently or have been overlooked during treatment.

In the last two sessions of treatment, therapist and patient work collaboratively on compiling a "therapy blueprint." The patient is usually asked to begin work on the blueprint for homework, which can be augmented in session. The blueprint contains an example of the case conceptualization, examples of positive beliefs about worry/rumination and threat monitoring, and evidence counteracting them. It includes statements that challenge negative beliefs about symptoms (e.g., "I learned that my symptoms are part of natural recovery, and not a sign I'm losing my mind"). It also consists of the final version of the new plan summary, which details new strategies for dealing with common triggers for the CAS.

Booster treatment sessions are usually scheduled for 3 and 6 months after treatment as an opportunity to monitor gains and reinforce the knowledge and strategies acquired in treatment.

PTSD TREATMENT PLAN

An overall 10-session treatment plan for implementing MCT in PTSD is presented in Appendix 16. This is intended as a guide to the structure and content of treatment and should be applied flexibly as individual circumstances require. The plan should be implemented with direct reference to the strategies described in this chapter.

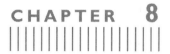

CHAPTER **8**

Obsessive–Compulsive Disorder

The principal feature of obsessive–compulsive disorder (OCD) is the occurrence of obsessions and compulsions. *Obsessions* are intrusive thoughts, images, and impulses that occur against the individual's will, and they are experienced as repugnant and uncharacteristic of the self. Obsessions are actively resisted. The person realizes that they are the product of his or her mind. Obsessional thoughts often have violent, sexual, or religious content or occur as doubts and ruminations concerning contamination. (*Note:* Ruminations may not occur against the individual's will or be actively resisted or repugnant. In the metacognitive model ruminations are part of the individual's strategy for detecting and preventing threat.)

Compulsions are overt or covert repetitive behaviors performed in response to obsessions. They are intended to reduce distress or discomfort or to prevent some dreaded event. Covert compulsions include counting, praying, or thinking in special ways, while overt compulsions include washing, ordering, checking, and repeating actions a specific number of times. Patients may have particular rules or systems for conducting their rituals. The DSM-IV-TR (American Psychiatric Association, 2000) diagnostic criteria for OCD are summarized in Table 8.1.

OVERVIEW OF MCT: OBJECT LEVEL VERSUS META LEVEL

The application of MCT to OCD requires greater therapist effort in actively maintaining focus on meta-level working when compared to the disorders described previously in this book. Some patients appear to be more rigidly fixed at the object level or in the object "mode." For instance, the patient with contamination fears typically believes that his or her problem is one of

TABLE 8.1. Diagnostic Criteria for OCD

Criterion A

The presence of either obsessions or compulsions.

Criterion B

At some time in the disorder, the person recognized that the obsessions or compulsions are excessive or unreasonable.

Criterion C

The obsessions or compulsions cause marked distress, take more than 1 hour a day, or interfere with functioning.

Criterion D

If another Axis I disorder is present the content of obsessions and compulsions is not restricted to it.

Criterion E

The obsessions and compulsions are not due to substances or a medical condition.

Note. Summarized from American Psychiatric Association (2000).

contamination by germs (object mode) rather than being one of thoughts concerning contamination (meta mode).

MCT focuses on patients' beliefs about inner experience—predominantly thoughts and feelings—and does not focus on beliefs about external domains.

For example, a 41-year-old woman presented with obsessional fears concerning being contaminated with feces. Treatment did not focus on challenging the belief about the probability of being contaminated, but focused instead on challenging her beliefs about the occurrence of the thought about feces.

This example represents the shift that is required from working at the object level to working at the metacognitive level. Some additional case examples will serve to illustrate this MCT focus:

A 27-year-old man experienced anxiety about traveling to and from work each day. Upon arrival at work or at home, he would spend a great amount of time washing his hands, so much so that he had developed dermatitis. In his route he had to follow a path alongside some old garages that he thought might contain rat poison. He was concerned that he would become contaminated with the rat poison, which would be harmful to himself and others. A traditional CBT approach would focus on challenging his beliefs about being contaminated and his sense of responsibility. It would use exposure and ritual prevention to facilitate habituation and/or as an experiment to test his belief in spreading contamination. However, in MCT the focus was on changing the patient's relationship with his thoughts about being contaminated and challenging his belief about the meaning of the intrusion.

The difference between the object-level and meta-level approaches is apparent in the types of questions the therapist asks in a Socratic dialogue. In CBT the therapist asks questions such as "Where's your evidence that the garage contains rat poison?" and "Where's your evidence that you will poison people?"

In contrast, in MCT the therapist might ask, "Is the problem that the garage contains rat poison or is the problem your thought that it does?" The primary question is followed by other questions that challenge the importance of the thought: "If you think it's contaminated, does that mean it must be so?" MCT treatment focused on how the patient related to and responded to these thoughts. In particular he held the implicit metacognitive beliefs: "Thoughts are facts, so if I think something is contaminated, then it must be contaminated" and "It's better to be worried about rat poison than to take a risk." Treatment focused on these metacognitions concerning the importance of thoughts.

A 36-year-old woman reported being distressed by sexual thoughts concerning animals. In this case the role of beliefs about thoughts was explicit from the outset. She attempted to suppress and avoid her sexual thoughts by thinking romantic thoughts about her boyfriend, but this oscillated, with deliberate sexual thoughts about animals, testing if she was "into bestiality." In order to determine her beliefs about thoughts, during MCT the therapist asked: "What does having these thoughts mean to you?" She believed that having the thoughts meant that she "was a pervert" or would "become a pervert" by thinking this way. Thus, it was necessary for the MCT therapist to change the way she related to these thoughts and to challenge her beliefs about them (i.e., prove that they did not mean she was a pervert and that they did not have the power to make her become one).

A 44-year-old man described his problem as having to repeatedly check his actions. In particular, he repeatedly checked his work in order to be sure that he had not made mistakes that could damage his company's reputation. He also repeatedly checked the journeys he made while driving his car to be sure that he had not collided with a pedestrian and killed him or her. In order to access the metacognitive level, the therapist asked: "When you have checked your actions, how often have you discovered that you have made a mistake?" The patient replied that it had rarely happened. This was followed by the question: "So is the problem that you are prone to mistakes or is the problem that you continue to believe that a thought about a mistake or a doubt means you must have made one?"

TWO TYPES OF METACOGNITIVE CHANGE

As we have seen in the treatment of disorders presented in earlier chapters, two basic types of metacognitive change are the focus of MCT. These are (1) how the patient relates to and experiences thoughts (e.g., nature of experiential awareness), and (2) what the individual believes about thoughts. These two factors are correlated but are not synonymous.

In each of the examples above, the patient is experiencing his or her thoughts as fused with reality and responds to them with the maladaptive CAS. At the level of beliefs about thoughts each patient believes that his or her thoughts, urges, or impulses are important and have special meaning or power.

MCT focuses on developing an alternative way of experiencing thoughts and modifies beliefs about the meaning and importance of thoughts and feelings. Treatment also focuses on modifying beliefs about rituals and the inappropriate internal criteria and strategies individuals with OCD appear to use to determine the level of threat in situations.

The model gives rise to some innovative treatment approaches that differ significantly from previous approaches. For instance, prolonged or repeated exposure is not necessary to produce cognitive and affective change. Exposure is configured metacognitively as a test of predictions based on metacognitive beliefs.

MCT focuses on changing the strategies that patients use to guide behavior and processing by rewriting subjective plans for action and cognition. Treatment challenges metacognitive beliefs about thoughts, and also the way in which individuals relate to their intrusive thoughts. In this latter respect it gives rise to new techniques such as exposure and response commission (ERC). In ERC, patients are encouraged to perform their rituals in a way that enables them to change the nature of their relationship with their thoughts.

More specifically, the patient is permitted to engage in rituals but is instructed to hold his or her obsessional thought in mind throughout his or her ritual. This activity provides a means of promoting DM and shifting to a metacognitive mode of experiencing. In parallel with these results, it can also weaken patient beliefs about the need to perform rituals. Furthermore, as described below, some rituals, such as checking, can be used to unambiguously show the patient how a thought is unimportant.

THE CAS IN OCD

In OCD the conceptual component of the CAS manifests as worry, rumination, and analytic thinking in response to thoughts or doubts. Threat monitoring consists of monitoring for certain unwanted thoughts or feelings or attending to possible threatening aspects of the environment (e.g., possible contaminants). The maladaptive coping strategies that constitute the CAS in OCD are thought suppression, overt and covert neutralizing, and ritual behaviors.

The CAS is problematic because it gives elevated importance to patient thoughts and inflates his or her sense of threat. For example, having a thought such as "I'm contaminated" becomes more threatening because the individual analyzes all of the situations in which he or she may have spread contamination and monitors for potential sources of harmful contaminants. These responses lock the individual into fusing the thought with material events rather than seeing the thought as simply an idea in the mind that can be let go.

Cognitive Perseveration: Rumination, Worry, and Covert Rituals

It is generally the case that patients engage in worry, rumination, and covert rituals as a means of avoiding threat or danger. These processes are the conceptual components of the CAS and are driven by metacognitive beliefs or rules about thinking and obtaining particular feeling states. Worry, rumination, and covert rituals are all examples of the individual's coping responses and are included in the formulation under "behavioral responses."

> Examples of this form of perseveration can be seen in the case of a female college student who reported an obsessional preoccupation with contaminating her books with bodily fluids. She continuously worried about contamination occurring and believed that worrying about it meant that she would be cautious and reduce the risk. Before settling down to work she had to plan the day so that she was sure that she could have an uninterrupted and pure work time that was not spoiled by impure thoughts or the risk of contamination. The mental planning alone could take several hours. It must not be interrupted by using the toilet as this would necessitate prolonged washing. She was concerned that the situation must be "just right" in order to use her books, otherwise she would spoil them and then she would become trapped in a "dead world" in which she was perpetually in a state of "unrest" when trying to study.

In this case, perseveration consisted of worrying about contamination and planning as a means of avoiding this outcome. The patient's rules and positive metacognitive beliefs about rituals were that she must not have impure thoughts and the study environment must conform to some status of being "just right."

[*Note:* Her negative metacognitive beliefs were that particular (impure) thoughts and feelings were important and had the power to trap her in a state of permanent unrest.]

Threat Monitoring

Threat monitoring in OCD is part of the person's coping behavior and takes different forms. For example, it can involve monitoring for possible signs of contamination, monitoring for certain "bad" thoughts in the stream of consciousness, monitoring for particular feeling states/emotions/sensations, monitoring for symmetry/lack of tidiness, and monitoring for memory phenomena.

> An example of memory monitoring can be seen in the case of a woman who checked her memory whenever she had an intrusive thought about her children being stabbed. She tried to remember everything that she had done since she last saw them. If there were no gaps in her memory, she could continue her routine without anxiety. However, any gaps meant she might have killed them and she would need to see her children to be sure she hadn't. In this example, the patient monitored for gaps in memory in response to a thought as a sign of the presence of threat.

Behaviors

Other unhelpful coping behavior in OCD appear as overt and covert rituals that are intended to reduce discomfort and prevent harm. Covert responses include magical sayings, praying, forming "safe images," retracing memory (memory monitoring [see above]), repeating words, counting, and so on. Overt responses often include washing, checking, ordering, repeating actions, tidying, aligning objects, and avoidance. These behaviors backfire because they:

1. Imbue intrusive thoughts/feelings with importance by maintaining belief in their power, meaning, and significance.
2. Prevent the person from strengthening a metacognitive mode of experiencing in which thoughts are seen as passing events in the mind.
3. Rely on inappropriate internal criteria that can exacerbate obsessional thoughts and contribute to perseveration. For example, we saw in the last case how the patient checked her memory for gaps and how these were interpreted as evidence that she might have murdered her children. The absence of a memory is not a normal criterion for deciding that one has done something; the

more a person checks his or her memory, the more aware he or she becomes of these normal memory gaps. So the criteria used to regulate coping and to appraise threat is often inappropriate and leads to further intrusions and distress.

METACOGNITIVE BELIEFS

Two domains of metacognitive beliefs are implicated in the model and treatment of OCD: (1) metacognitive beliefs about the significance or importance of thoughts and feelings and (2) metacognitive beliefs about the need to perform rituals.

Beliefs about Thoughts and Intrusions

Metacognitive beliefs about intrusive thoughts and/or feelings have been termed "fusion beliefs" (Wells, 1997), following the terminology introduced by Rachman (1993) as a label for cognitive distortions in OCD. In the metacognitive model (Wells, 1997) three domains of fusion meta-belief have been described, but these domains may not be exhaustive. These are:

1. *Thought–event fusion (TEF)*. TEF is the belief that an intrusive thought can cause a particular event to occur or the belief that an intrusive thought means that an event must have already occurred. For example, if one has the thought "Have I killed someone?," the thought itself leads to the belief that you probably have killed someone. Another example would be believing that having an intrusive image of a friend being involved in an accident will make the accident more likely to happen.

2. *Thought–action fusion (TAF)*. TAF is the belief that intrusive thoughts, feelings, or impulses have the power to cause one to commit unwanted and undesirable actions. For example, an individual who has an urge to stab someone while holding a knife will interpret this thought as if it will lead to commission of that uncontrollable act. Similarly, TAF can prompt the belief that a thought about shouting an obscenity in a public place will lead to that action. Another variety of TAF is the belief that performing an action while having an intrusive thought has the power to make that thought more real or more likely. For example, one patient believed that having the mental image of a murderer while stepping off the pavement would make the thought more tangible and more likely to push him to commit murder.

3. *Thought–object fusion (TOF)*. TOF is the belief that thoughts and feelings can be transferred into objects, the consequence of which is to make

thoughts and feelings more "real," more able to cause harm, to become inescapable, and/or to spoil objects. An example is the belief that "feelings of unrest" can be transferred into books, thus contaminating them such that the feeling can never be escaped when the infected books are used. Similarly, one patient described how he believed that having a thought of a pedophile while he was shaving had the power to transfer that thought into his razor such that future shaving would increase the risk of becoming a pedophile.

These beliefs may seem bizarre but they are simply exaggerations of beliefs that many people hold in some form. For instance, people carry lucky charms because they believe that they have protective power. In religious ceremonies objects are blessed, thus imbuing them with special purity, power, or significance. These behaviors are indicative of underlying fusion beliefs. Similarly, most people would feel uncomfortable wishing that a loved one be harmed and would resist this thought, an example of TEF (i.e., there is a fear that wishing this to happen could make it more likely).

Beliefs about Rituals (and Worry/Rumination)

Another important category of metacognitive belief concerns the need to conduct rituals and neutralizing behaviors. These beliefs usually reflect the importance of controlling thoughts, impulses, and feeling states such as arousal and anxiety (e.g., "I must check the stove; otherwise my feeling of discomfort will never end"). They include the need to maintain particular states of mind and body and can present as personal rules for self-regulation (e.g., "I must maintain a state of mental rest before I can work properly" and "I must discipline my mind in order to stay safe"). Beliefs about rituals constitute a plan for guiding coping responses. The goal of the plan is to obtain some desired state that acts as a stop signal for the ritual.

STOP SIGNALS

Since the importance and danger inherent in intrusive thoughts is subjectively determined by metacognitions and there is no readily discernable objective threat, the person with OCD is faced with trying to know when a situation is safe in the absence of objective evidence that it is so. For instance, how can a person know he or she has washed his or her hands enough when germs are invisible?

As a consequence the individual has an overreliance on internal and inappropriate signals that are the stop criteria (stop signals) for overt and covert rituals. For example, a person with contamination fears might stop washing when he can wash for 4 minutes without having an intrusive feeling or thought about contamination (i.e., all doubts are removed). The person fearful of having caused an accident might check her memory for gaps, since a gap could represent the time when the accident could have happened. In these cases if there are no doubts or no memory gaps, then there are no problems and rituals can be stopped. Unfortunately, these criteria are difficult to reliably achieve and they lead to further intrusions (doubts and worry about memory gaps) that maintain distress.

THE METACOGNITIVE MODEL OF OCD

So far I have illustrated how aspects of the CAS and metacognitive beliefs are made manifest in OCD. In this section we examine how they play out in the metacognitive model of OCD that forms the basis of case conceptualization and treatment. The metacognitive model (Wells, 1997) is presented in Figure 8.1.

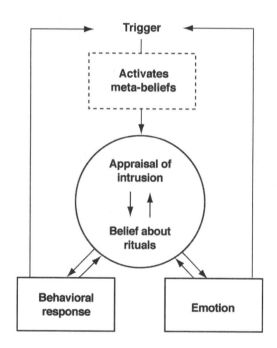

FIGURE 8.1. The metacognitive model of OCD. (Wells, 1997, p. 242). Copyright 1997 by John Wiley & Sons Limited. Reprinted by permission.

In the model the person with OCD becomes distressed in response to a trigger that is usually a thought, a feeling, or an urge. Thoughts include doubts or questions (e.g., "Have I hurt someone?") and intrusive images (e.g., image of an unwanted sexual act). Feelings include emotions and discreet states of tension or related symptoms. Urges include impulses to perform unwanted acts such as crashing into another car while driving at high speed. These intrusions occur normally. Indeed, obsessions are reported by the majority of individuals (e.g., Rachman & DeSilva, 1979).

Intrusions activate the person's metacognitive beliefs about their meaning and importance. In OCD these beliefs are erroneous and imbue intrusions with excessive negative importance. These beliefs are predominantly concerned with *fusion* in which particular inner experiences are believed to have a direct bearing on the outside world.

Specifically, these beliefs concern TEF (e.g., "Having a thought about an accident means that it must have happened"), TAF (e.g., "Having a thought about strangling the baby will make me do it"), and TOF (e.g., "Having bad thoughts and feelings will ruin objects and I'll never escape from the experience").

Activation of these dysfunctional metacognitive beliefs leads to negative appraisal of the intrusion as a sign of threat. This appraisal in turn leads to intensified negative emotions, predominantly anxiety, although other emotions such as guilt and anger also occur.

The change in emotion increases arousal and also increases the likelihood that thoughts and feelings will intrude into consciousness. The intensity and nature of the emotional response is affected by the person's beliefs about rituals and their appraised effectiveness in rendering the situation safe.

Once negative interpretations of intrusions occur, beliefs about rituals are activated and ritual/neutralizing behaviors are implemented in order to reduce threat.

Beliefs about rituals include rules concerning ways of controlling thoughts ("I must think of Jesus and we'll be safe"), ways of controlling feelings ("I must feel calm and clear, otherwise I'll make a mistake"), and ways of controlling behavior ("I must wash until I have no doubts"). In each case the rituals are implemented in accordance with specific internal rules and criteria/stop signals. Thus, beliefs about rituals form a metacognitive plan for guiding action and for appraisal of its success or failure.

The problem with these rules is that they do not set realistic or useful standards for judging the presence of threat and they are difficult and subjectively costly to achieve. In addition, they do not allow the patient to readily shift to experiencing thoughts simply as events in the mind. Therefore threat perceptions and negative emotion persists. For example, a patient with washing rituals had the belief "I must wash more this time than last time to be sure it is done properly." This belief and the rule it contained led to ever increasing washing periods that culminated in near-complete exclusion of other daily activities, ending in depression. The *"More to be sure"* metacognitive rule for guiding responses is particularly destructive in leading to an escalation of covert and overt rituals.

The activation of beliefs or rules about rituals gives rise to the performance of overt and/or covert behaviors. These behaviors serve the function of reducing threat, reducing distress, and controlling particular feelings. Overt behaviors include checking, ordering, repeating actions, washing, touching objects, following specified sequences, avoidance, and slowness. Covert behaviors include subvocalization of phrases or words, counting, concentrating, having neutralizing or "safe" images, and trying to suppress or remove particular thoughts from consciousness. The problem with these behaviors is that some of them backfire and lead to an increased awareness or intrusion of unwanted thoughts. For instance, a patient may try to determine if his or her coping response has worked by monitoring for signs of the intrusive thought remaining. However, the act of monitoring can be sufficient to produce the unwanted intrusion (e.g., try to monitor for the possible spontaneous occurrence of a thought about a pink tiger without having the thought right now).

A further problem with use of behaviors is that they prevent the individual from discovering that beliefs about intrusions (i.e., TEF, TAF, TOF) and beliefs about the need to perform rituals are inaccurate or unnecessary. For example, conjuring up positive images in response to a negative intrusive thought prevents the individual from discovering that the negative image does not have the power to cause negative outcomes. This is because the person can attribute the nonoccurrence of the feared event to use of the covert coping response rather than to the fact that the belief about the importance of the intrusion is faulty.

Another problem with the use of coping responses is that the person risks setting up a widening range of associations between the intrusion and situations. For example, if the person washes in response to a thought of being contaminated, the washing environment subsequently serves to remind the person of the intrusive thought about contamination.

Finally, a key problem with neutralizing is that the person repeatedly "acts as if" the thought is important and meaningful and therefore reinforces an object mode of processing and diminishes flexibility in experiential awareness. The person's metacognitive model and experience of his or her own cognition becomes increasingly constrained.

An example of a case formulation based on the model is presented in Figure 8.2. In this case the trigger consisted of intrusive thoughts about committing crimes.

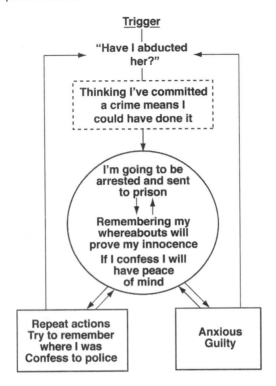

FIGURE 8.2. An idiosyncratic OCD case formulation.

THE MODEL IN ACTION

A closer look at these processes in a case of a woman suffering from contamination obsessions will serve to illustrate the model. The case conceptualization is presented in Figure 8.3.

   Her distress was repeatedly triggered in the kitchen at home. The trigger was looking at the kitchen floor and having the thought "a dead mouse
has been there." This thought was sometimes associated with a memory of
a dead mouse the cat had previously brought into the kitchen.

   This intrusive thought activated the implicit metacognitive belief that
thoughts about contamination are important and mean that things are
contaminated (TEF). In this case the patient believed: "Thinking the floor
is contaminated means it is contaminated." Although at the outset she was
unaware of this implicit belief, once the therapist had formulated it the
patient rated her conviction at 70%.

   Once activated, this belief gave rise to negative interpretations concerning danger, and the patient worried that she might spread germs and

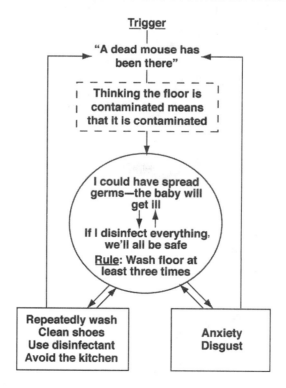

FIGURE 8.3. OCD case formulation of contamination obsessions.

cause her baby to become ill. This interpretation increased her anxiety and elicited feelings of disgust.

In association with the negative interpretation, beliefs about coping were activated. These concerned beliefs about remaining safe by disinfecting everything. But the problem the patient faces is knowing when the situation is safe since there is no objective measure of safety available. This problem was solved in this patient's case by the rule "Wash the floor at least three times." The third time constituted the stop signal for the ritual.

Her behaviors maintained her preoccupation with the thought of contamination and fed the intrusion. They linked the intrusion with other stimuli, such as her mop and bucket, which became cues for the intrusion subsequently. Her feelings and disgust also fed back into her appraisal of threat as symptoms themselves were misinterpreted as evidence of the presence of contamination. In addition, her behaviors maintained beliefs about rituals and appraisals of the importance of intrusions by preventing disconfirmation of them.

STRUCTURE OF TREATMENT

Treatment sessions are usually held on a weekly basis. Up to 12 sessions is typical although more may be required if OCD occurs in the context of perfectionistic personality traits. Treatment sessions are scheduled to last 45–60 minutes. An important early task in treatment is shifting the patient from an object mode to a metacognitive mode of processing. This is achieved via socialization and intensive use of DM and related strategies such as ERC. The stages of treatment are:

1. Case conceptualization
2. Socialization
3. Training detached mindfulness (and shifting to the metacognitive mode)
4. Modifying metacognitive (fusion) beliefs about intrusions
5. Modifying beliefs about rituals and stop signals
6. Reinforcing new plans for processing
7. Relapse prevention

CASE CONCEPTUALIZATION

Measures

Tools required during this stage are:

1. Obsessive–Compulsive Disorder Scale (OCD-S)
2. OCD Case Formulation Interview
3. Session checklists

The therapist usually administers the OCD-S to gain an impression of the patient's metacognitive beliefs and behaviors that should be explored and incorporated in the case formulation. The OCD-S is reproduced in Appendix 9. Other measures to consider that can be completed before sessions are the BAI (Beck et al., 1988) and the BDI-II (Beck et al., 1996) and specific OCD measures such as the Yale-Brown Obsessive–Compulsive Scale (Y-BOCS; Goodman, Price, Ramussen, Mazure, Fleischmann, et al., 1989), the Maudsley Obsessive–Compulsive Inventory (Hodgson & Rachman, 1977), and the Padua Inventory (Sanavio, 1988). For a more detailed assessment of metacognitive beliefs, the Thought Fusion Instrument (TFI; Wells, Gwilliam, & Cartwright-Hatton; see Appendix 3) should be considered.

Agenda of the First Session

The agenda for the first session should reflect the goals of mapping out a case conceptualization, increasing patient awareness of the factors maintaining disorder, and implementing the first strategies of metacognitive therapy. The first treatment strategy is introducing detached mindfulness as a new way of relating to obsessional thoughts and intrusions. In the introduction to the first session the therapist conveys the following:

> "In today's session I would like to explore a recent episode when you had intrusive thoughts and/or felt compelled to engage in a ritual. In doing so we can find the factors that are keeping your symptoms going and begin to examine ways that you can overcome your problem. I would also like to explain a little more about MCT and what you might expect from treatment. If there is time I will introduce you to a new way that you can respond to your obsessional thoughts and feelings. Is there anything you would like to put on the agenda and talk about today?"

Generating a Case Conceptualization

The therapist then proceeds with generating an idiosyncratic version of the metacognitive model that represents patient responses to a recent intrusive thought, impulse, or feeling.

One of the most efficient ways of generating the case formulation is to ask questions that follow a particular sequence as represented in the OCD Case Formulation Interview presented in Appendix 13.

This sequence consists of asking first about the recent occurrence of an obsessional thought or impulse or the occurrence of neutralizing. This is followed by asking about the emotion accompanying this trigger and then asking about the appraisal of the intrusion and belief about it. Finally, the therapist asks about the nature of behavioral responses and then beliefs about the need to engage in them. To add greater clarity, these steps are described in further detail below.

Step 1: Eliciting the Triggering Intrusion

The therapist begins by identifying an intrusion into consciousness that was associated with affect and/or the urge to neutralize:

> "Can you think back to the most recent time when you noticed a distressing intrusive thought or feeling? [If not: "Can you think of the last time you found yourself repeating things or having to do things in a special way?"] When was that? What was the internal event that triggered your emotion or behavior? Was it a thought, feeling, or urge?"

Step 2: Eliciting the Emotion

In the next step, as a route into exploring (often tacit) meta-appraisals of intrusions, the therapist asks about emotional responses and distress:

"When you experienced that triggering thought/feeling, what was your emotional reaction like? For example, did you feel anxious, apprehensive, guilty, or disgusted?"

Step 3: Eliciting the Appraisal of the Intrusion

Once the emotion or discomfort has been elicited, the therapist then questions the patient about the appraisal of the intrusion associated with emotion. To do this the therapist asks:

"It sounds as if having that thought/feeling meant something negative. What did it mean?" ("How much do you believe having the thought means that [insert patient's belief here]?")
"What's the worst that could happen if you continue to have that intrusion?"
"It seems as if the thought is important. What's important about it?"
"What's the worst that could happen if you continued to have the thought?"
"What does the thought say about you as a person?"
"Does the thought have any special significance or meaning?"
"Is having the thought harmful or dangerous? In what way?"
"Did any other thought enter your mind when you felt anxious?"
"Was there a sense of danger or threat?"

Step 4: Determining the Metacognitive Belief about the Intrusion

Once the appraisal has been obtained, next the therapist determines the metacognitive belief about the intrusion. This is usually a rephrasing of the appraisal to capture the overall belief about the intrusion:

"Do you believe these thoughts mean something?"
"So it sounds as if you think these intrusions are important and meaningful. In particular, you seem to implicitly believe that they [insert TEF, TAF, or TOF here]. How much do you believe that?"

Step 5: Eliciting the Nature of Rituals/Neutralizing

Next, the therapist determines the nature of overt and covert neutralizing and responses to the intrusion:

"Did you do anything to stop [negative outcome]?"
"When you thought that, what did you do to prevent [negative outcome]?"

Probe questions are useful to determine the scope of behavior. For example:

"Did you repeat things, do things in special ways, or avoid situations?"

"Did you try to control your thoughts, and if so, how did you do that?"

"How often do you engage in these responses and how much time do they take?"

Step 6: Eliciting Beliefs about Rituals and Stop Signals

Finally, the therapist determines the nature of beliefs about rituals and neutralizing responses, which is usually achieved by asking:

"What are the advantages of engaging in those responses? What's the worst that could happen if you didn't do these things?"

An important part of beliefs about rituals that contributes to their form as a plan for guiding action is the stop signal linked to them. The therapist determines the nature of the stop signal by asking:

"How do you know when to stop [e.g., checking, washing, neutralizing, repeating]?"

"How do you know it is safe to stop your ritual?"

"What is your goal in carrying out your ritual and how do you know when you have been successful?"

"Do you have a special rule that tells you how much to engage in your ritual?"

An example dialogue using these questions is presented below. The case conceptualization resulting from them is presented in Figure 8.4.

THERAPIST: When was the most recent time you were distressed by an intrusive thought or feeling?

PATIENT: This morning. I was worried about the children.

THERAPIST: What was the first distressing thought you had about them?

PATIENT: I couldn't hear them and I thought maybe I've harmed them.

THERAPIST: Was that a verbal thought or an image that you had?

PATIENT: It was a verbal thought.

THERAPIST: How did you feel emotionally when you had that thought?

PATIENT: I felt tense and scared.

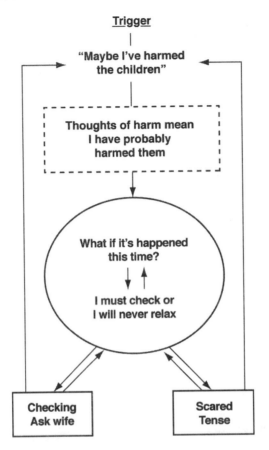

FIGURE 8.4. OCD case formulation of an obsessional ruminator.

THERAPIST: So it sounds as if having that thought meant something to you. What did it mean?

PATIENT: Well, it's a terrible thing if it happened.

THERAPIST: So did having the thought mean that it had probably happened.

PATIENT: Yes. Having the thought means it might have happened.

THERAPIST: How much do you believe having thoughts about harming your children means you have probably harmed them, on a scale of 0 to 100%.

PATIENT: Sixty percent.

THERAPIST: What worries went through your mind after you had the initial thought?

PATIENT: I thought, "What if it's happened this time?"

THERAPIST: What did you do to deal with the thought?

PATIENT: I went and checked to see if they were okay.

THERAPIST: Do you ever do anything else?

PATIENT: Yes, I ask my wife to check instead.

THERAPIST: How many times do you check?

PATIENT: I have to go back several times to make sure. It can be as many as four or five times.

THERAPIST: How do you know when to stop checking?

PATIENT: When I feel sure they are safe.

THERAPIST: How do you know they are safe?

PATIENT: I guess it's when I can walk away and not have another thought. Like sometimes I get an image of them suffocating in the pillow.

THERAPIST: What would happen if you didn't check?

PATIENT: I'd never be able to relax.

THERAPIST: It sounds like you have the belief I must check, otherwise I will never relax. Is that right?

PATIENT: Yes, I'd be overcome by anxiety.

SOCIALIZATION

After the case formulation has been derived, the next step is socialization. The aim of socialization is to introduce the idea that a central problem is not the occurrence of obsessional thoughts/doubts/feelings, but the meanings and responses that are applied to them.

At this stage it is helpful for the therapist to explain how obsessional thoughts are normally occurring phenomena and that approximately 80% of people experience them. The therapist emphasizes the idea that it is the patient's belief about these events and the way the patient relates to them that causes the problem of OCD. The therapist goes on to explain how it follows from this that changing beliefs about thoughts and feelings, and changing the way the patient relates to these inner events, can remove the problem.

The role of beliefs and behaviors leading to recurrent and frequent symptoms is explained with reference to the idiosyncratic case formulation. For example, the therapist says:

"Looking at your case formulation we can see that on this occasion you had an intrusive thought or doubt. It seems that you related to this thought in a special way. You acted as if it was true simply because you thought it. This is because you believe [e.g., 'Having a thought means something bad has happened']. If you no longer believed that your obsessional thoughts were important and meaningful, how anxious would you feel?

"So you see that what you believe about your obsessional thoughts affects the way you feel. What happens to the frequency or importance you give to your thoughts when you feel more anxious? So you see one of the vicious cycles maintaining your problem involves your beliefs about thoughts leading to anxiety, which makes danger seem more real.

"There is another vicious cycle, too. What happens when you try to get rid of the thought or stop your anxiety? Have you been successful yet? Engaging in your coping behaviors can cause problems. For example, trying not to think a thought can make the thought occur more. We can illustrate that with an experiment in a moment. There are other problems with behaviors, too. Some of them, such as checking, can reduce your confidence. Avoiding situations where thoughts might occur can set up associations so that the situation is more likely to induce the thought in the future. By checking or neutralizing, you fail to discover that these are just thoughts and you keep your belief about them alive. Each time you act as if the thought is important and meaningful. As a result, you do not develop alternative and better ways of relating to your inner experiences."

By questioning the consequences of coping behaviors the therapist helps the patient to see how aspects of his or her current response style contributes to a perpetuation of anxiety because it maintains a sense of the importance and meaningfulness of certain thoughts.

A useful question the therapist uses to illustrate the unhelpful nature of rituals and the erroneous nature of beliefs about them is: "If your rituals/behaviors are helping, why do you continue to have a problem with OCD?"

A related set of questions of value are: "How many times have you checked since you've had this problem?," "How many times has your checking revealed that your thoughts/doubts are correct?," and "Why have you not learned yet that your obsessional thoughts/doubts can simply be ignored?"

Socialization usually consists of behavioral experiments to illustrate the unhelpful effects of coping behaviors. Two useful experiments are thought suppression and thought monitoring. In the first, the patient is asked to try and suppress a thought, such as a thought of a white rabbit, to see how this is rarely completely successful.

In the thought-monitoring experiment the patient can be asked to monitor his or her thought stream for 1 minute, then to assume that a particular thought, such as the thought of a blue elephant, is harmful and it is important to monitor the stream of consciousness for such thoughts. The patient is then asked to monitor his or her thought stream again for a minute, and the therapist asks how many occurrences there were of the blue elephant. In this way it can be illustrated how monitoring for certain thoughts has the potential to increase them.

PRESENTING THE TREATMENT RATIONALE

We have seen how the therapist explains the persistence and escalation of symptoms in the context of the case formulation. The next step is to present an overview and rationale for metacognitive therapy that provides a bridge from formulation to learning to relate to obsessional thoughts in a new way.

The process of learning to relate to thoughts differently will later consist of developing DM, the modification of fusion-related metacognitive beliefs, and beliefs about the need to perform rituals. Before that, the therapist presents the overall rationale for MCT:

> "If we examine your case formulation, we can see that there are two important factors at the heart of your problem. The first concerns the implicit beliefs that you have about your intrusive thoughts, the second concerns the beliefs you have about having to act in response to them. These beliefs lead you to treat your obsessional thoughts as very important. In fact, you no longer treat these as thoughts; they have become fused with reality. If you could see them just as thoughts that had no special significance, how much of a problem would they cause you? The aim of treatment is for you to put these thoughts back into their appropriate place and see them simply as irrelevant and passing events in your mind."

ENGAGEMENT: NORMALIZING AND DESTIGMATIZING

It is important that the therapist gives his or her attention to effective engagement of the patient in the therapeutic process. Due to their content some obsessions are embarrassing and disclosure of their nature can be seen as threatening. At the outset it is useful for the therapist to decatastrophize and normalize the nature of obsessions and the disclosure of them as follows:

> "Obsessions are usually strange thoughts such as thoughts of harming children, or having sex with animals, or seeing images of a sexual or violent kind. You should not be worried about discussing the nature

of your obsessions, no matter how inappropriate they may seem to you. It is a fact that obsessional thoughts are like this, and I will not be surprised by what they are. You should know that most people have obsessional thoughts and the content of them is very broad."

DETACHED MINDFULNESS

The first step in metacognitive modification in OCD is training in DM. This helps to build the patient's skills of relating to intrusive thoughts in alternative and more adaptive ways and strengthens the metacognitive mode of processing. There are four components in OCD treatment:

Awareness

Initially, the therapist helps the patient to identify instances of obsessional thoughts. Depending on the nature of the presentation, individuals differ in their level of awareness of the initial thought, doubt, feeling, or impulse. For example, some patients do not identify a doubt (e.g., "Have I harmed someone?") as an example of an obsessional thought. To increase awareness the therapist reviews several recent episodes of neutralizing and distress and examines the specific intrusion(s) (thought or feeling) that occurred. The therapist helps the patient to identify this thought or feeling as a trigger to which DM should be applied. The patient is instructed to be aware of this trigger in the future.

Detached Mindfulness

Strategies for achieving DM are then implemented (see Chapter 5). This is first practiced with a neutral thought and then with an obsessional thought. For example, the therapist uses the free association task and introduces it in the following way:

> "I would like you to develop some experience of observing your thoughts in a detached way without the need to engage with them. We call this detached mindfulness. In a moment I'm going to slowly say a series of words and I want you to watch your thoughts without influencing them in any way. Perhaps nothing will pass through your mind, perhaps images or memories or feelings will pass through. I want you to watch the passage of events in your mind in a detached way without reacting to them in any way. Make yourself comfortable and try it with your eyes open. Let's start: tree . . . blue . . . bicycle . . . birthday . . . chocolate . . . sea . . . orange juice . . . friend. Were you able to watch your thoughts in a detached way without trying to influence them?"

The procedure may need to be refined and repeated, but when it has been successful the next step is to practice DM with an obsessional thought as follows:

> "Let's try detached mindfulness with an obsessional thought. Can you think of a thought that would cause you mild discomfort? I'm going to ask you to let your mind roam freely. Allow any thoughts to enter your mind including the obsessional thought. Don't do anything with your thoughts, just watch them in a detached way, allow your obsessional thought to enter, but remain detached from it. It may change but don't make it change, it may do nothing at all, it doesn't matter, just watch it in a detached way. See how you are the observer of your thoughts, how they are separate from you, a thought is just an event in the mind."

This step is followed by intensifying the experience of DM by attempting greater awareness of separation between the sense of self and the intrusive thought. This can be practiced first with a neutral thought and then with an obsessional thought as follows:

> "Close your eyes and have the thought of an apple. With that thought in mind, I want you to take a step back from it in your mind, but keep the thought present. It's as if you are moving away from it. Now focus on where you are in relation to the apple. Notice how you are separate from that thought: the apple is simply an event in your mind, but it is not part of you.
> "Let's now try that with an obsessional thought. Close your eyes and allow your obsessional thought to come into your mind. With that thought in mind, take a step back from it, but keep the thought present. Now focus on where you are in relation to the thought. Notice how your sense of self is separate from the thought. The obsession is simply an event in your mind, it is not an important part of you."

The application of DM is often more intensive in treating OCD than the other disorders presented in this book. Time is devoted to practicing DM to intrusions across several sessions.

Exposure and Response Commission

The next step consists of helping the patient to see how he or she normally reacts to obsessional thoughts with overt and covert rituals that are aimed at getting rid of thoughts or minimizing threat. However, these rituals simply give thoughts importance and fix the patient in the object mode. The therapist suggests that instead of getting rid of thoughts, one way to obtain distance from them and discover that they are unimportant events in the mind is to continue with rituals but to maintain the intrusion throughout. This technique is called exposure and response commission (ERC).

The therapist introduces the idea of actively engaging in rituals while maintaining intrusive thoughts. This can be done by visualizing the thought if it is an image or repeating it subvocally if it is verbal. For example, a patient with thoughts of the devil would perform a ritual of saying a prayer while cleaning the house. She was asked to constantly keep in mind the thought of the devil all the time she was saying the prayer. Similarly, a patient with contamination fears would wash and dry his hands repeatedly until he was able to wash and dry without having thoughts about contamination. He was asked to repeat continuously and covertly the thought "I'm contaminated with bacteria" for the duration of any washing.

In ERC the patient is allowed to perform rituals, but the goals of engaging rituals are modified. Rather than using his or her rituals to get rid of thoughts or to minimize danger, the patient should only use rituals in conjunction with maintaining awareness of his or her obsessional thoughts. In effect, the rules are changed so that the obsessional thought must be held in consciousness throughout performance of the ritual. This activity facilitates detachment from the thought and strengthening of meta-level experiencing of the intrusion.

Metacognitively Delivered Exposure and Ritual Prevention

Exposure and ritual prevention (ERP) is a traditional cognitive-behavioral treatment approach in OCD. It usually involves extensive exposure to feared stimuli or thoughts and the prevention of any rituals as a means of promoting habituation. In contrast, we saw above how in MCT rituals can be permitted and used to therapeutic advantage. However, ERP is also used in MCT but is presented in two ways: as a means of reducing the CAS that underlies the patient's overestimation of threat and as a behavioral experiment to challenge metacognitive beliefs in the domains of TEF, TAF, and TOF. Thus, exposure does not need to be prolonged or as extensive as that traditionally used in cognitive-behavioral approaches.

Reacting to alter threat or to dismiss thoughts with neutralizing responses is part of the CAS and prevents challenging of beliefs about the significance of thoughts. Therefore, such responses should be brought under control. This is done by the postponement or banning of any neutralizing or conceptual processing (i.e., worry/rumination) in the context of a behavioral experiment.

The therapist should undertake a detailed exploration of both overt and covert responses. Then the therapist suggests that the patient postpones all of these responses following the occurrence of the obsession and applies DM instead. Neutralizing responses should be postponed for as long as possible (a graded approach can be used to facilitate compliance where necessary), preferably until a set 10-minute period at the end of each day, which is designated as the ritual period. The therapist should emphasize that using the ritual period is not compulsory and that often patients do not use it.

Ritual prevention can be viewed as removing the CAS in MCT since rituals constitute maladaptive coping behaviors. In MCT prevention is extended to examining the patient's use of conceptual processes and threat monitoring, which are also banned. The removal of the CAS is a means of reducing the patient's overestimation of threat. For example, a patient with fears that she was contaminated with germs around her bottom did not allow her husband to touch that area of her body, washed excessively after visiting the toilet, and wiped all handles and faucets that she might have touched. The therapist discovered that the obsessional thought triggering her avoidance and cleaning behavior was "My bottom has harmful germs on it." The therapist and the patient discussed how this was likely to be a fact that many people might believe, but it is not a thought that promotes intense anxiety for most. The therapist asked the patient how she responded to the thought to give it such importance. The patient explained how she always attended to it and tried to analyze if she might have spread contamination (note that this is a worry/rumination response and is part of the CAS). This led to a discussion of whether analyzing and thinking about possible contamination resulted in a realistic or an exaggerated sense of threat. The patient realized that the process of washing, avoidance, and analyzing in response to her thought of contamination had caused her to attach a greater amount of threat to the situation. In order to prove that there was little or no threat, the therapist asked her to reduce her hand washing, ban wiping handles and faucets, and stop analyzing whether she might have spread contamination in response to intrusions. This was specifically operationalized as a test to see if refraining from these responses gave rise to sickness in the family over a 3-day period. If it didn't, then she could disregard her intrusive thought.

When ERP is used as a behavioral experiment the patient is asked to make a prediction based on metacognitive beliefs about thoughts and to test this prediction by having obsessional thoughts and refraining from enacting neutralizing responses. For example, a patient was concerned about having thoughts of a homosexual nature because she believed that these thoughts would transform her into a lesbian (TEF). To prevent this transformation she would normally respond to "lesbian thoughts" by imagining kissing her boyfriend and trying to hold onto a clear image of her and him kissing. The therapist worked with the patient to operationalize an experiment where, in response to lesbian thoughts, the patient tried to maintain an image of kissing a woman to see if this made her boyfriend seem less attractive to her.

INCREASING COMPLIANCE WITH ERP AND ERC

Giving up or postponing rituals is equivalent to removing a safety harness for most patients. Thus, it is not uncommon for relinquishing rituals to be met with resistance. Resistance can be minimized by presenting a clear rationale for these strategies that is based on an explanation of how existing behaviors give unnecessary importance to thoughts and imbue them with special significance. Initially, the therapist should aim to deal with resistance by revisiting the formulation and discussing the role of behaviors in problem maintenance.

Next, the therapist may find it helpful to run an advantages–disadvantages analysis of changing rituals. Commonly used advantages and disadvantages are presented in Table 8.2 to facilitate thinking about this process.

Patient compliance with homework is facilitated when he or she practices the desired behavior in the treatment session. This can be achieved by asking the patient to have an obsessional thought and to actively engage in ritualizing while the thought remains in consciousness (ERC). This step can be followed by a second one: the patient allows a thought to occur and postpones the neutralizing response to a designated 3-minute ritual period whose start and finish is signaled by the therapist.

The idea of deliberately evoking an obsessional thought can be met with anxiety and resistance, in which case the therapist should emphasize

TABLE 8.2. Advantages and Disadvantages of Changing Ritual Behavior in OCD

"What are the disadvantages of changing my rituals?"	"What are the advantages of changing my rituals?"
"It is difficult to accomplish change."	"I can discover if it really is difficult and make it easier."
"It will cause me distress."	"I will discover that the distress is only temporary."
"It could harm someone if I didn't perform them."	"I will discover that my beliefs about harm are untrue."
"I will never get rid of the thoughts."	"I will discover that I don't need to push thoughts away and they are not permanently distressing."
"Something bad will happen."	"I will discover that nothing happens and all thoughts are safe."
"I will become someone I don't want to be."	"I will discover that thoughts do not have the power to change me as a person."
	Outcome = ("Why I should change my rituals"):
	"My fear associated with thoughts is removed."

the rationale of "learning to relate to thoughts as benign events rather than things of immense significance." In a few cases some verbal challenging of beliefs about the significance and importance of thoughts is required (see next section) before returning to implementing the strategies described above.

CHALLENGING SPECIFIC METACOGNITIVE BELIEFS ABOUT THOUGHTS

Once the patient has successfully experienced obsessional thoughts in a way characterized by DM, treatment continues with modifying beliefs about the importance and power of thoughts. Thus, the focus of treatment moves from emphasizing metacognitive experiencing to modification of metacognitive appraisals and knowledge.

It is normally recommended that only two or three sessions focus on DM, since DM is simply a prerequisite for the belief modification that follows. It is important that DM does not become a neutralizing behavior (new ritual). The next stage focuses on beliefs concerning TEF, TAF, and TOF. Initially, verbal reattribution methods are used. These are followed with behavioral experiments.

Verbal Methods: Isolating and Verbalizing the Belief

It is useful for the therapist to consider that beliefs concerning obsessional thoughts are often implicit and may never have been articulated by patients. A common generic implicit belief is that intrusions are important and powerful in some way. The therapist should work with the patient to formulate the belief in a shorthand form. It can be explored by asking questions such as:

"Does thinking it make it so?"
"Are all thoughts about X meaningful?"
"Are thoughts about contamination always accurate?"
"Are all thoughts about X important?"

This analysis is augmented by examining the patient's responses on the OCD-S or the TFI, which provide an indication of important metacognitive beliefs.

Verbal Methods: TEF, TAF, and TOF

Strategies for challenging fusion metacognitions include the standard techniques of questioning the evidence for them, asking about the mechanism underlying fusion effects, and searching for counterevidence. Some examples to assist therapists are as follow:

> "What is the evidence that thoughts have the power to cause events?"
> "What is the evidence that your obsessional thought usually means something bad has happened?"
> "How many times have you checked to see if your thought was true, and what can that tell you about the significance of your obsession?"
> "How can a thought or a feeling be transferred to an inanimate object?"
> "How do only some of your thoughts have special power and not all of them?"
> "Is there any counterevidence you can think of that suggests thoughts alone do not have special power or significance?"
> "Have you ever had a thought and not been able to neutralize it? What happened, and what does that tell you about these thoughts?"

A further strategy is to induce dissonance or conflict in the patient's belief systems. This is done by searching for the presence of beliefs that when highlighted will conflict with beliefs about the power and meaning of obsessional thoughts.

> For example, a patient was asked how it was that his obsessional thoughts about harm occurring to his family had the power to cause such events. He stated that somehow God would punish him for thinking the thought. The therapist asked if he believed that God was all knowing, to which the patient replied he believed that God was. The therapist then asked how he could reconcile the belief that God is all knowing with the idea that God would not know that the patient's thoughts were merely obsessions. The therapist added further dissonance by pointing out that it appeared that the patient had the power to control God's behavior just by the power of his own thoughts.

Dissonance can also be activated between the patient's general self-beliefs and his or her metacognitive belief. This technique aims to show how the belief about the obsession is inconsistent with what the patient knows about him- or herself. The following dialogue illustrates this technique:

THERAPIST: What are you afraid will happen if you think of harming your daughter?

PATIENT: I'm worried that I may do something bad.

THERAPIST: What's the worst that could happen if you have the thought?

PATIENT: I'm scared that I will actually pick up a knife and slit her breasts.

THERAPIST: Let's look at the belief that you will act on the thought. What kind of person would you say you are generally? Are you a violent person?

PATIENT: No, I hate violence.

THERAPIST: Are you a person that really wants to harm his daughter?

PATIENT: No, not at all, that's the problem.

THERAPIST: Is it a problem that you don't want to harm her?

PATIENT: No, the problem is that I'm not like that but I can't help thinking it.

THERAPIST: What sort of person would harm his daughter in this way?

PATIENT: A madman who enjoyed hurting people.

THERAPIST: Is that the sort of person you are?

PATIENT: No, I'm not at all like that.

THERAPIST: So it sounds as if you know that you won't act on the thought because it isn't the kind of person you truly are. What would you say to that?

PATIENT: If I think about it in that way, then I know it's just a bad thought, but I still don't want it.

THERAPIST: Perhaps wanting it or not doesn't matter. You must begin to see it as simply a thought that has no real significance for you.

BEHAVIORAL EXPERIMENTS

Thought–Event Fusion

There are two subtypes of TEF, a prospective and a retrospective type. In the prospective type the patient believes that thinking a thought will cause a bad event to happen in the future (e.g., "If I think an accident will happen, then it will make it happen"). In the retrospective type the person believes that the occurrence of a thought means an event must have happened in the past (e.g., "If I think I've committed a murder, then I probably have committed it"; "If I think the floor is contaminated with feces, then it must be contaminated").

Prospective TEF can be challenged with behavioral experiments. When the threat is in the future, it is possible to manipulate the intrusion and observe any subsequent consequences. This can only be achieved when the time course of the catastrophe is within a testable period—for example, 1 or 2 weeks. When patients maintain that the negative event could happen at any time in the distant future, this can be an avoidance strategy. The therapist should deal with this avoidance by questioning the evidence to support the idea that the catastrophe would be delayed rather than more immediate and then proceed in running the experiment anyway. One strategy is to consider manipulating the content of the thought such that it contains direct reference to the event occurring within the next few days or on a specific planned day (e.g., "What are your plans for this Saturday? Let's see if we can think about your partner having an accident on that day").

To facilitate compliance with TEF experiments it is often beneficial to first introduce the idea of causing positive events through the power of thought. The therapist can ask the patient to try and win the lottery jackpot by thinking about it happening, or in a slightly more negative realm, try to make the therapist's car break down by imagining such an event.

When TEF is retrospective the therapist normally questions the evidence, reviews counterevidence, and elicits dissonance (e.g., "Is having a thought good evidence you have done something or would having a memory of doing it be better evidence? Are you the kind of person who would do such a thing?).

An experimental approach to dealing with retrospective TEF involves the use of "adaptive checking."

Adaptive Checking (ERC Revisited)

Checking behavior is considered to be maladaptive in cognitive-behavioral treatments of OCD. Thus, it is a behavior that is usually prevented. However, the metacognitive approach suggests that checking can be used to change metacognitive beliefs and facilitate detachment from obsessional thoughts. The way to use checking adaptively is to change the goals of checking behavior such that the goal becomes collecting data to evaluate the validity of metacognitive beliefs. More specifically, when there are retrospective fusion beliefs (e.g., "Thinking I've killed someone means that I have killed them"), checking can be used to collect data that unambiguously shows that "Thinking I've killed someone is simply an irrelevant thought."

When the threat is retrospective, the patient is encouraged to engage in checking behaviors that can provide evidence that the event has not occurred, and thus that the thought is only an event in the mind. Typically, the patient engages in checking strategies and does so with the intention of easing his or her worry and distress. By changing the explicit goal of checking, and if necessary, modifying the behavior itself so that it is appropriate for gathering evidence, it can be used to challenge meta-beliefs about the importance of intrusive thoughts.

Thought–Action Fusion

TAF beliefs concern the power of thoughts to cause the individual to perform unwanted actions. Behavioral experiments intended to modify these beliefs rely on evoking unwanted thoughts in the context of exposure to anxiety-provoking situations. The anxiety-provoking situation is one in which there is elevated subjective risk of performing the unwanted act.

A case example will serve to illustrate this process:

> A 28-year-old woman was concerned that she would stab someone with a knife, so she would check that all the knives were locked away in the kitchen before answering the door and before her children came home from school. For this patient, a mental image (obsessional thought) of stabbing someone activated the belief "Thinking this will make me do it." But this belief was only activated if she had access to knives. The therapist began the behavioral experiment by asking the patient to have the stabbing thought while holding a pen to see if this led her to stab the therapist. Next, the therapist asked her to use the "pen and thought" technique at home. The next week the therapist introduced a knife in the session and asked the patient to have the thought of stabbing the therapist while looking at the knife on the desk. For homework, she was asked to leave a knife on the kitchen worktop and to deliberately have set periods of thinking about stabbing her partner when he was home. In this way her belief that a thought would make her perform an unwanted act was effectively challenged.

> In a similar way a different patient was concerned that having thoughts of a naked child would cause him to molest children. So he avoided driving past schools or having any contact with children. After initially weakening this belief through verbal methods (questioning the evidence, inducing dissonance, questioning the mechanism), the therapist asked the patient to run an experiment. This consisted of driving past a local school while having the thought of a naked child.

Warning: It is important that there should be no doubt about actual risk. Thoughts should be clearly ego-dystonic and the behaviors are considered by the patient to be abhorrent, with no desire to act them out. These experiments should not be conducted if there is any doubt about the client's true motivations or risk.

Thought–Object Fusion

TOF is the belief that thoughts and feelings can be transferred to objects and places, meaning that it would be difficult to escape from them in the future, or that the connection of thought and object imbues thoughts with some greater influence or reality. In these cases behavioral experiments often focus on challenging predictions in the following areas: (1) that thoughts and feelings can be transferred into objects, (2) that under such circumstances thoughts and feelings will never end, (3) that such a process will lead to specific negative events.

To challenge the belief that thoughts/feelings can be transferred into objects, the therapist can ask the patient to guess the history of objects, such as who owned them and where they came from. It is useful to keep a collection of objects in the office such as old books, old pens, and so on, along with a description of their background and pictures of their previous owners. Patients can then be asked to describe the history of an object simply from touching the object, and the discrepancy between the true history and the patient's story can be demonstrated.

In one type of experiment the patient is asked to deliberately contaminate a blank card by placing a hand on the back of it while having obsessional thoughts. The card is marked on its unseen side with a small cross, and is returned to a stack of 50 identical unmarked cards. Finally, the patient is asked to close his or her eyes and try to identify the contaminated card by holding each one in turn.

In some instances it is appropriate for the therapist to conduct an experiment consisting of asking the patient to bring some contaminated objects to the treatment session along with some objects that are not contaminated. The challenge is for the patient to identify the contaminated objects reliably without being able to see them. For example, a patient concerned that her clothes were contaminated with a feeling of being "impure" was asked to bring to the session one sock that was contaminated and another one that was not. The therapist asked her to stand with her arms stretched out behind her back and systematically touched the back of her right hand with the unaffected sock. The patient was asked to state when she could "feel" the impure sock. On only one occasion was the "impure" sock used. The exercise was videotaped. After reviewing the videotape, the patient could see that she was unable to accurately detect when the "impure" sock was used. These results were discussed as evidence that clothing could not be contaminated and that the sense of contamination was simply a feeling of anxiety that the patient had when she had the obsessional thought "It's contaminated."

Challenging the belief that thoughts/feelings will never end so long as the patient has contact with the contaminated object is approached in several ways. One technique is to contaminate as many objects as possible with thoughts and feelings so that the patient can test what happens to the chronicity of emotional responses. Contrary to predictions, thoughts and feelings fade rather than become more consistent. This finding is inconsistent with the belief that thoughts and feelings can be transferred into objects since contaminating more objects eventually results in a decrease rather than a predicted increase in distressing thoughts and feelings.

The belief that fusing thoughts with objects will lead to negative outcomes can be tested by actively having "dangerous" thoughts or emotions while holding or being in contact with objects, and then waiting to see if catastrophes occur. For this approach to be successful it is important to operationalize the feared catastrophe in specific observable terms. For example, a patient believed that if she had blasphemous thoughts while reading her Bible then the Bible would become impure and this would lead anyone who touched the book to be harmed. The therapist worked with her to define the nature and time course of the catastrophe. It was decided that it would be possible to cause a negative outcome within a week by asking her daughter to touch the Bible after the patient had read it and had a blasphemous thought. This prediction was then tested.

CONTAMINATION FEARS: A SPECIAL CASE?

A question often asked by therapists learning MCT is how the metacognitive model deals with contamination-related OCD. Practitioners have some difficulty immediately understanding how the model fits this subtype. However, this subtype is not a special case for which the model requires modification. A question to ask patients is simply: "Is your problem that things are contaminated or is your problem that you keep thinking that they are?"

More specifically, the problem is conceptualized in terms of the implicit metacognitive beliefs that are held about the significance of the contamination-related thought or need to worry in this way. Typically, such thoughts are significant in two ways: "I think it, therefore it must be so" (TEF) and/or "I need to think it's contaminated in order to remain vigilant and safe" (that is, this is a worry process). The following dialogue illustrates this line of questioning:

THERAPIST: You repeatedly have the thought that public seating is contaminated with saliva or bodily fluids, is that right?

PATIENT: If I see a stain or it doesn't look clean, then I think that could be bodily fluids.

THERAPIST: So is your problem that seating is contaminated in that way or is your problem that you keep thinking that it could be?

PATIENT: Well, I keep thinking it, but it could be contaminated, so both, I suppose.

THERAPIST: Was there a time you didn't think like that?

PATIENT: Yes, I didn't always avoid things or wash my clothes so much. I used to act like anyone else.

THERAPIST: So what has changed? Is there more bodily fluid around these days or has your thinking changed?

PATIENT: (*Laughs*) No, it's obviously what I'm thinking about.

THERAPIST: It sounds to me, then, that the problem is what you believe about these thoughts about contamination. Have you been treating them just as thoughts or have you been treating them as facts?

PATIENT: I've been treating them as real, but it would be dangerous to ignore them.

THERAPIST: If they are nothing more than thoughts, how could ignoring them be dangerous?

PATIENT: Because I could contaminate my family if I pick up some disease.

THERAPIST: Are you treating them just as thoughts right now, or are you defending them as real?

PATIENT: I'm seeing them as real again, aren't I?

THERAPIST: Yes, that's a useful discovery you've just made. You seem to have the implicit belief that these thoughts about contamination are important and that you must act on them. I wonder, do you ever deliberately have these thoughts? I mean, question if something is contaminated?

PATIENT: Yes, that's part of the problem. I go around asking myself, "Is it or isn't it contaminated?" That's something you don't want to get into because then everything gets worse.

THERAPIST: So you believe that having the thought probably means it is so, but also you actively question if things are contaminated, which means you have the thought in order to be safe. That sounds to me like you have a real problem with your thinking. How can you ignore these thoughts if thinking them means it is contaminated and you must continue to think it to be safe?

PATIENT: By washing and throwing my clothes away.

THERAPIST: Has that stopped you thinking this way yet?

PATIENT: No.

THERAPIST: So we need to change how you think. What about having thoughts about bodily fluids and looking at them just as thoughts in your mind, rather than something that you must act on. Also, what about banning your questioning of whether something is or isn't contaminated?

This example illustrates how the patient's problem is with implicit beliefs about thoughts and the need to have particular thoughts as part of a safety strategy. It is apparent that the problem is one of metacognitions about thinking and not a problem with the concept of harm resulting from contamination. However, the patient's awareness of the nature of the problem is often firmly anchored in the object level of processing. The challenge is to shift the individual to the metacognitive level.

The Magical Spray

Contamination fears have been treated traditionally through exposure to contaminants coupled with ritual prevention. Exposure approaches have been quite ingenious including the making of magical contaminated sprays that facilitate wide-ranging and difficult-to-neutralize contamination of the environment. For example, faced with a fear of contamination from germs, the therapist can dab a piece of paper against a toilet bowl and then dip it into a spray bottle containing clean water, thereby producing a "contaminated" solution. The therapist or patient can then lightly spray the solution onto clothing, around the office or the house, and even onto his or her hair. This facilitates exposure to feared contamination and makes complete cleaning difficult, thus facilitating response prevention.

The metacognitive application of this exposure exercise is one in which it is used as an experiment to (1) challenge beliefs about the permanence of thoughts and feelings and/or (2) to shift patients to a metacognitive level of processing. When used in the former case, the therapist asks the patient to spread contamination widely in order to discover what happens to worries, doubts, and anxiety when this is done. The experiment can be configured where appropriate to test specific beliefs about losing control of emotions or being paralyzed with worry.

When the experiment is used to shift to meta-level processing, the therapist asks the patient to use the spray as a means of testing whether the problem is thoughts about contamination or a problem with actual contamination. For example, the therapist says: "You need to be sure that the problem is simply what you believe about having a thought rather than a problem of dangerous contamination. To do this I want you to spray this contaminant everywhere in order to find out if there is a true danger or if it is just a matter of thinking there is."

MODIFYING BELIEFS ABOUT RITUALS

Beliefs about rituals should be examined and challenged during the course of MCT. This is normally done after initial work on beliefs about intrusions, but may be required earlier to increase engagement with behavioral experiments requiring ritual prevention.

The Rationale

The therapist normally begins by reminding the patient of the unhelpful role that rituals play as depicted in the case formulation. The therapist then proceeds to a Socratic dialogue aimed to expand the patient's awareness of the unhelpful consequences of rituals, as follows:

THERAPIST: In the case formulation we can see how the use of rituals is linked to obsessional thoughts and to negative beliefs about your thoughts. Do you remember what happened a few sessions ago when I asked you to suppress the thought of a white rabbit?

PATIENT: Yes, I found it hard to do.

THERAPIST: That's right, which shows that engaging in some rituals, such as trying to control your mind or prevent thoughts, doesn't work and can sometimes backfire. There is another problem with your rituals too. If you constantly do something to counteract the power of a certain thought, does that allow you to discover that the thought is unimportant?

PATIENT: No, I suppose not.

THERAPIST: Can you discover that nothing bad really happens if you believe you have saved the situation with your ritual?

PATIENT: Well, I'm sure I'd feel worse if I did nothing.

THERAPIST: So do you believe that your rituals are helpful?

PATIENT: Yes, they can be.

THERAPIST: How long have you been using them?

PATIENT: A long time, for about 5 years.

THERAPIST: So why haven't they worked yet? Why do you still have OCD?

PATIENT: Well, I can see that they work in the short term, but maybe they don't work completely.

THERAPIST: That's right, you believe they remove immediate danger, but that prevents you from discovering that your thoughts or emotions are not dangerous or meaningful anyway. What do you believe would happen if you abandoned your rituals?

PATIENT: I'd become a bad person. My thoughts would change my personality.

THERAPIST: So you believe that the rituals stop you from becoming a bad person?

PATIENT: I don't know, maybe.

THERAPIST: Looking at the evidence we've just discussed, how much do you believe that your rituals help you?

PATIENT: I'm not sure.

THERAPIST: How much do you think they could contribute to your OCD?

PATIENT: Well, I'm sure they are a problem.

THERAPIST: What would happen if you abandoned your rituals?

PATIENT: I'm not prepared to do that. It will become a mess in my mind.

THERAPIST: It sounds risky right now. So first let's look at the advantages and disadvantages of using your rituals.

Advantages–Disadvantages Analysis

Reviewing the advantages–disadvantages of rituals offers a means of raising awareness of the problems caused by these behaviors. The therapist aims to reinforce awareness of a range of disadvantages and to challenge the validity of the advantages to motivate change. The following questions are used to elicit disadvantages:

1. "Can you think of any problems caused by your rituals?"
2. "Have your rituals enabled you to overcome your OCD?"
3. "How might your rituals keep your OCD going?"
4. "What negative effect are your rituals having on your environment?"
5. "What are the negative effects of your rituals on you?"
6. "Can you discover the truth about thoughts and emotions so long as you avoid them by using your rituals?"
7. "What's the worst that can happen if you continue with your rituals?"
8. "Even if your rituals reduce distress in the short term, do they reduce it in the long term?"
9. "Can your rituals stop you seeing the situation realistically?"
10. "How do your rituals affect the quality of your life?"

Reframing Advantages

To elicit the advantages of rituals, the following questions are normally used in conjunction with an appropriate "reframe" question in which the therapist challenges the validity of the appraised advantage:

1. "What are the advantages of performing your rituals?"
   (Reframe: Is this a short-term or a long-term solution?)
2. "In what other ways do your rituals help you?"
   (Reframe: How might they keep your problem going?)
3. "Can you think of anything positive about your rituals?"
   (Reframe: Is there some other way you could achieve that?)

4. "Do you believe your rituals prevent harm?"
   (Reframe: Have you tested if the harm is real or imagined?)
5. "Do you believe your rituals stop you from losing control?"
   (Reframe: Was there a time you couldn't perform them? What happened?)
6. "Do your rituals give you peace of mind?"
   (Reframe: If your rituals work, you should be free of worry in the long term. Is that the case?)

BEHAVIORAL EXPERIMENTS AND BELIEFS ABOUT RITUALS

Experimental strategies provide a means of modifying strongly held beliefs about the need to perform rituals, and they strengthen alternative strategies for relating to intrusions. These experiments are designed principally to test predictions concerning the consequences of not performing rituals.

Patients often believe that if they do not perform their rituals, then this will lead to exposure of self or others to (unrealistic) threat, the experience of unremitting emotions or worry, and an inability to function properly. For example, failure to wash one's hands for 5 minutes in hot water will lead to contaminating the children with poison. Not aligning objects so that they point toward the hospital will lead to overwhelming and unending worry about the health of the family. Failure to control one's mind will result in mental chaos and an inability to perform one's job.

In each of these examples, the therapist aims to expose the patient to the situation that triggers distress and the urge to engage in the ritual. The therapist determines the obsessional thought or feeling that triggers the urge, and then asks the patient to refrain from the ritual. Exposure and response prevention experiments (discussed earlier) can challenge beliefs about obsessions and at the same time beliefs about the need to perform rituals. However, beliefs about rituals can exist as separate packets of knowledge that are distinct from beliefs about obsessional thoughts and feelings. For example, one patient believed that having thoughts of a homosexual nature could make her become a lesbian. She neutralized these thoughts by replacing them with images of her boyfriend. While her metacognitive belief about the power of the thought to change her sexual preferences was effectively challenged during MCT, she reported that she had a more general and pervasive tendency to classify her thoughts as good or bad in order to "keep her mind pure and uncluttered." She predicted that if she failed to do this it would spoil her activities and she would not enjoy them in the future. This tendency predated her preoccupation with sexual thoughts, and appeared to exist as a separate set of beliefs about mental rituals (strategies). Treatment focused on getting her to ban the strategy of classifying her thoughts. The therapist asked her to induce a cluttered mind while engaging in pleasurable activities such as reading and watching television. In this way the patient discovered that she could enjoy activities even if she did not classify her thoughts.

NEW PLANS FOR PROCESSING: STOP SIGNALS AND CRITERIA FOR KNOWING

The metacognitive model proposes that patients use inappropriate internal criteria to guide behavior and appraisals. Rituals in OCD are performed until specific internal criteria are achieved.

> A 56-year-old patient was repeatedly concerned with the thought that he might have engaged in sexual relations with his boss. In order to put his mind at rest and prevent the need to resign from work, he would review his entire memory of the office party to ensure that it was clear and there were no memory gaps. If there was a gap, he interpreted this as the time at which he could have had sex.
>
> In this instance the memory-check routine was the patient's preemptive strategy for dealing with doubts and possible worry by trying to know that he had not engaged in a particular behavior. The therapist worked with scripting a new set of strategies that involved a ban of memory checking, deciding on appropriate criteria for knowing if the event had occurred (remembering the incident rather than an absence of memory), and applying detached mindfulness to doubts or intrusions.

Aside from dysfunctional memory criteria, some individuals use attentional strategies as part of their plan for reducing or minimizing threat. For example, they monitor for signs of dirt or contamination (e.g., stains on seats) or for certain mental events. These strategies backfire because they lead to enhanced detection of the stimulus, leading to a greater sense of threat and an escalating urge to neutralize and perform rituals. The metacognitive perspective draws attention to the necessity of modifying attentional priorities in anxiety-provoking situations in order to rewrite habitual processing plans.

> For example, a 40-year-old male patient would check in the mirror to see if he looked like a particular rapist he had seen in the news. This patient was troubled by intrusive images of the rapist's face and he believed that having the thought meant he might begin to take on the rapist's features. His old plan for processing was to check his reflection but to do so quickly and with a fleeting glance because he must do so without having the obsessive thought. The therapist discovered that

when the patient looked in the mirror he was not so much processing his own reflection as he was processing the presence or absence of the image of the rapist. The new plan consisted of looking full-on into the mirror and seeing his whole reflection while allowing himself to have the thought. He was instructed to "look through" the thought at the outside image (see "Metacognitive Guidance," Chapter 5).

Another observed form of dysfunctional monitoring is paying too much attention to or expending great mental effort in performing an action, in an attempt to be sure that it has been completed and/or as an attempt to obviate all doubts/intrusions.

For example, a patient explained how he would check that he had closed all doors and windows by trying to get a "standing solid" feel for the action. In this way he could be certain that he had performed the action properly. The therapist worked with him in developing an alternative plan that consisted of "seeing that" rather than "feeling that" he had closed the doors and windows, banning checking, and applying detached mindfulness to any subsequent doubts. Later the therapist used ERC, in which the patient was asked to check the door and windows while constantly doubting that he had done it properly.

In each of these examples patients and therapist develop an alternative plan or script for attention, behavior, and processing of intrusions/doubts, which should be practiced in place of the original plan. An example of an old plan and a new plan is given below:

Old (OCD) Plan

- "I focus entirely on locking the car door and try to remember the feel of it."
- "I try to remember the feel of it as I walk away."
- "If I cannot remember the feel vividly I interpret this as meaning I haven't done it properly."
- "I go back and check, and try to create the feel of it."

New Plan

- "I focus momentary attention on seeing that I am locking the door."
- "I ban trying to remember if I have done it as I walk away."
- "I tolerate any doubts and tell myself they are only thoughts, not facts."
- "I apply detached mindfulness to any remaining thoughts."

RELAPSE PREVENTION

In the final two sessions of treatment, work on the therapy blueprint commences. The blueprint consists of an example of the case formulation, a list of the patient's metacognitive beliefs about intrusions, and a summary of evidence challenging them that has been obtained through verbal and behavioral methods. The blueprint consists of summary statements concerning the disadvantages of performing rituals and a detailed exposition of the old and new plan for processing/behavior.

The therapist checks for residual fusion beliefs and the presence of rituals/avoidance as markers for remaining dysfunctional beliefs or plans that require further modification. The OCD-S is normally used as a guide to these factors.

OCD TREATMENT PLAN

An overall 10-session treatment plan for implementing MCT in OCD is presented in Appendix 17. This is intended as a guide to the structure and content of treatment and should be applied flexibly as individual circumstances require. The plan should be implemented with direct reference to the strategies described in this chapter.

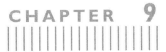
Major Depressive Disorder

The metacognitive model and treatment of major depressive disorder (MDD) is focused on understanding the causes of rumination and then removing this unhelpful process. Rumination is a key feature of the CAS activated in response to negative thoughts, sadness, and loss experiences. The CAS prolongs sadness and negative beliefs, leading to depressive episodes.

MDD is characterized by one or more major depressive episodes. A major depressive episode is defined in DSM-IV (American Psychiatric Association, 1994) as "a period of at least two weeks during which there is either depressed mood or the loss of interest or pleasure in nearly all activities" (p. 320). In addition, there must be at least four further symptoms from a list including changes in appetite or weight, insomnia or hypersomnia nearly every day, restlessness or being slowed down that can be observed by others, fatigue or loss of energy, feeling worthless or excessive guilt, diminished ability to think or indecisiveness, recurrent thoughts of death, or suicidality. Symptoms must persist for most of the day, nearly every day for at least 2 consecutive weeks. The DSM-IV-TR (American Psychiatric Association, 2000) criteria for a major depressive episode are summarized in Table 9.1.

If untreated, major depressive episodes (MDE) typically last 6 months or longer. In most cases there is complete remission, but in approximately 20–30% of cases some symptoms insufficient to meet full MDD criteria remain for months or even years. Individuals may experience repeated depressive episodes during their lifetimes. Some episodes can become unremitting; they are classified as chronic when criteria for MDE has been met for at least the past 2 years.

TABLE 9.1. Diagnostic Criteria for MDE

Criterion A

At least 5 of the following symptoms present for the same 2-week period, most of the day, nearly every day (that must include 1 or 2):

1. Depressed mood

2. Diminished interest or pleasure in most activities / weight loss or gain / insomnia or hypersomnia / agitation or retardation / fatigue or loss of energy / worthlessness or guilt / difficulty thinking / recurring thoughts of death or suicide

Criterion B

Criteria for a mixed manic and depressive episode are not met.

Criterion C

Symptoms cause significant distress or impairment.

Criterion D

Symptoms not due to substance.

Criterion E

Symptoms not better accounted for by bereavement.

Note. Summarized from American Psychiatric Association (2000).

RUMINATION AND DEPRESSIVE THINKING

Rumination is a central feature of the CAS in depression. It has been defined in a variety of ways, but broadly speaking it refers to difficult-to-control repetitive thoughts about personal problems. Nolen-Hoeksema (1991), in her response styles theory of depression, views rumination as repetitive and passive thinking about symptoms of depression and the possible causes and consequences of those symptoms. According to the theory, rumination consists of "repetitively focusing on the fact that one is depressed; on one's symptoms of depression; and on the causes, meanings, and consequences of depressive symptoms" (Nolen-Hoeksema, 1991, p. 569).

Martin and Tesser (1989, 1996) use the term "rumination" more broadly to refer to any class of thought that has a tendency to recur. They suggest that "rumination is a class of conscious thoughts that revolve around a common instrumental theme and that recur in the absence of immediate environmental demands requiring the thoughts" (1996, p. 7).

In summary, rumination has been defined in different ways as a broad class of repetitive thoughts linked primarily with depression (e.g., Papageorgiou & Wells, 2004). The theoretical account of disorder offered by the metacognitive approach (Wells & Matthews, 1994) views both rumination and worry as voluntary and active coping strategies consisting of repetitive thoughts aimed at dealing with emotion and threatening events. *Rumination* can be seen as mental processing aimed at understanding the reasons for sadness and working out ways of dealing with disturbing thoughts and feelings. In contrast, *worry* is directed at anticipating danger and planning ways to avoid or deal with it. Rumination seeks answers to questions such as "Why do I feel this way?," "What does this mean about me?," and "How can I feel better?" In comparison, worry seeks answers to questions such as "What should I do in the future?," "How can I avoid danger?," and "How can I be prepared?"

According to the metacognitive model, both types of thinking are strategies aimed at self-regulation triggered by internal events such as negative thoughts and emotions. For instance, worry is usually triggered by danger-related thoughts such as "What if I get attacked?," while rumination is typically triggered by thoughts such as "No one likes me." An important distinction is made between negative automatic thoughts and the worry or ruminative response that follows them. In MCT, negative automatic thoughts, which are deemed particularly important in traditional CBT, are seen merely as triggers for dysfunctional processing styles (e.g., rumination) that are the greater cause of pathology and the focus of treatment.

Although there are overlaps between worry and rumination, there are some differences, as exemplified by the types of questions each process attempts to address. Rumination appears to be more past-oriented, while worry is more future-oriented. Worry concerns avoiding or preventing danger, while rumination appears to be concerned more with establishing understanding and meaning. Both appear to be associated with avoidance of negative experiences.

Empirical evidence supports the overlap. Measures of rumination and worry are correlated, with overlaps of 16–21% (e.g., Segerstrom, Tsao, Alden, & Craske, 2000). In an exploration of the similarities and differences of worry and rumination, Papageorgiou and Wells (1999a, 1999b, 2004) found in nonpatients that in comparison to worry, rumination was lower in verbal content, and was associated with lower compulsion to act, lower effort, and lower confidence in problem solving. However, rumination was more past-oriented than worry. In a clinical sample, rumination in patients with MDD was compared with worry in patients with panic disorder. In comparison with the worry of individuals in the panic group, the rumination of individuals in the depressed group was longer in duration, less controllable, and less dismissible, and was also associated with a lower effort to problem-solve, lower confidence in problem solving, and a greater past orientation. However, after adjustment for multiple comparisons, the only differences remaining were effort to problem solve, confidence in problem solving, and past orientation.

Fresco, Frankel, Mennin, Turk, and Heimberg (2002) factor-analyzed items from the Penn State Worry Questionnaire and the Ruminative Response Styles Questionnaire. They revealed two rumination factors they labeled "dwelling on thoughts" and "active cognitive appraisal," and two worry factors they labeled "worry engagement" and "absence of worry."

In summary, rumination and worry are overlapping but distinguishable subtypes of repetitive, negative, and self-relevant thinking strategies that are aimed at coping with events, thoughts, and emotions. They are the conceptual processes described in the CAS, and they draw from similar metacognitions. It follows from all this that treatment of worry and rumination will share several similarities.

THE CAS IN DEPRESSION

As the foregoing suggests, a central feature of the CAS is rumination. However, worrying is also a component of the syndrome in depression. Some patients worry about the reoccurrence of depressive symptoms and catastrophize about their ability to cope in the future (e.g., "What if my depression never ends?"; "What if this symptom is a sign of illness again?"). The following example illustrates a rumination/worry sequence:

> "I feel terrible. Why do I feel like this? I worry that it might never end. I just feel that I can't face anything, I have nothing to look forward to, it's just the same as it always is. Everyone is getting on with life, but I just can't. Why has this happened to me? What does that say about me? I must be abnormal. I should be happy, but I'm not. Why do I feel this way? I don't seem to be able to find a solution, I don't have an answer. It's like a disease taking me over. I don't think I'm going to get rid of it."

In this example, the patient repeatedly questions her reasons for feeling depressed, what it means, and how to find an answer. The process is circular and leads to a negative conclusion that may be viewed as hopelessness.

Aside from rumination, a further component of the CAS is threat monitoring. In depression this occurs in the form of focusing on the symptoms of depression and mood changes. For example, patients monitor their energy levels or check for signs of fatigue as they attempt to gauge the severity of their problem and assess their ability to cope.

Maladaptive coping behaviors include avoidance of activities and social contact. Activities are reduced to make more time for rumination or to increase rest under the mistaken belief that these efforts will provide valuable recovery time. Substances may be used as a means of attempting to regulate mood. In some cases self-injury or self-punishment is used to try and connect with alternative feelings to sadness or loss of affect.

THE METACOGNITIVE MODEL OF DEPRESSION

The metacognitive model that forms the basis of case conceptualization is presented in Figure 9.1. Key features of this model are (1) positive meta-cognitive beliefs about the need to ruminate as a means of overcoming depressed feelings and finding answers to problems; (2) negative meta-cognitive beliefs about the uncontrollability of rumination, the psychological vulnerability of the self, and the danger of depressive experiences; (3) diminished meta-awareness of rumination; and (4) the CAS (rumination, threat monitoring, and unhelpful coping behaviors).

The model is intended to represent the metacognitions and processes that maintain a depressive episode, but within each episode periods of

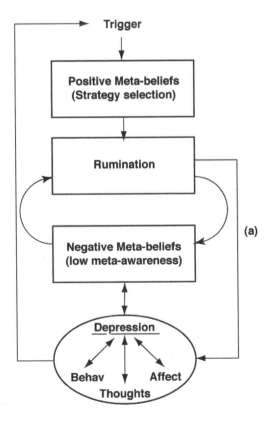

FIGURE 9.1. The metacognitive model of depression.

exacerbation of sadness or greater loss of interest, that are superimposed on the general level of negative affect, can normally be identified. The model captures these exacerbations as state-like responses to individual "triggers."

Depression is maintained and intensified by activation of rumination and unhelpful response patterns. A typical trigger is a negative thought about the self, the future, or the world, or a symptom such as feeling fatigued, unmotivated, or sad. The trigger activates positive metacognitive beliefs about the need to engage in sustained mental processing or rumination (brooding) about the meaning and causes of this event. Positive metacognitions also concern the importance of monitoring for signs and symptoms, which are seen as threatening because they signal depression. In some cases the individual's beliefs concern the usefulness of maintaining flattened affect as a means of avoiding stronger emotional fluctuations. For example, a patient described how he tried to maintain a low level of sadness because it was safer to do so than to run the risk of coping with a descent from happiness. Examples of positive metacognitive beliefs include:

"Thinking about the causes of sadness will help me prevent it."
"If I dwell on my past mistakes, I can be a better person."
"Thinking about how bad I am will make me snap out of it."
"Thinking pessimistically will stop me being disappointed."
"Thinking about how bad I feel is the punishment I deserve."
"It's better for me to be pessimistic than it is to be disappointed."
"Focusing on feeling sad keeps me stable."

Positive metacognitive beliefs give rise to sustained brooding on the meaning and causes of symptoms and one's life circumstances. This has the effect of prolonging and intensifying depressive symptoms. This direct effect is important in maintaining mood disturbances, especially in the early stages of depression (signified by the arrow labeled "a" in Figure 9.1).

As a result of the persistence of symptoms and psychosocial factors (e.g., what the patient learns about depression through contact with the medical system), negative metacognitions are activated or reinforced. These beliefs contribute to a persistence of rumination and unhelpful coping behaviors because the person believes that he or she is no longer in control. They concern the idea that depressive thoughts and symptoms are uncontrollable and the idea that they are symptoms of disease. Examples include the following:

"I have no control over my mind and mood."
"My mind has changed; I am not myself."
"I'm losing control—I have an illness in my brain."

"I am defective for being like this."
"All I can do is wait and hope it goes away."
"It's impossible to stop myself from ruminating."

Negative metacognitions also consist of a reduced awareness of the process of ruminating as the continuation of the process renders it a familiar habit with few dangerous consequences to draw the person's attention to it. In contrast, the person begins to see depression itself as an increasing danger. Other processes too may reduce an individual's awareness of the extent of his or her rumination such as disruption in metacognitive monitoring and attentional control that are side effects of depression.

Depressive responses such as reductions in behavior, loss of motivation, and changes in thinking patterns that accompany depression contribute to rumination. Some patients reduce their activities to give themselves more time to think about their problem, but such loss of activity and failure to deal with problems can have social consequences that increase negative thoughts. For example, feelings and thoughts of guilt and inadequacy resulting from failure to complete tasks can act as widening triggers for rumination.

Once a depressive episode has occurred the person can become fearful of subsequent episodes, a fear that is underpinned by negative metacognitions (e.g., "My mind can't take too much stress") and is associated with beliefs about the need to be vigilant for early symptoms and signs of depression. This is the source of worry about recurrence that contributes to a mixed anxiety–depression presentation. It increases sensitivity to triggers for rumination and depression, as normal variations in levels of energy, mood, stress, or motivation are misinterpreted as a sign of the return of a "depressive illness."

THE MODEL IN ACTION

A presentation of the model for a rumination episode will serve to illustrate how these components operate.

An increase in rumination is triggered by a negative thought, memory, or emotion. If there is a clear external precipitant, the precipitating event is followed by a negative intrusive thought or emotion that is the internal trigger for positive metacognitive beliefs leading to sustained rumination.

The negative thought that acts as a trigger is often a negative self-statement such as "I'm a failure," "I'm useless," "I don't feel right," "I'll never succeed," "No one likes me," and "I'm unattractive." In the example depicted in Figure 9.2, the patient reported getting dressed for a party and her mother stating "You've put on weight." The mother's statement immediately prompted the negative intrusive thought "I'm fat."

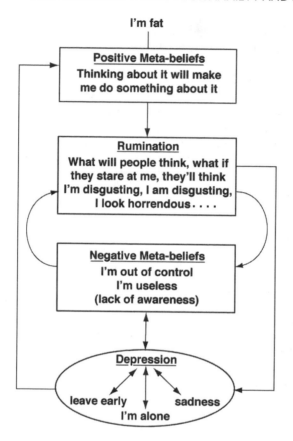

FIGURE 9.2. An idiosyncratic depression case formulation.

This negative intrusive thought activated positive metacognitive beliefs about rumination as a means of finding answers to the problem of being overweight. In this case the positive metacognition was "Thinking about how fat I am will help me do something about it." This metacognition was followed by a sustained rumination process: "What will people think? What if they stare at me? They'll think I'm disgusting. I am disgusting. I look horrendous."

During the rumination sequence negative emotions (sadness) intensified, which activated the negative metacognitive belief that "I'm out of control, I'm useless," which fed into the continued rumination cycle. The patient attempted to cope with her negative thoughts and feelings by avoiding people at the party, leaving early, and returning home to sleep. All these activities provided additional time for ruminative thinking and gave rise to other negative thoughts about being "alone" that acted as new triggers for sustaining rumination.

The patient was not aware of the extent or problem of rumination because she had used this strategy for many years to deal with her negative feelings and it had long since become a means of attempting to change herself. Thus, diminished awareness of the nature and consequences of rumination were apparent. The patient held the negative metacognitive belief that she was "out of control," but in essence she was using the wrong type of control (rumination and avoidance) because she held the mistaken belief that rumination and avoidance should restore her control and motivate her to change.

STRUCTURE OF TREATMENT

The stages of MCT for depression are set out below. Treatment incorporates the attention training technique (ATT) as a means of promoting meta-awareness, increasing flexible control, and recovering cognitive resources from depressive thinking styles. The programmed practice of the ATT also serves to counteract depressive inertia by providing a discreet set of daily exercises. MCT also focuses on removing rumination and modifying positive and negative metacognitive beliefs. Treatment typically ranges from 5 to 10 sessions and comprises:

1. Case conceptualization
2. Socialization
3. Attention training and detached mindfulness training
4. Challenging negative metacognitive beliefs (uncontrollability, disease model)
5. Challenging positive metacognitive beliefs about rumination
6. Removing residual behaviors and threat monitoring
7. Reinforcing new plans for processing
8. Relapse prevention

CASE CONCEPTUALIZATION

Measures

Tools required during this stage are:

1. Major Depressive Disorder Scale (MDD-S)
2. Depression Case Formulation Interview
3. Session checklists

The therapist begins by administering the MDD-S and examines the negative and positive metacognitive beliefs the patient endorses in order to obtain a preliminary impression of the types of beliefs and thinking styles that should be explored and incorporated in the case formulation. The MDD-S is reproduced in Appendix 10. This scale also provides an impression of the types of behaviors engaged during low mood. Other measures typically considered for completion before the session are the BAI and the BDI-II. For a more comprehensive assessment of rumination, the Ruminative Response Scale (Nolen-Hoeksema & Morrow, 1991) can be used. Further measures of positive and negative beliefs about rumination are the Positive Beliefs about Rumination Scale (PBRS; Papageorgiou & Wells, 2001a, 2001b) and the Negative Beliefs about Rumination Scale (NBRS; Papageorgiou, Wells, & Meina, 2008).

Agenda of the First Session

The therapist sets out the agenda for the first session in the following way:

"In today's session I would like to explore a recent episode when your mood worsened or you found yourself dwelling on how bad you felt. We can identify the factors that keep depression going and begin to examine ways that you can overcome your problem. I would also like to explain a little more about metacognitive therapy and what you might expect from treatment. I will also introduce you to a technique called 'attention training' that I would like you to practice. Is there anything you would like to put on the agenda and talk about today?"

Generating a Case Conceptualization

The therapist proceeds with generating an idiosyncratic version of the metacognitive model that represents the events in a recent distressing rumination episode. Because the patient's awareness of rumination may be limited at first, the therapist can consider a recent period of worsening sadness (an affect shift) as a marker for intensified rumination. The therapist asks, "Was there a time recently when your sadness worsened— for example, you became tearful?" In some cases an affect shift is difficult to identify because the patient reports a general unremitting level of sadness or a general flattening of affect. In these circumstances the therapist can use periods of behavioral inactivity as a marker for investigating rumination processes or ask direct questions about the nature of the patient's thinking.

The therapist specifically asks:

"Was there a time recently when you did nothing and just spent time brooding about your feelings and your situation?"

"Have you recently found yourself dwelling on how you feel and how bad your situation seems?"

"While going about your usual activities have you found that your mind has been preoccupied with thinking negative thoughts about yourself and your situation?"

Having identified experiences that are used as a prime for generating the case formulation, the therapist asks a sequence of questions as depicted by the numerical sequence in the Depression Case Formulation Interview in Appendix 14.

First, the therapist looks for an internal trigger associated with the affect shift or period of rumination. This is typically a negative automatic thought, examples of which include "What's the point, I've failed," "No one cares," "I'm ugly," "I'll never get what I want," "I have no energy," and "I'm weak."

After the therapist has identified the patient's negative automatic thought, his or her next step is to identify the rumination response. The therapist asks, "When you had that thought what did you next think about?" A brief description of the chain of ruminative thoughts is obtained by repeating the question "What did you think next?," as in the example dialogue given below. The therapist obtains an impression of the duration of the ruminative sequence by asking "How long did you go on thinking this way?"

THERAPIST: After you had the thought "I'm ugly," what did you go on to think about?

PATIENT: I thought everyone will stare at me.

THERAPIST: What did you think next?

PATIENT: I thought they would think I was a freak.

THERAPIST: What did you think next?

PATIENT: I just thought that I was ugly and a failure.

THERAPIST: What did you think next?

PATIENT: I'm not sure—it was just how I'd never sort myself out and how pathetic I am.

THERAPIST: Chains of negative thinking like this are called "rumination." How long did you go on thinking in this way?

PATIENT: It lasted all night until eventually I fell asleep.

Next, the therapist asks about the effect of rumination on emotion with the aim of showing that it intensifies or prolongs sadness: "When you were thinking like that what happened to your emotions?" The therapist specifically asks about the effect of thinking on feelings of sadness/depression: "What happened to your feelings of depression as a result of dwelling on those thoughts?" Depression is divided into its salient components. To this end the presence of avoidance/withdrawal behaviors, cognitive symptoms, and affective symptoms are elucidated and incorporated in the formulation.

The therapist uses the patient's account of emotion as a pathway into exploring negative beliefs concerning the uncontrollability of rumination and the patient's illness model: "It sounds as if ruminating made you feel worse. Is that something you could stop doing?" and "How much control do you believe you have over ruminating?" The illness model is explored by directly asking: "Do you believe you can do anything about your symptoms? Do you think your depression is biological or psychological?"

Following the elicitation of negative metacognitions concerning uncontrollability, the therapist explores positive beliefs about rumination: "Are there advantages to ruminating?" "Are there any advantages to repeatedly analyzing your problems and how you feel?" "What is your goal in ruminating?" "Can ruminating in response to a negative thought or feeling help you in any way?"

An example dialogue using this complete range of questions is presented below. The case conceptualization resulting from the dialogue is depicted in Figure 9.3.

THERAPIST: Was there a time recently when you found yourself dwelling on how wretched you felt?

PATIENT: Yesterday morning I felt terrible.

THERAPIST: What was the first thing you thought as you began to dwell on your feelings?

PATIENT: I just thought I don't have the energy to go to work.

THERAPIST: So the thought was "I don't have the energy." Is that right?

PATIENT: Yes, I just felt exhausted.

THERAPIST: When you had that thought and feeling, what did you then go on to think about?

PATIENT: I thought I had nothing to look forward to. What do I do about it? I thought that it would be like this until I die, and why is everyone happier than me?

THERAPIST: What did you think next?

PATIENT: I don't know, I was just focusing on why I felt like this.

THERAPIST: This type of thinking is called "rumination." How long did it go on?

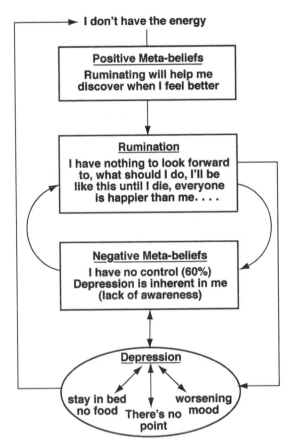

FIGURE 9.3. Depression case formulation arising from the dialogue.

PATIENT: Until I got to work and had to deal with people.

THERAPIST: What was the effect of ruminating on your emotions?

PATIENT: It made me feel worse—even more depressed.

THERAPIST: What did you end up thinking?

PATIENT: That there was no point to anything. Why should I go on?

THERAPIST: How did that affect your behavior?

PATIENT: I just went to bed when I got home—I didn't bother to eat or anything.

THERAPIST: It seems that ruminating makes things worse. Could you stop doing it?

PATIENT: I'm not sure, it's like it just comes over me like a cloud.

THERAPIST: How much do you believe it's uncontrollable on a scale of 0 to 100%.

PATIENT: Sixty percent.

THERAPIST: Do you think you can do anything about your depression?

PATIENT: My father had it, and I'm afraid I have it from him—it's inherited.

THERAPIST: Are there any advantages to ruminating?

PATIENT: No, I'm not sure there is. I'm hoping that one day I'll wake up and find that I feel better.

THERAPIST: What would happen if you didn't ruminate?

PATIENT: I guess I would feel better, but maybe I wouldn't know it.

THERAPIST: So, will rumination let you know when you're better?

PATIENT: Yes, it will help me discover when I feel better.

SOCIALIZATION

The therapist begins the process of socialization by tracing out the case conceptualization and drawing the patient's awareness to ruminative thinking. A core aim at the outset is to help the patient begin to recognize the central role that rumination has in "feeding" depression. A useful metaphor is the "dig yourself out of a hole" metaphor. The therapist can say: "Is it possible to dig yourself out of a hole and at the same time make the hole smaller? Rumination is like trying to dig yourself out of a hole. The hole gets bigger the more you dig. Because rumination can take you deeper, it's not a good way out of depression."

The therapist uses metaphors as a means of illustrating the role of rumination and provides a basis for building meta-awareness. It is important that the patient begins to construct a model of the significance of thought processes rather than being focused on the reality or otherwise of depressive thought content.

The therapist reviews the case formulation to explain how the model works. The therapist says the following:

"Looking at the diagram we have mapped out it is possible to see some important factors that allow us to understand the causes of your depression. In particular, we can begin to see what it is that feeds depression and keeps it going. An important factor is the tendency that you have to dwell on and brood about negative thoughts and feelings. This type of thinking is called 'rumination,' and it appears that you have some beliefs about the need to ruminate in order to understand and solve your experiences. However, you also have limited awareness of this process and you have doubts about how controllable it is. Another factor keeping your depression going is your behavior. Depression is associated with reduced activity and this can create its own problems as difficulties begin to pile up and you have more time on your hands to sink into a state of rumination.

"Rumination deepens and prolongs your depression and leads you to an increasingly negative place. For example, how often have you arrived at a happy conclusion to your rumination? Does it lead you to feel better or worse about yourself? So you see, by ruminating you strengthen unhelpful negative beliefs about yourself and your situation."

Socialization to the model is aided by using questions that illustrate the effects of rumination, metacognitive beliefs, and behavior. Frequently used socialization questions are:

"How long have you been ruminating about your problems? Has it solved your problems yet? How much longer do you anticipate it will take?"

"You believe that rumination helps to solve your depression. That sounds promising because it means that all you need to do is ruminate more and you should get better. How much do you believe that?"

"It seems that you have been trying to think yourself better by ruminating. Why hasn't it worked yet?"

"It seems that you have been trying to think yourself better by ruminating, but is rumination a balanced and evenhanded way of viewing the situation you're in?"

"What happens to your sadness if you are distracted from ruminating, say, when you have to do something else? What does that say about the role of rumination in affecting your feelings?"

ENHANCING MOTIVATION

Some depressed patients are ambivalent about improving their mood and giving up rumination. They view depression as a form of punishment that they deserve or they have personality traits that support a more pervasive overconceptual and analytical approach to emotions and activities. In these circumstances the therapist aims to enhance dissonance both as a socialization technique and as a means of enhancing motivation to modify rumination. For example, the therapist says the following:

"It seems you believe you deserve to be depressed as a form of punishment. Does this punishment fit the crime? If you continue to punish someone, will he or she change? How will you decide when you have had enough punishment?

"It appears that you are of two minds about rumination. On the one hand, you believe it is a beneficial thing to do, but, on the other, you believe it is uncontrollable and much of the time you are not aware of it. How helpful can it really be if you can't control it and you have limited awareness of its occurrence?"

In some cases low levels of patient motivation and engagement in treatment are associated with high levels of perceived hopelessness in which the patient believes that his or her problem cannot change. In such cases the therapist should assess for suicide risk and elicit and reinforce deterrents where necessary. Hopelessness is challenged by introducing the idea that the problem is that the patient responds to thoughts about hopelessness without testing out these thoughts. The therapist works with the patient to show how new ways of responding to these thoughts with structured activity rather than with rumination can give a more accurate sense of the possibilities for change. By responding to thoughts of hopelessness with rumination and inactivity the patient effectively closes off opportunities for change, a process that should be reversed.

Hopelessness and low levels of motivation can often be traced to negative metacognitive beliefs such as the belief that depression is an uncontrollable illness or that it is impossible to control depressive thoughts. In each case of hopelessness the therapist focuses on modifying hopelessness at the beginning of treatment.

HELPING PATIENTS UNDERSTAND THE ROLE OF BEHAVIORS

It is very important that patients develop an understanding of the unhelpful role that their own behaviors play in the maintenance of depression.

By questioning the effects of behavior, the therapist can help patients discover that their behavior has not been effective in alleviating sadness and symptoms of depression. We have seen how covert coping behaviors such as rumination are a problem. So too are overt behaviors such as reduced activity and social avoidance. We saw above how the therapist uses a range of questions to help the patient understand that rumination is problematic. Similar questions can be used to help patients understand the problem with overt behaviors:

"How effective have your behaviors been in getting rid of your depression?"

"What happens to your mood if you increase your activities?"

"What happens to your rumination when you decrease your activities?"

"Do you feel better when you do more or when you do less?"

ATTENTION TRAINING

Following socialization the therapist proceeds with an overview of treatment and introduces attention training. Attention training is used because it helps the patient to develop awareness and more flexible control of ruminative thinking.

Patients are instructed to treat internal intrusions of thoughts or sensations (triggers) as "noise" during the flexible control of attention. The procedure is not used as distraction from triggers, but as a means of maintaining awareness of them without allowing attention to be bound up with ruminative responses. A typical rationale for the ATT is given as follows:

"As we have seen, when you become depressed there are changes in your pattern of thinking. For instance, your concentration is poor. This is because rumination takes center stage or it goes on in the background even when you are trying to go about your usual business. It comes to the forefront when you are actively trying to find answers to your problems. You are not always aware of this rumination and even when you are aware it seems that it is uncontrollable. The first thing to do is to help you regain awareness, flexibility, and control in your thinking. For this purpose you will learn a technique called attention training, which you will be asked to practice each day."

The therapist then presents the ATT. This involves patient ratings of self-focused attention before and after practice and the setting of ATT daily practice for homework. The protocol for ATT is presented in detail in Chapter 4. ATT is practiced for approximately 12 minutes at each treatment session. (A recorded version of the ATT is available at *www.mct-institute.com*.)

DETACHED MINDFULNESS
AND RUMINATION POSTPONEMENT

At the same time that the ATT is introduced, the therapist introduces responding to the triggers for rumination with detached mindfulness

(DM). The therapist explains how DM should be applied by the patient at times when triggers occur between the ATT practice sessions. The idea is that patients apply DM to cognitive and affective reactions that are normally the trigger for rumination. The patient's aim is to be aware of the trigger in the absence of sustained conceptual analysis of it or its meaning. DM is normally introduced along with rumination postponement in the following way:

> "I would like you to practice a new way of responding to the thoughts or feelings that act as triggers for ruminating. When you notice a negative thought or feeling, for example, [insert patient example from case conceptualization], I would like you to acknowledge it and choose not to engage with it. Perhaps you can say to yourself: 'There's a negative thought, I'm not going to deal with it now, I'm not going to activate my rumination.' Allow the thought to do its own thing, don't push it away, and don't try to work it out. Instead, postpone the rumination and any further thinking until a specific rumination time later in the day. Postpone your rumination until later and then if you must do so, allow yourself 10 minutes for ruminating on your problems, say, between 7:00 and 7:10 P.M. But you don't have to use that rumination time. Most people decide in the end that they don't need it."

The therapist needs to check to make sure that the patient does not confuse postponing the rumination process with thought suppression: "The aim is not to get the original negative thought/feeling out of your mind, but to choose not to engage with it with sustained rumination. Can you see the difference between trying to rid your mind of thoughts versus disengaging the subsequent rumination process?"

IMPLEMENTING DM TECHNIQUES

Several techniques for illustrating the concept of DM and providing experiential awareness of the state were described in Chapter 5. One or a combination of these techniques is used both to illustrate the meaning and nature of DM and to provide some experience of DM after the concept is introduced. For example, the therapist can use free association to give a sense of DM:

> "I would like you to experience what it feels like to apply detached mindfulness to events in your mind and body. By doing this you can begin to relate to these internal events in a new way without ruminating. In a minute I will say some words, and I would like you to allow

your mind to roam freely. Do not control the content of your thoughts, just passively watch what they do. You may find that nothing happens or you may find that you experience images, sensations, or memories. It doesn't matter what happens—just watch these events without influencing them in any way. I'm going to say some words now (*pause*): apple, bicycle, summertime, chocolate, birthday, roses, clouds. What did you notice when you watched your thoughts? The idea is that you should allow yourself to experience your negative thoughts and feelings that trigger rumination in this way. Just allow them to be there without getting caught up in them."

If the difference between getting "caught up" in thoughts and DM remains unclear to the patient, the therapist illustrates the difference with a recent thought that triggered rumination. For example, one patient noted that her rumination started with the thought "I'm a failure." The therapist asked her to close her eyes and induce this thought in the session. The therapist then instructed the patient to take a step back from the thought and to observe it from a distance. While doing so the therapist asked her to be aware of herself existing separately from the thought as merely an observer. Next, the therapist asked her to become caught up in the thought and to ruminate by analyzing all the ways in which she was a failure. This was followed by a repeated process of stepping back and interrupting the process of rumination.

MODIFYING NEGATIVE METACOGNITIVE BELIEFS

The therapist typically begins metacognitive belief change by exploring and modifying beliefs about the uncontrollability of rumination. The following steps are normally undertaken in this process:

Step 1: Verbal Method

The therapist reviews the evidence and counterevidence for the belief that rumination is uncontrollable, and then summarizes the evidence that rumination can be controlled. For example, if the postponed rumination period has already been implemented successfully, then this success can be used as evidence that rumination is under control. When the patient presents evidence that rumination is uncontrollable the therapist reinterprets this evidence. For example, a patient argued that the presence of her depression was evidence that she had no control over her thoughts. The therapist helped her to see how she had not used the most appropriate form of control and how her depression was inadvertently maintained by using the coping strategies of inactivity and brooding.

When there is persistence in the belief that rumination is uncontrollable, the therapist asks the patient if he or she thinks it would be possible to increase rumination. If the patient learns that it can be increased, then the patient must admit that it must be subject to personal control. Some patients find that it is useful to distinguish between *beliefs* about control and *experiences* of control because these are not the same thing. For example, a person may not believe that a process is controllable simply because he or she has rarely attempted to control it; often the patient has made few attempts at controlling rumination.

The therapist asks questions that generate evidence that rumination is controllable. For example, "If rumination is truly uncontrollable, how does it ever stop?" This is followed by questions such as "If you are ruminating and an emergency happens that you have to deal with, what happens to your rumination? Is this evidence that it is controllable or uncontrollable?"

Step 2: Rumination Modulation Experiment

The therapist introduces a rumination modulation experiment as a means of testing the patient's belief in uncontrollability:

> "One of the problems is that you have engaged in rumination as a way of dealing with problems and you have not effectively interrupted the process. This keeps your belief that rumination is uncontrollable going. I would like us to try an experiment right now. In a minute I will ask you to ruminate and I will then ask you to suspend your rumination and bring your mind to a state of watchful stillness.
>
> "Can you think of a recent trigger for rumination? I want you to allow yourself to have that trigger right now. When you notice that trigger, can you ruminate about it? Ask all of your usual questions and try to find an answer. When I say 'Let your mind be still' I'd like you to suspend your rumination but let your awareness of the trigger or any related thought remain. Let's try that now."

This experiment is refined and repeated if further challenging is required. In particular, the therapist asks the patient to repeat the process of rumination, but this time gives the instruction to try to increase the intensity of rumination and lose control of the activity. Throughout these exercises the therapist rates the patient's degree of belief in uncontrollability. These experiments are followed up with a continuation of rumination postponement for homework.

Once beliefs concerning the uncontrollability of rumination have been effectively challenged (this can be determined by verbal belief ratings and by examining scores on the MDD-S), the therapist next explores metacognitive beliefs about the meaning of symptoms.

The therapist addresses any patient tendency to misinterpret changes in motivational state, energy levels, fatigue, or affect as a sign of illness, mental deterioration, or abnormality.

Verbal and behavioral reattribution methods are used to weaken these negative beliefs. The therapist questions the evidence that symptoms are always a sign of depressive illness, and aims to reattribute the causes of symptoms to normal daily fluctuations in mood, motivation, or energy levels.

Some patients report that they have low energy levels that act as a trigger for rumination. Therapists should review the relationship between activity levels and feelings of energy. Energy levels normally fluctuate in response to diet and blood glucose levels. Low levels of activity can lead to low levels of energy and feelings of fatigue; similarly, very high levels of physical and mental exertion can contribute to fatigue. The therapist illustrates a range of alternative benign explanations for symptoms. Tracking symptom patterns for homework and equating fluctuations with daily hassles can be used to counteract beliefs that all symptoms are caused by an intractable abnormality of the brain.

The therapist discusses the fact that mood fluctuation is a normal and natural occurrence. Pie charts can be used to explore a range of explanations of mood fluctuation. For example, a recent patient believed that changes in his mood were a sign that he was vulnerable to "serious mental illness." The therapist worked with him to construct a list of a range of potential explanations for mood fluctuation as follows:

THERAPIST: One of your beliefs is that daily changes in your mood are a sign that you must be vulnerable to serious mental illness. Have you considered other explanations for mood fluctuations?

PATIENT: No, I just don't think it's normal for my emotions to fluctuate so much.

THERAPIST: Let's see if we can generate a list of causes of fluctuation in emotion. What do you think causes your mood to go down?

PATIENT: I don't know. I've always thought it was because I'm ill.

THERAPIST: We've looked at rumination. What about that?

PATIENT: Yes, rumination can make it worse.

THERAPIST: Good, I'll put that on the list.

PATIENT: But the rumination doesn't give me the feelings in the first place, does it?

THERAPIST: What about other things that make your mood dip? What about hearing something negative?

PATIENT: Yes, if I'm criticized that makes me feel bad.

THERAPIST: Good, I'll put criticism on the list. What about feeling tired?

PATIENT: Yes, feeling tired can affect my mood.

THERAPIST: What about feeling hungry? Some people feel moody when they have low blood sugar.

PATIENT: Yes, that's definitely me, I get really irritable.

THERAPIST: What about drinking alcohol?

PATIENT: No, that doesn't really affect me, as I hardly drink.

THERAPIST: What about not living up to the standards you set yourself?

PATIENT: It's more when other people don't live up to my standards.

THERAPIST: Do you think mood changes can just be normal fluctuations?

PATIENT: I suppose they can. But do other people experience them?

THERAPIST: We could try and find out with a survey later. For the time being, can you think of anything else?

PATIENT: No.

THERAPIST: What about paying attention to your feelings? Is that something you do a lot?

PATIENT: Yes, I check how I feel in the morning, and I feel tired even when I've just got out of bed.

THERAPIST: Fine, I'll add to the list that you check your feelings. Anything else for the list?

PATIENT: No, I don't think so.

THERAPIST: Finally, I must add your original explanation to the list: "I'm vulnerable to serious mental illness." Looking at this list of causes, how much do you now believe that your mood fluctuations must be a sign of serious mental vulnerability?

PATIENT: Well, maybe I'm just considering the worst. But I'm still not sure other people feel like this.

THERAPIST: We can find out. Let's do a minisurvey and ask some people if they ever notice their mood changing and have difficulty knowing why.

The strategy outlined above was followed by asking the patient to conduct a minisurvey for homework. To accomplish this, first the therapist and the patient made up a short series of questions that the patient would ask that would be useful in evaluating his belief that mood fluctuation was a sign of serious illness and therefore abnormal. Three questions were generated:

1. "Do you have fluctuations in your mood, energy, or interest in things?"
2. "Do you sometimes feel sad or down and don't know why?"
3. "Do you feel tired even when you wake up in the morning?"

The patient agreed to ask these questions with five people that he knew and to report back on the results at the next treatment session. The patient was surprised to discover that everyone he interviewed reported fluctuations in energy and levels of tiredness. Most of the people also reported that they felt sad at times and sometimes they were not sure why.

MODIFYING POSITIVE METACOGNITIVE BELIEFS

Positive metacognitive beliefs are conceptualized as propositional beliefs (e.g., rumination helps me find answers), and also as proceduralized knowledge or plans for processing. It is necessary to modify these positive beliefs because they underlie motivation to engage rumination in response to triggers. It is also necessary to strengthen new and alternative plans for guiding thinking styles and behavior in response to subsequent triggers. We will return to these issues in the next section.

Several strategies are available to the therapist for modifying positive metacognitive beliefs about rumination. These can be combined into a sequence as outlined below. Initially, it is recommended that verbal strategies be used to weaken beliefs; these should be followed up with behavioral experiments. The following steps are usually undertaken:

Step 1: Advantages–Disadvantages Analysis

The therapist undertakes an advantages–disadvantages analysis of rumination. He or she reinforces the disadvantages by examining the evidence showing that rumination is a problem. Following up, the therapist challenges the validity of any advantages elicited from the patient and if necessary explores alternative methods by which the same advantages can be achieved other than by the process of rumination.

For example, a patient stated that he believed that he must ruminate about his problems because otherwise he would not be thinking about them. The therapist asked if it was possible to think about problems in a way that was different from rumination. A useful discussion followed about how the patient had a black-and-white view of rumination—that is, he believed it was rumination or nothing. Interestingly, he did not ruminate about performing his job but could normally focus on what needed to be done even in the face of unhelpful distractions. The therapist asked if he could apply the same thinking strategy to his symptoms, that is, focus on the tasks that needed to be done even in the face of his symptoms, rather than analyzing their meaning.

Step 2: Questioning the Evidence

The therapist asks the questions: "If rumination helps, why haven't you recovered or solved your problems of depression yet? What does this suggest about the usefulness of rumination?"

Additionally or as an alternative, the therapist asks about the mechanism underlying the proposed beneficial effects of rumination: "How does rumination work? How does it allow you to solve problems and find out the causes of your sadness?"

If preferred, less direct questioning can be used by asking about the evidence that rumination helps to solve problems and find appropriate meanings (e.g., "Do you have any evidence that rumination helps you to overcome your difficulties?").

The therapist also questions the patient about his or her goals in ruminating. Questions such as the following are normally used for this purpose: "What do you aim to achieve when you ruminate?" "How effective is rumination in achieving this goal?" "If it is effective, why do you need to continue with rumination?" "How will you know when you have ruminated enough?" "How close has rumination got you toward overcoming your depression?"

Step 3: Rumination Experiments

The therapist then introduces behavioral experiments to test the usefulness of rumination. For example, the patient can be asked to ruminate more on one day and then to ban rumination on the next day in response to a symptom or thought. The therapist instructs the patient to observe if problems are solved and mood is improved on the day that rumination occurred compared to the day it was abandoned. This is a rumination modulation experiment that is similar to the worry modulation experiment described in Chapter 6 that is used to challenge positive beliefs about worry in GAD.

MODIFYING THREAT MONITORING

Unhelpful attentional strategies in depression often involve focusing on symptoms as a means of judging personal ability to cope on a daily basis. For example, one patient described how she focused on whether or not she had a feeling of "emptiness" on waking each morning to determine if she needed to remain in bed to try and feel better. Similarly, a young depressed mother frequently checked her thinking processes to determine if her head "felt like cotton wool" as a means of determining if she could cope with taking care of her children. A 40-year-old patient reported how he repeatedly checked for the presence of "how I used to feel" (i.e., contented) as a means of determining if his depression was improving.

During MCT the therapist explores the presence and nature of threat monitoring and aims to counteract it. Having identified the process and made the patient aware of it as a factor that might contribute to depression, the therapist implements an advantages–disadvantages analysis. The disadvantages are reinforced and the patient is asked to ban the activity.

MALADAPTIVE COPING WITH MOOD FLUCTUATION

In addition to ruminating and threat monitoring, patients have a tendency to respond to mood variations with unhelpful overt behaviors. These behaviors typically include reduced activity levels, prolonged sleeping, overeating, using alcohol, or self-injurious responses. The therapist elicits and reinforces the disadvantages of these responses and provides explicit instructions to change them.

Formal activity scheduling and scheduling of pleasurable activities may be used to counteract reduced activity levels and provide patients with a greater daily structure. The therapist explores the metacognitive beliefs that support the patient's need to respond to sadness with lowered activity levels. For instance, one patient believed, "I must reduce my work level when feeling sad because my mind can't take it." This belief reinforced her sense of vulnerability and maintained her vigilance for feelings of sadness. The therapist questioned this belief and set the experiment of increasing her work rate the next time she felt sad. Contrary to the idea that her mind couldn't take it, the patient discovered that working more actually improved her mood.

NEW PLANS FOR PROCESSING

Once the patient's negative and positive metacognitive beliefs have been modified, the final step of treatment, which contributes to relapse prevention, is consolidating and strengthening alternative metacognitive plans that can be used to control responses to depressogenic triggers in the future. We have seen how rumination can be a long-standing strategy over which the patient has limited initial awareness. To reduce activation in the future, alternative more adaptive replacement plans should be strengthened that compete for control over thinking.

Strengthening of replacement plans requires repeated practice of new processing strategies. Of particular importance is that the patient maintains awareness of rumination and unhelpful coping behaviors such as reduced behavioral activity. The new plan for processing should reflect responses that are incompatible with rumination and behavioral avoidance/diminished activity. The therapist compiles an idiosyncratic plan on the basis of the patient's formulation of maladaptive response patterns. To facilitate this process a "plan summary" (Appendix 19) is constructed to represent the maladaptive old plan and to summarize the new responses to be repeatedly practiced in response to idiosyncratic triggers.

Implementation of this strategy has three important components. First, a comprehensive range of patient triggers for symptoms must be elicited so that patient awareness of these triggers can be enhanced. Second, a detailed set of statements written in the first person is scripted on the summary to capture the old plan and the new plan to be practiced. Third, the patient is encouraged to repeatedly implement the new plan as an alternative to the old plan. Each of these components is considered below.

My Triggers consists of a list of typical internal events that activate old styles of processing and coping. Typical examples include negative thoughts (e.g., "I'm no good"), energetic symptoms (e.g., energy levels, lack of motivation), cognitive symptoms (e.g., difficulty concentrating), and physical symptoms (e.g., aches and pains). Triggers can also include external events (e.g., receiving criticism, being ignored by someone), even though this will be linked to an internal trigger for maladaptive styles such as an initial thought: "What have I done wrong?"

Thinking style consists of a directive behind the old ruminative and negative brooding thought process. For example: "I must dwell on and analyze why this has happened to me, why I feel this way, what this means about me as a person, why I'm such a failure." The new plan should capture an instruction that encapsulates alternative responses learned in treatment: "I must interrupt any dwelling on the issue and postpone analyzing it. If negative thoughts occur, I will apply detached mindfulness and continue with what I am doing."

Behaviors consist of a statement summarizing old responses of avoidance and diminished activity contrasted with new responses. For instance, "I must avoid meeting people, try to sleep more, and leave the daily chores" becomes "I must continue working and meeting people even if I don't feel like it because I must have confidence to function even when I feel sad."

Attention focus refers to the old tendency to monitor for signs of threat which should be replaced with a new attention plan. For instance, a patient explained how she would check her feelings of fatigue each morning as a means of deciding whether or not she was going to have a "bad day." She would also postpone tasks until she "felt like doing them." Her old strategy was one of checking her level of motivation as a means of deciding what she could or could not manage. The old plan was written as "I must check my tiredness levels to decide if the day will be bad. I must check if I feel like doing things before doing them." The new plan was: "I must ban checking my tiredness. I must focus on a positive aspect of myself each morning. I must focus on actually doing things, not on how I feel about doing them. I must prove to myself I can do things even when feeling tired."

RELAPSE PREVENTION

The formulation of the replacement plan is a component of relapse prevention. A further component is a review of residual scores on the MDD-S, paying particular attention to the frequency and duration of rumination and negative and positive beliefs. Residual elevated scores on these dimensions should be explored and modified because they are potential relapse factors.

The therapist usually checks for other subtle forms of rumination or similar perseveration processes that may have developed more recently or have been missed during treatment.

In the last two sessions of treatment, the therapist and the patient work collaboratively in compiling a "therapy blueprint." The patient is usually asked to begin work on the blueprint for homework, which can be augmented in session. The blueprint should contain an example of the case conceptualization, examples of negative and positive beliefs about rumination, and evidence counteracting them. It should also consist of the final version of the plan summary, which outlines new strategies for dealing with common triggers (e.g., thoughts, symptoms, sadness).

Booster treatment sessions are scheduled for 3 and 6 months after treatment as an opportunity to monitor gains and reinforce the knowledge and strategies acquired in treatment.

FEAR OF RECURRENCE

Future deviations in mood and occurrences of sadness are reframed as normal occurrences. Mood disturbances should be interpreted as an opportunity to practice the strategies learned in treatment. Each practice offers an opportunity to strengthen alternative and more helpful responses.

The final part of the plan summary consists of a "reframe" that aims to interpret symptoms in a positive and normalizing way. Each experience of symptoms is seen as an opportunity to practice implementation of the new plan. The reframe consists of statements such as "Changes in mood are normal, I will not complicate them by responding with the old plan.

Each experience is an opportunity to practice and strengthen my new way of responding."

A NOTE ON SUICIDALITY AND SELF-INJURY

In cases marked by self-injurious behaviors or suicidal intent an appropriate risk assessment is undertaken and deterrents to these responses are elicited and strengthened. Self-injury can be conceptualized as a behavior occurring as a result of protracted rumination. In some instances it offers a means of exiting from the feelings and thoughts produced by rumination. This function should be conceptualized and alternative means of postponing rumination and modulating feelings are explored.

Hopelessness is an important factor in suicidality and therefore should be reduced. In MCT hopelessness is conceptualized as a manifestation of rumination on the theme that things cannot change and the patient is powerless. The therapist draws the patient's attention to this as another manifestation of rumination and asks the patient to suspend the activity. Patients are asked to redirect attention away from rumination and onto alternative activities such as taking specific steps to solve problems or to organize important aspects of their lives that may have been neglected.

When risk is an issue, appropriate steps are taken to reduce risk and other health professionals are involved as necessary.

DEPRESSION TREATMENT PLAN

An overall eight-session treatment plan for implementing MCT in depression is presented in Appendix 18. This is intended as a guide to the structure and content of sessions and should be applied flexibly as individual circumstances require. The plan should be implemented with direct reference to the strategies described in this chapter.

||||||||||||||||||||

CHAPTER 10

The Evidence for Metacognitive Theory and Therapy

This chapter reviews the evidence base supporting the role of the CAS and metacognitions in psychological disorder as proposed by the present theoretical approach. Evidence of the effects of specific treatment techniques and outcome data for the treatment packages is also presented. This review is intended to be an overview rather than an in-depth discussion of studies, which could constitute a volume on its own. Furthermore, my intention is to remain within the objectives of this volume, which is to provide a more practical guide to MCT.

In organizing the evidence, I first review the studies that have linked aspects that are features of the CAS with psychological disturbance. These aspects are worry, rumination, attentional threat monitoring, and metacognitive coping strategies. Next, I review evidence of links between metacognitive beliefs and psychological disorders. Finally, I summarize studies of the effects of metacognitive manipulations, attention manipulations, and evaluations of effectiveness of full treatment.

THE EXISTENCE AND CONSEQUENCES OF THE CAS

Worry and Rumination

There is a large database supporting the idea that repetitive styles of thinking in the form of worry or rumination are deleterious for emotional well-being. Early work on worry was conducted in the area of test anxiety (e.g., Wine, 1971; Sarason, 1984) where anxiety has been divided into two subcomponents: emotionality and worry. Numerous studies suggest that the worry component has a deleterious impact on test performance, an effect attributed to the fact that it uses up attentional resources. These data are consistent with the view that worry is attentionally demanding and can interfere with task-oriented behavior and processing.

There can be little doubt that perseverative forms of thinking figure prominently in psychological disorders. For instance, worry has been identified as a process in a wide range of disorders including panic (DSM-IV; American Psychiatric Association, 1994), social phobia (Clark & Wells, 1995; Mellings & Alden, 2000), health anxiety (Bouman & Meijer, 1999), traumatic stress (Holeva, Tarrier, & Wells, 2001), and generalized anxiety (DSM-IV; American Psychiatric Association, 1994). A similar process of rumination has been identified in depression (e.g., Nolen-Hoeksema, 1991).

In the metacognitive model, worry has deleterious effects on self-regulation because it blocks emotional processing; uses cognitive capacity, giving rise to performance difficulties; and focuses processing on threat. Research on the negative effects of worrying and rumination support these negative effects. Early exploration of the effects of worrying outside of the test-anxiety field examined the effects of brief worry periods in high and low worriers. Brief periods of worry appear to lead to more anxiety, more depression, less task-focused attention, and more negative thoughts in a subsequent breathing task in high, compared with low, worriers (Borkovec et al., 1983).

Hazlett-Stephens (1997) explored the effects of worrying in speech-anxious subjects asked to give five consecutive speeches. Subjects in the control conditions displayed habituation of subjective anxiety over repeated exposures, while subjects in the worry condition who worried prior to each exposure, did not.

Mellings and Alden (2000) examined postevent worry/rumination in high socially anxious subjects and found it predicted recall of negative self-relevant information, negative bias in self-judgments, and recall of anxiety sensations on a subsequent occasion involving anticipation of a social interaction.

The idea that worry might interfere with other processes such as those needed for emotional processing is central to metacognitive theory and has been directly tested. Butler, Wells, and Dewick (1995) and Wells and Papageorgiou (1995) showed participants a gruesome and stressful film and asked them to engage in different types of thinking during a brief postfilm thinking period. Some of the participants were asked to worry; those that did showed significantly more intrusive images concerning the film over a subsequent 3-day period. Since intrusive images are thought to be an index of failed emotional processing (e.g., Rachman, 1980), it may be inferred that worrying blocks emotional processing.

A process similar to worry is that of rumination. These processes overlap in many respects as demonstrated in comparative studies, but there are also some differences (Papageorgiou & Wells, 1999a, 2004). As far as the metacognitive model is concerned, they both have negative effects on self-regulation and emotional well-being.

There is a substantial amount of evidence of the negative effects of rumination on emotion and psychopathology (see Lyubomirsky & Tkach, 2004; Nolen-Hoeksema, 2004, for reviews). Nolen-Hoeksema and colleagues have conducted much of the initial groundbreaking research in the area of rumination. Rumination has been shown to prolong depressed mood following stressful life experiences (e.g., Nolen-Hoeksema & Morrow, 1991; Nolen-Hoeksema & Larson, 1999). In a large longitudinal study of over 1,100 community adults those that showed clinical depression and a ruminative thinking style at initial assessment had more severe and longer-lasting depressive symptoms 1 year later, were less likely to show remission, and were more likely to have anxiety symptoms (Nolen-Hoeksema, 2000). Rumination not only affects mood but also biases thinking and influences behavior (Spasojevic, Alloy, Abramson, Maccoon, & Robinson, 2004).

Overall, these studies provide a compelling level of support for the notion that thinking styles characterized by preservative processing, specifically worry and rumination, contribute to symptoms of emotional disorder. Since some of these studies have used experimental manipulations or prospective analyses of effects of these thinking styles, they are consistent with a causal role of these styles in the development of disorder. There is an even greater database of self-report and cross-sectional studies that show that individual differences in worry and rumination are positively correlated with measures of vulnerability to psychological disorder as assessed by constructs such as neuroticism and depression proneness (e.g., Matthews & Wells, 2004). Furthermore, as described later, the use of worry to control thoughts has been examined specifically as a factor associated with psychological disorder and emotional vulnerability.

Attentional Threat Monitoring

When we first presented the S-REF model (Wells & Matthews, 1994), the grounding of the metacognitive approach, we focused on explaining attention and performance data as well as data on psychological disorder.

In the metacognitive model abnormality in selective attention consisting of an excessive tendency to focus on personally relevant threatening information is a feature of the CAS.

A wide range of studies have demonstrated such bias experimentally, often by use of the emotional Stroop task. This task requires the subject to name the colors that words with emotional or threatening content are printed in. Typically, patients are slow to name the colors of the words that are congruent with their disorder. For example, individuals with GAD are slow to color-name threatening words (Mathews & MacLeod, 1985), individuals with depression are slow on negative emotion words (Gotlib & Cane, 1987), and Vietnam veterans are slow to name the colors of negative combat-related words (Kaspi, McNally, & Amir, 1995).

Debate about the nature of attentional bias in emotional disorder has focused on the concept of automaticity. A cognitive process is considered automatic if it meets three criteria: (1) initiation and termination are involuntary, (2) few or no attentional resources are required for processing, and (3) processing is not amenable to consciousness (Schneider, Dumais, & Shiffrin, 1984). Automatic processing can be contrasted with controlled processing, which is voluntary, capacity-limited, and partially accessible to consciousness (Schneider et al., 1984), although a rigid dichotomy between these processes is probably unhelpful.

Bias in Stroop tasks has been attributed to involuntary and largely automatic mechanisms (e.g., Williams, Watts, MacLeod, & Mathews, 1988). However, the S-REF model and the metacognitive theory of disorder proposes an alternative: that bias primarily reflects strategic processing.

What evidence is there in support of this counterproposal? We (Wells & Matthews, 1994; see also Matthews & Wells, 2000) have previously reviewed several lines of evidence. Studies of priming effects show that in depressed individuals prior presentation of self-relevant material increase interference (Segal & Vella, 1990). Similar effects have been found in non-clinical subjects exposed to a self-focus manipulation. These effects appear to operate over time intervals that are equated with voluntary processing (e.g., Richards & French, 1992). Furthermore, there appears to be an effect of presenting similar types of Stroop material together rather than different types in pseudorandom order. Richards, French, Johnson, Naparstek, and Williams (1992) found bias effects related to trait anxiety only in trials that were blocked by word type, suggesting bias might depend on expectancy of threat. Matthews and Harley (1996) used a connectionist simulation of the emotional Stroop test to explore two possible automatic mechanisms and a strategic mechanism. Simulations did not support automatic mechanisms analogous to hard-wired sensitivity to threat or analogous to repeated exposure effects. The strategic simulation tested a continuation of monitoring for threat while performing other tasks. Only this manipulation produced impairment of color-naming emotional words. These data are consistent with the hypothesis that bias can be explained as a result of a strategic threat-monitoring mechanism.

The proposal of strategic threat-monitoring effects does not rule out influences of emotion on automatic processing. Both automatic emotion-related biasing and strategic threat-monitoring effects probably operate together. However, the data reviewed do support a particular threat-monitoring and expectancy-related response as predicted by the metacognitive approach.

The precise threat-monitoring strategy seen in each disorder may depend on the particular disorder experienced. Eysenck (1992) equates generalized anxiety as being associated with hypervigilance for threat. Obsessional patients show heightened cognitive self-consciousness, the tendency to monitor thought processes (Cartwright-Hatton & Wells, 1996). Patients with health anxiety and panic often tend to monitor their own bodily symptoms for signs of ill health.

Metacognitive Coping Strategies

It is generally accepted that coping strategies such as avoidance and self-medication with uncontrolled drugs and alcohol can have negative consequences and exacerbate psychological dysfunction. These are examples of maladaptive coping behaviors that are part of the CAS. In addition, the metacognitive theory asserts that many coping behaviors are metacognitive in nature and these should be of particular interest in contributing to disorder. For example, the suppression of unpleasant thoughts has been shown to lead to enhancement or rebound of the suppressed thought, so that the strategy is counterproductive in the long term (Purdon, 1999; Wegner, Schneider, Carter, & White, 1987; Wenzlaf & Wegner, 2000). There is a large literature on the effects of thought suppression but it has produced equivocal results in terms of the reliability of immediate or delayed effects of trying to suppress a target thought. However, the overriding conclusion is that trying to suppress a thought is not entirely effective. This generally supports the idea that metacognitive thought control strategies aimed at removing thoughts from consciousness are likely to be inefficient, yet this is the strategy often reported by patients.

A central idea of the model is that worry and rumination can be used as coping strategies. This implies that they can be differentiated from worry as simply a symptom of anxiety. Wells and Davies (1994) developed the Thought Control Questionnaire (TCQ), a measure of individual differences in use of a range of thought control strategies and included worry and punishment as important and potentially counterproductive strategies. As we saw in Chapter 2, the TCQ has five subscales. Consistent data have emerged demonstrating that worry and punishment are positively associated with emotional disorder. Worry and punishment are closely related to the CAS (punishment involves negative self-evaluation). Worry and punishment differentiate motor vehicle accident survivors with acute stress disorder from those without (Warda & Bryant, 1998). Patients with OCD use more worry and punishment (Amir et al., 1997; Abramowitz et al., 2003). These thought control strategies predict lower levels of recovery from depression and PTSD (Reynolds & Wells, 1999). The use of worry to control thoughts is cross-sectionally correlated with stress symptoms in college students (Roussis & Wells, 2006).

Morrison, Wells, and Nothard (2000) examined nonpatients scoring above and below the median on a measure of proneness to hallucinations. High hallucinators endorsed greater use of punishment and greater reappraisal TCQ strategies.

Longitudinal studies show that TCQ worry measured soon after a trauma predicts the subsequent development of PTSD (Holeva et al., 2000), and is associated with greater traumatic stress symptoms following discharge from intensive care units (Knight, 2004).

Because the use of thought control strategies is linked to metacognitive beliefs about the harmful and positive consequences of negative thinking, the metacognitive theory predicts conflict or vacillation in attempts to engage with or get rid of worry or rumination. Purdon (2000) examined the *in vivo* negative appraisal of worrying in nonpatients and found that it was associated with greater attempts to get rid of thoughts. However, positive beliefs about worry emerged as simultaneous predictors of a reduced motivation to get rid of them.

Overall, the available data clearly show that some (but not all) thought control strategies, when assessed as trait variables, are positively associated with psychological disorder. Moreover, it is the worry-based and punishment-related strategies that emerge consistently, as predicted by the metacognitive model.

METACOGNITIVE BELIEFS

The Metacognitions Questionnaire (MCQ; Cartwright-Hatton & Wells, 1997) and its shorter derivative, the MCQ-30 (Wells & Cartwright-Hatton, 2004), were developed to test the metacognitive theory of psychological disorder, especially the hypothesized role of beliefs about worry. A large number of studies have used these instruments to demonstrate relationships between metacognition, emotion disorder symptoms, and psychological disorders. Erroneous metacognitions appear to be associated with trait emotion (Cartwright-Hatton & Wells, 1997), anxiety and its disorders (Wells & Carter, 2001), depression (Papageorgiou & Wells, 2001a, 2001b), psychotic symptoms and disorders (Morrison et al., 2002; Stirling, Barkus, & Lewis, 2007), alcohol abuse (Spada & Wells, 2005, 2006; Spada, Zandvoort, & Wells, 2007), and stress in the context of medical conditions (Allott, Wells, Morrison, & Walker, 2005).

Cartwright-Hatton and Wells (1997) reported positive correlations between all MCQ subscales and trait anxiety (ranging from .26 to .73). Each subscale also correlated positively with obsessions (.40–.73), checking (.28–.47), and social and health worries (.20–.69). Overall, negative beliefs concerning uncontrollability and danger of worrying showed the strongest correlations across a range of vulnerability measures. Regarding unique predictors among the MCQ subscales, obsessional thoughts were independently associated with positive beliefs about worry, negative beliefs concerning uncontrollability and danger, and poor cognitive confidence. Obsessional checking was uniquely associated with positive beliefs about worry and cognitive confidence. In each equation the inclusion of the MCQ subscales significantly increased the variance accounted for by 12–27% over and above that attributable to trait anxiety. This is a substantial amount, especially when considering that the MCQ is not a metacognitive measure designed to be specific to obsessive–compulsive symptoms.

Wells and Papageorgiou (1998b) examined relationships between metacognitive beliefs, trait worry, and obsessive–compulsive symptoms. They controlled for the overlap between worry and obsessions in examining the metacognitive predictors of each cluster of symptoms in nonpatients. Each MCQ subscale was positively correlated with compulsive checking, obsessional thoughts, and pathological worry. In regression analyses two MCQ subscales, positive beliefs about worry and negative beliefs about uncontrollability and danger, were individual predictors of pathological worry. A range of MCQ subscales also emerged as specific and unique predictors of obsessive–compulsive symptoms.

Other investigators have provided evidence of reliable links between metacognition and obsessive–compulsive symptoms. For instance, Janeck, Calamari, Riemann, and Heffelfinger (2003) found that heightened cognitive self-consciousness, that is, the tendency to monitor thoughts, differentiated OCD from a mixed anxiety disorder comparison group. Hermans, Martens, De Cort, Pieters, and Eelen (2003) compared individuals with OCD with nonanxious control participants and found differences on several metacognitive belief dimensions. Participants with OCD held higher negative beliefs about the uncontrollability and danger of mental events, they reported more negative beliefs about the harmful consequences that might follow from having specific thoughts, they monitored their thoughts more, and they had lower confidence in their cognitive abilities. Lower cognitive confidence appeared to be present on three dimensions: (1) memory for actions, (2) discriminating actions from imaginations, and (3) resistance to distraction. In a different line of research on the effects of behavior on metacognition, Van den Hout and Kindt (2003a, 2003b) showed that repeated checking did not affect the accuracy of memory but it did affect meta-memory. Specifically, checking reduced confidence in memory.

Bouman and Meijer (1999) used the MCQ to explore beliefs about worry in hypochondriasis. These researchers addressed the question of whether hypochondriacal individuals are more concerned about their illness-related worries than they are about worrying, thereby also addressing the question of whether these individuals show content-specific metacognitions. These authors substantiated previous findings of significant associations between the MCQ factors and proneness to pathological worry as assessed by the Penn State Worry Questionnaire. Furthermore, they showed that a measure of hypochondriasis was positively associated with two MCQ dimensions: (1) negative beliefs about uncontrollability and danger and (2) the need to control thoughts including themes of superstition, punishment, and responsibility.

Davis and Valentiner (2000) showed that subjects with generalized anxiety had higher scores than individuals in nonworried anxious groups on negative metacognitive belief dimensions; uncontrollability and danger, and negative beliefs concerning the need to control thoughts including superstition, responsibility, and punishment.

Spada and Wells (2005) examined the relationship between the MCQ-30 and two measures of alcohol use and problem drinking. Positive beliefs about worry and negative beliefs concerning uncontrollability and danger were positively associated with a measure of the quantity and frequency of alcohol consumption in the last 30 days, and with an alcohol disorders screening measure. Low cognitive confidence and beliefs about need to control thoughts were also positively associated with a quantity and frequency measure. Beliefs about need to control thoughts significantly predicted alcohol use even when anxiety and depression were controlled.

In a semistructured interview study of 10 patients with problem drinking, metacognitive profiling revealed that all patients reported positive metacognitive beliefs about using alcohol as a cognitive, emotional, and self-image regulation strategy. Six patients endorsed negative metacognitive beliefs. Nine out of 10 patients reported that they did not know when they had achieved their self-regulatory goal while drinking and that their stop signal was becoming ill or blacking out, suggesting metacognitive monitoring anomalies (Spada & Wells, 2006). In an endeavor to further test the metacognitive theory applied to alcohol abuse, Spada and Wells (2008a) developed the Positive Beliefs about Alcohol Use and Negative Beliefs about Alcohol Use Scales. These measures are correlated with alcohol misuse measures, with positive beliefs explaining variance in alcohol misuse measures over and above alcohol expectancies (Spada, Moneta, & Wells, 2007).

Despite the fact that the metacognitive approach was developed initially to account for emotional disorder, it also appears to apply to psychotic symptoms. The relationship between metacognitive beliefs and proneness to auditory hallucinations has been tested in several studies. Morrison et al. (2000) adapted the Launay–Slade Hallucination Scale to measure predisposition to auditory and visual hallucinations and relationships with metacognition in a nonpatient population. Positive beliefs about unusual perceptual experiences were the best predictor of predisposition to hallucinations. Those participants who scored higher on predisposition had higher scores on the MCQ subscales of uncontrollability and danger, need for control involving superstition, punishment, and responsibility, and cognitive self-consciousness.

Lobban, Haddock, Kinderman, and Wells (2002) investigated differences on a modified version of the MCQ between schizophrenic patients who were currently experiencing auditory hallucinations and those who had never had hallucinations. Control groups included a group of patients with anxiety disorders and a group of nonpatients. Current hallucinators differed from never-hallucinating schizophrenic patients on beliefs that thoughts needed to be consistent. Other differences between groups were found on cognitive self-consciousness, where hallucinators had higher scores than nonpatients. Current hallucinators also had higher scores on uncontrollability and danger than the anxiety control group.

In a nonclinical study of predictors of proneness to auditory hallucinations, Morrison et al. (2002) found that MCQ positive beliefs about worry and positive interpretations of voices individually predicted predisposition to hallucinations when trait anxiety and other MCQ subscales were entered.

Stirling et al. (2007) sought to determine whether healthy individuals distinguished in terms of hallucination proneness or level of schizotypy could also be differentiated on subscales of the MCQ. Schizotypy is regarded as a trait that reflects the extent to which an individual is prone to psychosis. Two versions of the MCQ were used: the original scale and a modified scale that replaced items relating to worry with items relating to thinking or reflecting on thinking. Highly significant differences were obtained between groups of individuals categorized in terms of high, medium, or low proneness to hallucinations on four out of five MCQ subscales and three out of four modified subscales. Higher hallucination-prone individuals scored higher on uncontrollability and danger, lower on cognitive confidence, and higher on negative beliefs concerning need to control thoughts. Schizotypy correlated positively and significantly with all five of the MCQ subscales. Thus, high schizotypes simultaneously have stronger positive and negative beliefs about worrying, have doubts about their cognitive functioning (cognitive confidence), and have concerns about the negative consequences of not controlling thoughts.

These data on relationships between metacognitive beliefs and psychotic symptoms demonstrate a reliable positive association with metacognitive domains. However, the precise domain varies, perhaps depending on whether the sample is a clinical group or not, and depending on the symptom measure utilized. The data support the idea that positive and negative metacognitive beliefs are linked to psychological vulnerability by extending this finding to psychotic experiences.

Apart from the data examining metacognitive vulnerability to anxiety, worry, alcohol abuse, and psychosis, studies have tested links between metacognition and depression and trait measures of depressive rumination. Papageorgiou and Wells (2001a) used a semistructured interview to explore the presence of metacognitive beliefs about rumination in patients with DSM-IV recurrent MDD. All patients reported both positive and negative metacognitive beliefs about rumination. The content of positive beliefs reflected the theme that rumination was a coping strategy, while the content of negative beliefs focused on rumination being uncontrollable and harmful. The beliefs elicited in this study were the basis of two subsequent measures developed to assess positive and negative beliefs about rumination.

Tests of the metacognitive model of depression have used the Positive Beliefs about Rumination Scale (PBRS; Papageorgiou & Wells, 2001b) and the Negative Beliefs about Rumination Scale (NBRS; Papageorgiou, Wells, & Meina, 2008). The PBRS is positively correlated with rumination ($r = .53$) and with depression ($r = .45$) in nonclinical samples (Papageorgiou & Wells, 2001b, 2001c, 2003), and in individuals with clinical depression (Papageorgiou & Wells, 2003). Similarly, negative metacognitive beliefs have been found to correlate positively with rumination and depression in nonclinical (Papageorgiou & Wells, 2001c, 2003) and clinically depressed ($r = .54$) individuals (Papageorgiou & Wells, 2001c). Furthermore, positive and negative metacognitive beliefs distinguish patients with recurrent major depression from patients with panic disorder, agoraphobia, or social phobia (Papageorgiou & Wells, 2001b).

Taken together, these studies demonstrate consistent positive relationships between metacognitive beliefs, emotional vulnerability, and a wide range of psychological disorders. Relationships exist for both positive and negative metacognitions as implicated in the metacognitive model. Beliefs about the uncontrollability and danger of thoughts appear to be particularly important.

INTERIM SUMMARY

In summary, there is a large body of evidence supporting the existence of the CAS in psychological disorder. Furthermore, worry and rumination appear to have negative consequences for self-regulation, as predicted by the metacognitive model. Attentional bias can be identified with strategic processing and the patient's strategy for anticipating and coping with threat, consistent with predictions. Metacognitive regulation strategies can be distinguished that appear to relate to increased vulnerability and to play a causal role in the development of traumatic stress symptoms. Consistent with the effects predicted by the model, perseverative strategies of worry and punishment are associated with emotional disorder. Finally, positive and negative metacognitive beliefs have been identified in semistructured interviews, and measures of these beliefs are consistently and positively correlated with a wide array of indices of vulnerability to emotional and psychological disorder.

CAUSAL STATUS OF THE CAS AND METACOGNITIONS

Earlier in the chapter evidence was reviewed supporting a causal role of the CAS in psychological disorder. To recap, longitudinal studies of the effects of rumination following stressful life events show that this aspect of the CAS is associated with greater levels of subsequent stress symptoms and depression (e.g., Nolen-Hoeksema, 2000). Furthermore, laboratory manipulations of rumination and mood have demonstrated that rumination can prolong dysphoric mood responses (see Lyubomirsky & Tkach, 2004, for a review).

Experimental manipulations that increase the experience of worry have been shown to lead to greater intrusive thoughts during a subsequent nonworry task (Borkovec et al., 1983). The induction of brief periods of worry following exposure to stressful material is associated with an increase in intrusive images over a subsequent 3-day period (Butler et al., 1995; Wells & Papageorgiou, 1995).

Further data of relevance to the causality question is available. Rassin, Merckelbach, Muris, and Spaan (1999) investigated the effects of experimentally induced metacognitive beliefs on obsessional thoughts in nonpatients. In this study participants were led to believe that an EEG apparatus to which they were connected would detect the occurrence of the thought "apple," and on detecting that thought would deliver an electric shock to another participant the subject had just met. Subjects were informed that they could interrupt the electric shock by pressing a button within 2 seconds after the word "apple" had surfaced in their consciousness. In a comparison condition subjects were told that the EEG could detect the thought "apple" but no information about shocks was given. The manipulation of metacognitive beliefs resulted in more intrusions, greater discomfort, more internally directed anger, and greater efforts to avoid thinking.

Nassif (1999) conducted a prospective study of the development of generalized anxiety and pathological worry. She demonstrated that negative metacognitive beliefs about uncontrollability and danger predicted the development of generalized anxiety several weeks later. Yilmaz, Gencoz, and Wells (2007a) showed that metacognitive beliefs measured at time 1 predicted the development of symptoms of anxiety or depression 6 months later even after controlling the effect of stressful life events.

A large number of studies have investigated the effects of manipulating thought suppression. These studies have shown that thought suppression can lead to an increase in the occurrence of the unwanted thought.

However, the results are inconsistent with some studies showing an imme-diate effect during suppression and others showing a delayed rebound of the unwanted thought once suppression ceases or no effect at all (e.g., Wegner et al., 1987; Merckelbach, Muris, van den Hout, & de Jong, 1991; Lavy & van den Hout, 1990; Muris, Merckelbach, van den Hout, & de Jong, 1992; Roemer & Borkovec, 1994). These differences have been attributed to methodological differences between studies, but taken together it seems safe to say that suppression appears to be an inconsistent strategy.

In a longitudinal study of the development of PTSD Holeva et al. (2001) demonstrated that the tendency to use worry as a means of con-trolling thought intrusions predicted the subsequent development of PTSD following motor vehicle accidents. Roussis and Wells (2008) showed that use of worry as a thought control strategy predicted stress symptoms approximately 3 months later in college students.

Overall, the studies summarized here are consistent with the view that the CAS and metacognitions play a causal role in the persistence and devel-opment of emotional symptoms and in impairments or inefficiencies in self-regulation.

DOES METACOGNITION CONTRIBUTE TO DISORDER ABOVE ORDINARY COGNITION?

In metacognitive theory, metacognitive appraisals of thoughts are consid-ered to make a contribution to disorder independently of ordinary cogni-tive appraisals or topological features of thoughts. For instance, negative interpretation of worrying (meta-worry) is considered more important in GAD than the nature of the worry. Several studies provide data relating to this prediction.

Wells and Carter (1999) tested the relative contribution of meta-worry and Type 1 worry to individual differences in pathological worry as mea-sured by the Penn State Worry Questionnaire. Meta-worry was uniquely associated with both pathological worry and the level of problem with wor-rying, and this relationship was independent of the content of worry, trait anxiety, and uncontrollability.

Nassif (1999, Study 1) tested the contribution of meta-worry to patho-logical worry in a Lebanese sample while controlling for trait anxiety and the content of worry. The strongest individual contribution to pathological worry was made by meta-worry. In a follow-up study Nassif (1999) screened nonpatients for the presence of DSM-III-R generalized anxiety and found that meta-worry was significantly higher in the group with GAD than in a nonanxious group.

Nuevo, Montorio, and Borkovec (2004) extended the study by Wells and Carter (1999) by examining the relationship between meta-worry and worry in an elderly Spanish sample. Meta-worry consistently emerged as a predictor of pathological worry and interference from worry, relationships that held when the general (nonmetacognitive) content of worry, trait anxiety and uncontrollability of worry were partialed-out.

In a study of the specificity of negative meta-beliefs and appraisals to GAD Wells and Carter (2001) showed that patients with GAD had significantly higher beliefs in the uncontrollability and danger domain than other selected patient groups. When Type 1 worry frequency was treated as a covariate, these effects remained, suggesting that differences in negative metacognitions are important discriminators and are not simply a function of worry frequency.

A study by Ruscio and Borkovec (2004) examined differences in the experience of worry and the appraisal of worry in high worriers with and without GAD. This study addressed whether the presence or absence of GAD can be attributed to differences in worry, to differences in metacognitions about worry, or to both. The study groups showed similar experiences and consequences of worry, but substantial differences in beliefs about worry. The GAD group showed higher negative beliefs about the uncontrollability of worry and the danger of worry.

Yilmaz, Grencoz, and Wells (2007b) tested the unique contribution of cognition and metacognition to depression. Cognition (belief) was measured with the Dysfunctional Attitudes Scale while metacognitive beliefs were measured with the Positive Beliefs about Rumination Scale and the Negative Beliefs about Rumination Scale. Results showed that the two metacognitive measures individually explained variance in depression symptoms but that subscales of the Dysfunctional Attitudes Scale did not. These results are consistent with the view that metacognitive beliefs may contribute more to depressive symptoms than do dysfunctional beliefs (schemas) in the "cognitive" domain.

Several researchers in the area of obsessive–compulsive symptoms have demonstrated specific contributions of metacognitive beliefs to symptoms over and above the contribution made by other nonmetacognitive belief domains. Gwilliam et al. (2004) tested whether metacognitive beliefs or responsibility-related cognitions predicted obsessive–compulsive symptoms in nonpatients. Both the cognitive (responsibility) and the metacognitive (fusion-related) belief domains were positively correlated with symptoms. However, the metacognitive domains were the strongest correlates and the relationship between responsibility and symptoms was no longer present when metacognitions were accounted for.

Myers and Wells (2005) also examined the relative contribution of metacognitions and responsibility cognitions to obsessive–compulsive symptoms. Both subtypes of belief were positively correlated with symptoms even when overlap with worry was controlled. The association between metacognition and symptoms remained when responsibility and worry were simultaneously included in the equation, but relationships between responsibility and symptoms did not.

The studies reviewed so far in this section are cross-sectional and do not address the relative causal roles of cognition and metacognition in the development of psychological symptoms. However, a study by Nassif (1999, Study 2) examined the longitudinal predictors of pathological worry and GAD over a 12–15-week interval. Meta-worry, but not Type 1 worry, predicted the presence of GAD at Time 2 when GAD status at Time 1 was controlled. As for pathological worry, negative metacognitive beliefs predicted worry at Time 2 when worry at Time 1 was accounted for. These results suggest that it is not cognition (i.e., Type 1 worry) but metacognition (i.e., Type 2 worry and negative beliefs about thoughts) that predicts the development of GAD.

In summary, the studies reviewed support the view that metacognitions contribute to emotional vulnerability and symptoms beyond the contribution made by cognitive constructs. Furthermore, in several instances the cognitive constructs measured did not explain additional variation in symptom measures above metacognition.

MODEL TESTING: DATA FROM PATH ANALYSES AND STRUCTURAL EQUATION MODELING

Several studies have set out to directly test the disorder-specific metacognitive models using path analysis and structural equation modeling (SEM) techniques. These studies have shown that the metacognitive models have either an acceptable fit to the data with no modifications or fit following minor theoretically consistent modifications.

Papageorgiou and Wells (2001b) examined the relationships between positive metacognitive beliefs about rumination, rumination, and depression. The S-REF model proposes that positive beliefs give rise to the CAS, which gives rise to psychological disturbance. Translating this account into a testable form gives rise to a path diagram where positive beliefs about rumination lead to rumination, which in turn leads to depression. The relationship between positive metacognitions and depression should be fully or partially mediated by rumination. Papageorgiou and Wells (2001b) showed that this was the case for both state and trait measures of depression in nonpatients.

Papageorgiou and Wells (2003) tested the fit of a more complete metacognitive model of rumination (incorporating positive and negative metacognitive beliefs) in two samples: a sample of depressed and a sample of nondepressed participants. In the depressed sample the model was a good fit to the data. In this model positive belief about rumination led to rumination, which led to negative metacognition and to depression. The relationship between rumination and depression was mediated by two negative metacognitive belief domains: uncontrollability and danger, and social consequences. In the nondepressed group the model did not fit the data well. Tests suggested that the fit of the model could be improved in the nonclinical sample by including direct and indirect paths between rumination and depression. The indirect path was mediated by negative metacognitions about the social consequences of rumination. These results suggest that direct and indirect effects of rumination on depression might depend on whether or not individuals are currently depressed. Overall, the data show that the metacognitive model incorporating prespecified theory-based pathways involving positive and negative metacognitive beliefs and rumination fits the data of depressed individuals.

Subsequently, Roleofs et al. (2007) tested the depression model in Dutch undergraduates. They found that following some theoretically consistent modifications the model was an adequate fit to the data. The results were consistent with the metacognitive model of depression in which there are both direct and indirect links between rumination and depression involving negative metacognitions. Furthermore, these authors added a link to the structural model by including self-discrepancies activating positive beliefs about rumination, as implicated as a mechanism in the original S-REF model. Evidence was found for positive beliefs about rumination partially mediating the relationship between self-discrepancies and rumination. These results extend the depression model and bring it further in line with the founding S-REF model by supporting links between self-discrepancies and thinking styles that are mediated by positive metacognitive beliefs.

Similar analytic strategies have been applied to testing the specific metacognitive models of traumatic stress symptoms, obsessive–compulsive disorder, generalized anxiety, and alcohol abuse.

Roussis and Wells (2006) tested path models of relationships between metacognitive beliefs, thought control strategies of worry, and traumatic stress symptoms as predicted by the metacognitive model of PTSD. The relationship between positive metacognitive beliefs about worry and symptoms was mediated by the tendency to use worry as a thought control strategy. However, the relationship between negative beliefs about worry and stress symptoms was not mediated by the use of worry. This pattern of results is consistent with the metacognitive model in which symptoms activate negative beliefs and interpretations of symptoms, while positive metacognitive beliefs exert their effect through the person's coping strategies. In a subsequent study (Roussis, 2007), structural equation modeling confirmed the fit of a model in which positive beliefs exert an effect on symptoms via strategies of worry. Negative beliefs were involved in a cyclical relationship, with symptoms feeding back into them via negative interpretation of the occurrence of thoughts.

Work on obsessive–compulsive symptoms has shown that the metacognitive model depicting the relationship between thought fusion beliefs, appraisal, and beliefs about rituals and symptoms fits the data well in nonpatients. Tests of alternative rival models of relationships among these variables did not fit the data (Myers, Fisher, & Wells, 2007).

In generalized anxiety, the relationship between negative metacognitive beliefs and group membership (GAD vs. non-GAD) is mediated by the frequency of meta-worry (Wells, 2005). Thus, pathological worry fits a model in which negative metacognitive belief leads to a greater frequency of meta-worry and GAD.

Alcohol abuse also appears to fit an S-REF-based model. Spada and Wells (2008b) specified a model in which emotion activates positive metacognitive beliefs about using alcohol as a self-control strategy. However, diminished self-monitoring occurs with drinking, which constitutes an indirect link between positive beliefs and drinking. Problem drinking is also associated with negative beliefs about uncontrollability, which have a cyclical relationship with drinking behavior.

In a test of relationships between emotion and smoking dependence, Spada, Nikcevic, Moneta, and Wells (2007) showed that metacognition partially mediated this relationship. Without metacognition, the model linking emotion with smoking dependence no longer fitted the data.

SUMMARY OF EVIDENCE ON THEORY

In summary, there is clear evidence of a CAS across psychological disorders of the kind specified in metacognitive theory. Furthermore, clear deleterious consequences of worry and rumination and metacognitively focused coping behaviors have been demonstrated. A small proportion of the research has sought to manipulate worry and rumination and to explore the longitudinal consequences of these strategies. These studies show that conceptual processing and metacognitive control of this kind has the predicted negative consequences for emotion, adaptation, and performance.

The evidence supports the view that coping strategies are associated with disorder, and that metacognitively focused coping strategies contribute to the development of disorders following stress. Attentional bias data fits a model of individuals strategically maintaining anxiety on sources of threat. Although not reviewed here, the literature is also replete with data on links between elevated self-focused attention (a marker for the CAS) and psychological disturbances (e.g., Ingram, 1990; Wells & Matthews, 1994).

Tests of metacognitive models of specific disorders, namely, PTSD, GAD, depression, and OCD, support relationships with metacognitions. The relationships also appear in alcohol abuse, smoking dependence, and psychoses. Testing of fully specified models suggests that the data generally fit the models.

The theory and models behind MCT appear to be supported by a growing database using a wide range of methodologies on patient and nonpatient samples. Overall the findings are consistent across a range of anxiety, mood, psychotic, and addiction-related disorders.

The Evidence on Treatment

In the remainder of this chapter I describe the studies that have examined the effectiveness of specific metacognitive treatment techniques and of overall treatment, beginning with attention training.

Effectiveness of Attention Training

The effects of attention training have been evaluated using formal single-case experimental designs and trial methodologies. These studies support the positive effects of the ATT as a stand-alone procedure on anxiety and mood. Studies have also examined the impact of the ATT on underlying mechanisms of worry/rumination and metacognitive beliefs. Despite the fact that the ATT was not intended originally to be a treatment in its own right, preliminary evidence suggests that the effects of the ATT are surprisingly large.

Wells (1990) reported the first study of the ATT in a single case of a patient with Panic Disorder and relaxation-induced anxiety. After a no-treatment baseline period, the ATT was associated with a reduction and eventual elimination of panic attacks in the first ATT treatment phase. This was followed by a phase of autogenic training aimed at reversing external focus and reinstating body focus. This phase was associated with a recurrence of panic attacks, which then ceased following reintroduction of the ATT. Treatment gains were maintained at 3- and 12-month follow-up. The contrasting effects of the ATT versus autogenic relaxation suggest that ATT effects are not simply due to relaxation, but are more likely to reflect reductions in self-focused rumination or monitoring of symptoms.

In a subsequent systematic replication series across patients, Wells, White, and Carter (1997) tested ATT effects in two panic disorder cases and one social phobia case. A "true-reversal" methodology was used in the social phobia case in which an initial phase of the ATT was followed by instructions to engage in a phase of body-focused attention, after which the ATT was reintroduced. By reversing ATT mechanisms and reinstating symptoms, it was possible to ensure that the ATT produced treatment effects if reintroduction of the ATT ameliorated symptoms once again. In this case the ATT was associated with reductions in anxiety and negative beliefs. This effect was reversed by the self-focus manipulation, but the beneficial effects were reinstated with a reintroduction of the ATT. In the two panic cases, which did not involve reversals, the ATT was associated with significant decreases in panic attacks and reductions in negative beliefs. In all cases gains were maintained at 3- and 6-month posttreatment assessments.

Papageorgiou and Wells (2000) examined the effects of the ATT across four consecutive cases of recurrent MDD. The duration of the current MDD episode ranged from 4 to 11 months, and the number of previous MDD episodes ranged from two to four. Patients were allocated to 3–5-week no-treatment baselines and the ATT was delivered over five to eight sessions. Each case showed marked improvements in anxiety and depression. Treatment gains were maintained at 3-, 6-, and 12-month posttreatment follow-up. Diagnostic screening at 12-month follow-up showed that none of the patients met criteria for MDD. This study included measures of automatic thoughts, rumination, self-focus, and metacognitions. Substantial reductions were shown in all of these parameters following treatment and were maintained over follow-up.

Papageorgiou and Wells (1998) tested the effects of the ATT across three patients with hypochondriasis. No-treatment baselines were extended until stability was observed in the outcome measures. The three patients reported that they had suffered from hypochondriasis for 11, 20, and 35 years. All patients showed a large reduction in the frequency of health-related worry, illness beliefs, and body-focused attention associated with treatment. Improvements persisted over the 3- and 6-month follow-up interval. Patients also showed large reductions in scores on the Somatosensory Amplification Scale (Barsky, Wyshak, & Klerman, 1990), a measure of the tendency to exaggerate and misinterpret bodily sensations.

A randomized controlled trial of the ATT was conducted by Cavanagh and Franklin (2000). They allocated hypochondriacal patients to six sessions of the ATT or to a no-treatment condition. The control group showed no improvement in symptoms. However, the ATT-treated group showed significant improvements in a range of outcome measures. There were substantial improvements in degree of health worry, disease conviction, and behavioral measures at posttreatment and at 18-month follow-up. The researchers concluded that the ATT appears to be a clinically effective treatment for hypochondriasis.

Attention training has been incorporated in a "cognitive control" training package by Siegle, Ghinassi, and Thase (2007). Depressed patients were randomly allocated to the attention treatment plus treatment as usual or just treatment as usual. Outcome was assessed in terms of effects on depressive symptoms and rumination. In a subsample the neuropsychological effects were examined using fMRI and pupil dilation. Patients who received 2 weeks of the attention treatment showed significantly greater improvements in depression and rumination than those receiving treatment as usual. Improvement after 2 weeks of the attention treatment was greater than the average change in depression associated with the usual 6-week treatment program. Preliminary fMRI data showed neuropsychological changes in amygdala activity in the attention treatment group. From pre- to posttreatment right amygdala responses increased in response to positive words and decreased in response to negative and neutral words.

Valmaggia, Bouman, and Schuurman (2007) examined the feasibility of using the ATT to treat auditory hallucinations in a patient suffering from schizophrenia who had not responded to earlier psychological intervention. They appeared to find an improvement in symptoms during the ATT, but the design precludes conclusions because of the absence of a baseline. Nevertheless, the data do show that the ATT might be used with this client group and sets the stage for studies in this direction in the future.

In summary, the data on effects of the ATT appear to be reliable across a range of disorders. The effects are clearly replicable and suggest that a brief attention modification is associated with a reduction in symptoms of anxiety and depression. The technique appears to impact on worry, rumination, and negative metacognitive beliefs. Data from controlled trials is limited at the present time but is available in a study of hypochondriasis and a study of depression. These studies show that the ATT alone or in combination with treatment-as-usual was effective.

Effectiveness of Metacognitive Exposure Strategies

In addition to more intensive treatment techniques such as the ATT, metacognitive therapy incorporates a range of specially devised treatment strategies that are intended to facilitate cognitive and emotional change. These techniques are part of metacognitively delivered exposure.

Metacognitively delivered exposure is brief, has an explicit metacognitive rationale, and utilizes techniques such as in-situation attention focusing and detached mindfulness to enhance change. What is the evidence that these approaches are more effective than brief exposure alone?

Wells and Papageorgiou (1998a) examined the relative effects of brief exposure presented with a habituation rationale against exposure with a rationale emphasizing shifting away from self-processing and onto the features of the external social environment. In a repeated measures cross-over study, patients with social phobia showed significantly greater reductions in anxiety and negative beliefs in the attention condition compared with the exposure condition. These results support the enhanced effects of metacognitively delivered exposure in which the style of attention is manipulated in order to facilitate learning.

In a different evaluation of metacognitively delivered exposure in OCD, Fisher and Wells (2005) tested the relative effects of brief exposure and response prevention configured as a metacognitive experiment against exposure and response prevention with a habituation rationale. Exposure consisted of listening to obsessional thoughts played on a closed-loop tape. The habituation rationale emphasized staying with the thoughts rather than avoiding them through neutralizing so that the patient could discover that anxiety decreases. The metacognitive rationale emphasized that the patient believed that obsessional thoughts were important and a way to discover this was not true was by abandoning rituals in response to them. Both rationales were seen as equally credible. The metacognitively delivered exposure and response prevention produced significantly greater reductions in anxiety, urge to neutralize, and negative beliefs than the habituation condition.

These initial findings are consistent with the view that specific metacognitive techniques such as situational attentional refocusing and metacognitive experiments can produce significant changes in anxiety and beliefs. Moreover, these effects are not simply attributable to nonspecifics such as credible rationales and expectancies or the effects resulting from brief exposure to feared stimuli. Metacognitively delivered exposure appears to have an effect beyond the effects of brief exposure alone.

Effectiveness of Full MCT

To date, several studies of the effectiveness of MCT have been completed, and other studies are ongoing. These studies have evaluated the effects of MCT in GAD, social phobia, PTSD, OCD, and MDD.

In an open trial of patients suffering from DSM-IV generalized anxiety disorder, Wells and King (2006) treated patients with 3 to 12 weekly sessions of MCT, with each session lasting 45–60 minutes. The sample was recruited from referrals made to a psychological service by general practitioners and psychiatrists. Fifty percent of the patients had more than one diagnosis, with 40% meeting criteria for an additional depressive disorder. None of the patients were screened for Axis II problems. The duration of GAD ranged from 2 to 60 years. Pretreatment scores on trait anxiety and worry measures were comparable to those in other trials. All patients improved during the course of MCT and these improvements were large and statistically significant. Posttreatment effect sizes were very large: BAI

= 1.82, trait anxiety = 2.78, meta-worry = 1.47, social worry = 1.13, health worry = 1.12, and BDI = 1.41. These effect sizes were of similar magnitude at 6- and 12-month follow-up. Using clinically significant change criteria on trait anxiety showed that 87% of patients were recovered at posttreatment and all patients met criteria for clinically significant improvement. At 6- and 12-month follow-up 75% of patients remained recovered.

In a randomized trial MCT was compared with applied relaxation in the treatment of patients suffering from GAD (Wells, Welford, King, Papageorgiou, Wisely, & Mendel, 2008). The results showed that MCT was superior to applied relaxation in producing improvements in anxiety, worry, and negative metacognitive beliefs. Effect sizes for MCT were very large, and recovery rates for MCT were 80% at posttreatment and 70% at 6- and 60% at 12-month follow-up as assessed by trait anxiety. Recovery rates were 80% at posttreatment and 70% and 80% at follow-up as assessed by the Penn State Worry Questionnaire. These rates are higher than the aggregated recovery rates for previous trials of applied relaxation, cognitive therapy, or CBT (see Fisher, 2006).

Turning to social phobia, studies have evaluated the Clark and Wells (1995) cognitive treatment of social phobia, which is based in part on the metacognitive model. These studies show that the treatment is effective. Clark et al. (2003) compared the treatment to the selective serotonin reuptake inhibitor fluoxetine plus exposure or placebo with exposure. At posttreatment the cognitive treatment performed significantly better than the other two conditions on measures of social phobia; this effect was maintained at 1-year follow-up. However, in its original form as evaluated in these studies the treatment is multimodal and also incorporates more traditional CBT techniques alongside MCT strategies.

With a view to enhancing and abbreviating the social phobia treatment, Wells and Papageorgiou (2001) returned to examining the metacognitive basis of the treatment and tested a more focused metacognitive form. In a single case replication series across six patients with social phobia the brief treatment appeared to be effective, with all patients showing substantial improvements. Gains were maintained over follow-up. Mean level of improvement in Fear of Negative Evaluation was 13.8 (57%) and in Social Avoidance and Distress 12.8 (62%). This was achieved in a mean of 5.5 treatment sessions (range four to eight) each of 45–60 minutes duration.

The effectiveness of MCT for PTSD has been examined in several studies. Wells and Sembi (2004b) treated six consecutive patients with DSM-IV PTSD using an A-B with follow-up direct replication. Follow-up assessments were conducted at 3- and 6-month posttreatment and at the longer term of 18–41 months. The patients had been exposed to sexual or violent crimes and had been suffering from PTSD for a period of 3–10 months. In all cases treatment was associated with large reductions in traumatic stress, anxiety, and depression symptoms. The mean level of improvement in symptoms measured by the Impact of Events Scale (IES) was 83%, and as measured by the Penn Inventory, 69%. A further two consecutive cases were added to the series and posttreatment effect sizes ranged from 3 to 5. None of the patients met criteria for PTSD at the 3, 6, and longer-term follow-up assessments.

In a subsequent open trial of chronic PTSD, Wells, Welford, et al. (2008) treated 12 patients in a mean of 8.5 sessions. In these cases the duration of PTSD ranged from 6 to 39 months. Large and statistically significant improvements were found in traumatic stress symptoms, anxiety, and depression. The gains were maintained over 3- and 6-month posttreatment follow-up. The application of standardized recovery criteria showed that at 6-month follow-up 89% of patients were reliably improved or recovered as measured by the IES.

Colbear and Wells (2008) conducted a randomized controlled trial of MCT for PTSD. Patients were randomly allocated to either a wait list or an MCT treatment condition. The patients in the control group showed little or no improvement in symptoms during the wait period, while the treated group showed significant improvement in all symptom measures. Examination of clinically significant change showed that 80% of the treated patients recovered and 10% reliably improved in the MCT condition compared with only 10% of patients who improved and none who recovered in the wait list condition on the basis of the IES.

MCT has been evaluated in the treatment of OCD in adult and child populations. Fisher and Wells (2008) used a direct replication series to examine the effects of treatment in four patients with DSM-IV OCD. Patients were assigned to no-treatment baselines of 3–4 weeks until stability in baselines were clear. Following baseline MCT was delivered weekly for 12–14 sessions and patients were followed up for 3 and 6 months after treatment. In all cases posttreatment and follow-up scores on OCD and metacognition measures showed substantial levels of improvement. All four patients met standardized recovery criteria at posttreatment (Yale-Brown Obsessive–Compulsive Scale [Y-BOCS] cutoff = 14, reliable change = 10). One patient no longer met recovery criteria at 6 months but was still reliably improved. Six-month data was not available on another patient, but the other two patients retained their recovery status.

Simons, Schneider, and Herpertz-Dahlmann (2006) examined the effects of metacognitive treatment for OCD in children and adolescents. A total of ten children and adolescents were randomly allocated to either MCT or exposure and response prevention conditions. The treatment combined the metacognitive treatment described in this book with elements of CBT, so it is not possible to disentangle the relative contribution of modalities. However, the data suggested that this treatment might be a useful alternative to exposure and response prevention.

Rees and van Koesfeld (2008) conducted an open trial of group MCT for patients suffering from OCD. Outcome was assessed using the Y-BOCS and metacognitions were assessed with the MCQ-30. Statistically significant improvements were found in OCD symptoms measures at posttreatment. Gains continued to be made over the 3-month follow-up. Reductions were also found in some metacognition subscales, especially beliefs about need to control thoughts that were maintained over follow-up. The posttreatment and follow-up effect sizes for the Y-BOCS were 2.28 and 3.57, with a mean reduction of 62% on the Y-BOCS by follow-up. Using cutoff criteria on the Y-BOCS, 40% of patients were recovered as posttreatment; this increased to 95% meeting criteria for recovery at 3-month follow-up. The study is limited by the lack of a comparison control condition, but the significant improvement over follow-up is intriguing and may capitalize on random fluctuation or spontaneous recovery. However, the results are consistent with a large effect associated with MCT.

Turning to MDD the results of two studies provide preliminary evidence of the effects of MCT. In an A-B multiple baseline study, patients were treated with six to eight weekly sessions of MCT (Wells, Fisher, et al., 2008). Large improvements were seen in depression, anxiety, and metacognitions. For example, mean pretreatment BDI score was 24.35 and mean posttreatment score was 6.5. At posttreatment and 3-month follow-up all patients met standardized recovery criteria on the BDI. At 6-month follow-up one patient fell outside the cutoff for recovery but continued to show statistically reliable improvement. Although preliminary and based on a limited sample, the data support further evaluation.

This multiple baseline series was followed by an open trial of MCT for patients suffering from MDD (Wells, Fisher, et al., 2008). Treatment was associated with very large improvements in depression and anxiety symptoms assessed by self-report and interviewer ratings. Treatment was associated with large reductions in rumination and maladaptive metacognitive beliefs. Using formal criteria for clinical significance of change and for recovery showed that 75% of patients were recovered at posttreatment and 66% were recovered at 6-month follow-up, based on the Hamilton Depression Scale in an intent-to-treat sample.

In summary, a growing number of studies have explored the effects of individual MCT techniques and full MCT. These studies have used formal single-case series, open trial, and randomized comparative trial methodologies. The overall conclusion that may be drawn is that MCT appears to be an effective treatment approach. The effects have been found across a range of disorders, effect sizes are large, and gains are stable over 6- or 12-month posttreatment. Limitations of the treatment outcome data are the relatively small number of randomized evaluations, but several studies are currently in progress. Longer-term stability of treatment effects is yet to be examined.

CONCLUSION

In this chapter the evidence base for metacognitive theory, techniques, and treatment has been briefly presented. Overall, there is a large database. However, not all studies have been reviewed here. For example, there is a large literature not reviewed demonstrating that self-consciousness (a proposed marker for the CAS) and its state equivalent, induced self-awareness, are positively associated with emotional vulnerability and psychological disorder (e.g., Carver & Blaney, 1977; Fenigstein & Vanable, 1992; Ingram, 1990; Wells, 1985).

There is currently a greater amount of data supporting the theory than there is data supporting treatment. Moreover, the treatment data is based mainly on small experimental evaluations. This is an inevitable consequence of the systematic approach we have taken to treatment development and evaluation.

Our strategy has been to combine theory building based on the scientific literature with clinical observation as a starting point. This has been followed by testing of the basic metacognitive theory, model building and evaluation, developing and evaluating specific treatment techniques, and constructing and evaluating treatments through single case studies before progressing to outcome trials. This approach is consistent with the progressive model of clinical research (Agras & Berkowitz, 1980).

Treatment studies clearly show effects associated with MCT. The majority of patients show reliable improvement or recovery during treatment. The effects appear to be consistent across a range of disorders, thereby establishing generalizability.

Taken as a whole, the database provides a strong case for the continued application and evaluation of MCT. It is a new and emerging approach that has been born out of systematic model building and hypothesis testing, leading to theoretically grounded techniques and applications. Further controlled studies should seek to determine the effectiveness of the treatment when conducted away from its site of origin and determine its effects over longer follow-up intervals.

CHAPTER **11**

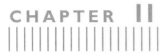

Concluding Thoughts

The principles and treatment presented in this book are the culmination of research and development aimed at producing a scientifically based understanding and treatment of psychological disorder. This approach grew out of dissatisfaction with existing psychotherapeutic approaches that do not capture important characteristics of maladaptive thinking and the factors that control it.

Psychological treatments have usually consisted of combinations of methods from a wide range of sources. Therapists have used what appears to work based on experience. While this system offers a pragmatic approach to developing intervention packages, it is not noted for producing consistent advances in understanding disorders and developing effective treatments. Significant advances could be made by basing treatments on models of how cognition is controlled and becomes locked into dysfunction. A dynamic model of maladaptive processing and mental control like that offered by metacognitive theory provides the basis for the development of theory-driven treatment techniques that might be more precisely targeted at well-specified causal psychological mechanisms and processes.

For instance, we have seen how the attention training technique (ATT) and detached mindfulness (DM) have been developed to facilitate greater metacognitive control over processing, to disrupt perseverative self-focused worry and rumination, and to strengthen alternative metacognitive experiences of thoughts. Furthermore, specific techniques have been developed, as described throughout this book, that modify erroneous and unhelpful metacognitive beliefs and plans for processing.

The metacognitive approach identifies a general style of thinking, the cognitive-attentional syndrome (CAS), across psychological disorders. The CAS is comprised of worry and rumination, attentional monitoring of threat, and coping behaviors that backfire because their effects interfere with effective self-regulation and prevent corrective learning experiences. The CAS has a range of damaging effects on emotional recovery and repair. It impairs normal emotional processing, locks cognition onto perceived sources of internal and external threat, and strengthens negative appraisals and beliefs.

For most people instances of negative thoughts and emotions are fleeting experiences. While the CAS may be activated, it is quickly brought under control and alternative and more adaptive coping is implemented. Psychological disorder involves a failure to bring the CAS under control and a lack of flexibility in implementing alternative thinking and response styles. The CAS is activated to deal with thoughts, emotions, and self-discrepancies and flexibility is impaired because of a lack of metacognitive awareness of the activity and because of metacognitive beliefs. Of particular importance, the vulnerable individual becomes locked into the CAS because of a combination of positive metacognitive beliefs (e.g., "I must worry in order to avoid threat") and negative metacognitive beliefs (e.g., "I have no control over worrying"). Positive metacognitions support the persistent and frequent use of maladaptive styles such as worry and rumination, while negative metacognitive beliefs lead to failures to attempt to exert effective control and to the perception of inner events as threatening (thereby further contributing to distress).

I have described how the CAS is an online strategic form of processing and coping. It embodies the person's strategies for dealing with threat. Thus, the concept of coping and a specific thinking style links the person's beliefs to emotional disorder. Many of the coping strategies used in psychological disorder are metacognitive strategies involving the control of thoughts by suppression or avoidance and the use of attention and perseverative conceptual strategies.

Both positive and negative metacognitive beliefs contribute to appraisals of threat. For example, the positive belief "I must pay attention to danger in order to be safe" maintains a sense of threat, while the negative belief "I have no control over my thinking" interferes with the individual's ability to give up unhelpful thinking styles. Furthermore, negative beliefs such as "thinking these thoughts will make me lose my mind" contribute to the sense of current and escalating danger. So each of these metacognitive belief domains contributes to sustained processing of threat or self-discrepancies, which maintains negative emotions.

The metacognitive theory shares with more traditional cognitive (schema) theory the idea that the individual's beliefs influence mental processing. But it also differs considerably from schema theory in several ways, most notably by specifying the specific role of metacognitive beliefs.

While schema theory identifies disorder with general social beliefs, metacognitive theory specifies that metacognitive beliefs are the major influence on thinking and on psychological disorder. Other differences are also clear. Schema theory focuses on the content of thoughts, whereas metacognitive theory focuses on the style of thinking and formulates a specific cognitive-attentional syndrome. Treatment based on schema theory does not explicitly focus on training metacognitive ways of experiencing inner events, whereas metacognitive therapy focuses on the how of experiencing them. In schema theory a cognitive architecture differentiating between levels of information processing is not specified, but in metacognitive theory it is. This is potentially important because the location of disorder within the architecture of a mental subsystem has implications for the development of treatment techniques. In particular, the identification of disorder with predominantly top-down mechanisms gives rise to greater optimism and specific approaches to modifying processes such as worry and rumination. It also opens the way for generating predictions concerning the effects of strategic processes on low-level (sub-cortical) activity.

Schema theory does not distinguish between cognitive and meta-cognitive subsystems, but metacognitive theory makes this distinction a grounding of theory whose treatment is aimed at the metacognitive level. Schema theory focuses on declarative beliefs, while metacognitive theory considers beliefs to exist in declarative and procedural forms in which the latter are not directly verbally expressible. Schema theory characterizes disordered conscious appraisals as negative automatic thoughts (NATs), while metacognitive theory focuses on chains of conceptual processing and brooding that are intermeshed with more telegraphic intrusive thoughts. Metacognitive theory views NATs as triggers for the CAS and not as the most proximal cause of disorder. As this point illustrates, metacognitive theory differentiates between types of conscious thought that have different functional relationships with knowledge and emotional outcomes. A distinction between different types of thinking is not generally made in other cognitive-behavioral treatments.

Although the metacognitive approach is based on the principle that there are core similarities in pathological mechanisms across disorders, it also recognizes that there is content specificity at the cognitive and meta-cognitive levels. For example, generalized anxiety disorder (GAD) consists of negative beliefs about the uncontrollability and danger of worrying. However, obsessive–compulsive disorder (OCD) consists of negative meta-cognitive beliefs about the meaning and power of intrusive thoughts. Thus, fusion-related beliefs are more characteristic of OCD than of GAD.

As the disorder-specific models show, metacognitive theory assumes that the CAS plays out in slightly different ways in different disorders, which are best captured by specific formulations. Despite this variety, the metacognitive approach also lends itself as a transdiagnostic treatment approach. In our early exposition we (Wells & Matthews, 1994) argued for developing a single generic treatment that might be applied as a first-line intervention for all emotional disorders. In the next section I outline the nature of such a hypothetical approach, although at the present time it remains untested.

Specifications of a Transdiagnostic Treatment

One implication of the metacognitive approach is the possible development of a single standard treatment that is effective across disorders. This would have the advantage of simplifying treatment: only one model would be used as a basis for formulation and treatment could be applied more prescriptively. While this might not generate optimal treatment effects, which would require specific model-based formulations, it could provide a first-line approach in a stepped-care model of treatment delivery, especially in cases of mild and subthreshold disorder. Patients with mild disorders could be offered a standard (generic) treatment first and, if necessary, specific treatments later.

The disadvantages of such an approach might be outweighed by a greater accessibility to treatment. However, it is prudent to remember that a generic approach of this kind has not been evaluated and is speculative. A potential danger is that failure of any standard treatment might build resistance to subsequent specific MCT interventions.

A single generic treatment should focus on modifying the CAS. What would a general treatment targeted at the CAS look like? It is likely that it would consist of the following elements:

1. Use of a universal model for case formulation
2. Socialization into the role of the CAS in problem maintenance
3. Training detached mindfulness (DM) and Attention Training (ATT)
4. Removal of worry and rumination
5. Removal of attentional threat monitoring
6. Removal of maladaptive coping
7. Repeated implementation of new thinking styles

The removal of the CAS would be achieved through a combination of techniques that should include:

1. Development of metacognitive awareness and metacognitive experiencing skills through DM and the ATT
2. Challenging metacognitive beliefs about uncontrollability
3. Challenging positive beliefs about strategy use
4. Challenging negative beliefs about the danger of thought/emotion
5. Postponement and banning of worry/rumination

6. Banning/reversing threat monitoring
7. Reversing maladaptive coping in a way that increases the flow of corrective information into experience (e.g., P-E-T-S)

A Universal Formulation

If the aim is to treat the CAS, then a formulation is required that captures the causes and consequences of the CAS in a manner that is appropriate for explaining the maintenance of all disorders. Since the disorder-specific models are grounded in the basic metacognitive (S-REF) model, a reasonable place to start would be to return to the S-REF model and present its central features in a form suitable for use as a generic case formulation. To satisfy the goals of formulation a clinical model must effectively explain the maintenance of disorder, and it must do so in a way that can be readily communicated to clients in a manner that can be used as a basis for change.

There is a trade-off between accuracy and simplicity in developing a generic formulation when compared with the disorder-specific models described in this book. The generic model is therefore better considered as a clinical heuristic rather than as a tightly specified model.

A tentative universal case formulation diagram based on the S-REF is presented in Figure 11.1. There are four elements in the formulation diagram: metacognitive beliefs, the CAS, emotion, and self-/worldview.

Metacognitive belief consists of negative beliefs about the uncontrollability of thoughts and the danger of thoughts and emotions. It also contains positive beliefs about the importance of controlling thoughts and engaging in worry/rumination and threat monitoring.

The CAS consists of the usual worry and rumination, attention to threat, and unhelpful coping behaviors.

Emotion consists of affect (anxiety, depression, anger) and its associated symptoms: physical (e.g. sweating, fatigue), cognitive (e.g. poor concentration, dissociation), and behavioral (e.g. sleep disturbance, restlessness).

The self-/worldview consists of beliefs about the self and the world outside of the metacognitive content domain. Examples include: "I'm vulnerable," "The world is dangerous," "People will ridicule me," "The future is hopeless," "I have a weak heart." This knowledge shapes the content of worry/rumination but does not drive the process, which emerges from the metacognitions.

What do the arrows represent in this model? The bidirectional arrow linking metacognitive beliefs to the CAS represent the influence of metacognitive beliefs on thinking style. The CAS is determined by accessing positive and negative metacognitions. For example, beliefs about the posi-

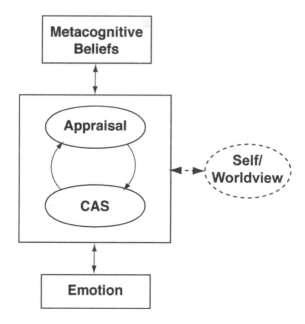

FIGURE 11.1. A potential universal case formulation diagram.

tive value of worrying and beliefs about lack of control over the process will contribute to the selection and persistence of the CAS. In turn the activity of the CAS can strengthen or modify metacognitions. For example, repeated worrying may prolong the perception of threat or block emotional processing, leading to more intrusive thoughts, feeding the sense of loss of control.

The bidirectional arrow linking emotion to appraisal/the CAS signifies that emotion activates self-regulatory processing such that appraisals/the CAS can increase, maintain, or decrease emotion. For instance, maintaining attention on potential sources of interpersonal danger maintains activation of the anxiety program.

The cyclical relationship between appraisals and the CAS signifies that negative appraisals are maintained by and can be the output of the attentional and perseverative thinking processes.

An example of this formulation for a patient with health anxiety and panic attacks is depicted in Figure 11.2. In this example, anxiety is heightened and maintained by the CAS, which consists of worry in the form of thinking about possible future panic attacks and the situations that might induce them. Threat monitoring consists of focusing on bodily sensations/responses, in this case, breathing patterns. The patient believes that by monitoring breathing it will be possible to detect fluctuations and restore regular patterns. There are beliefs about the need to control panic-related thoughts, and a positive belief about the importance of negatively inter-

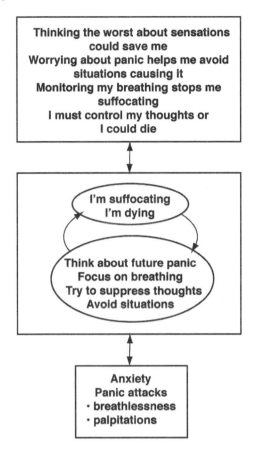

FIGURE 11.2. An example case formulation of health anxiety with panic attacks.

preting bodily sensations (e.g., "Thinking the worst about sensations could save me").

In the case presented in Figure 11.2 our hypothetical treatment focuses on removing the CAS, challenging metacognitions, and changing the processes maintaining misinterpretations. Catastrophic misinterpretations are generated or sustained via the CAS. So blocking this process in the patient and teaching him or her to engage with spontaneous inner sensations with DM should be a focus of treatment. The style of misinterpreting symptoms is also associated with positive metacognitive beliefs about "thinking the worst," and therefore such metacognitions should be targeted in treatment.

As in standard CBT, treatment might involve exposure to bodily sensations but the exposure would have the metacognitive goal of changing the

way the individual relates to symptoms as an adjunct to or instead of challenging belief. Important differences include the direct targeting of worry
and rumination processes that are seen as separate from more discrete
misinterpretations of symptoms. Thus, patients learn to experience and
respond to their misinterpretations and symptoms with lower levels of conceptual activity and with a view to abandoning attempts to remove threat.

What types of questions should the therapist ask to obtain the relevant material for the standard formulation? Some suggestions are set out
below. In constructing the formulation the therapist might first ask about
emotional symptoms, next the CAS, then metacognitive beliefs, and finally
determine the self-/worldview. This sequence might be operationalized
with questions similar to the following:

Emotion

"How have you been feeling emotionally?"
"What symptoms have you noticed?"
"What physical symptoms have you noticed?"
"What mental symptoms have you noticed?"
"Has your behavior changed?"

CAS

"Have you been worrying about your symptoms? What is that like?"
"Have you been focusing more attention on the things that concern
    you? How do you do that?"
"Have you been trying to control your thoughts and emotions?
    How?"
"Have you been interpreting events negatively?"
"Have you been dwelling on particular symptoms or concerns?"
"What have you been doing to remove danger or threat?"

Metacognitive Beliefs

"Is worrying helping you?"
"Can you stop yourself worrying?"
"Are there advantages to thinking about symptoms/anxiety/situa-
    tions?"
"Are there advantages to paying attention to threat/your body/sensa-
    tions?"
"Why is it important to control your thoughts/emotions/bodily func-
    tion?"
"What are the advantages of thinking negatively about your symp-
    toms/self/world?"

"What's the worst that could happen if you continue to feel this way/ have these thoughts?"

"What are the advantages of worrying/ruminating?"

Self-/Worldview

"When you worry/dwell on problems what do you believe/think about yourself?"

"When you worry/ruminate what conclusion do you reach about yourself or your situation?"

In Figure 11.1 metacognitive beliefs are represented separately from the "self-/worldview" which is intended to represent more general non-metacognitive beliefs. This element will not be necessary in all cases.

Neurobiology and MCT

What does the S-REF model suggest about the neurobiology of emotions and the structures and processes involved in emotional disorder? First, it predicts that emotion is an emergent property of interactions between conscious cortical processing and reflexive processing. We should find evidence of emotional networks biasing higher-level cognitive processes and of higher processes in turn activating and modulating emotional processing networks in the brain.

The amygdala has been identified as a center of emotional processing, particularly in relation to fear. As such, evidence should be found that links amygdala activity to biasing of encoding, metacognition, attention, and judgments. Similarly, evidence should be found linking changes in metacognition and conscious strategies to changes in amygdala activity in response to negative or fearful stimuli.

Since it is assumed that fear responses naturally cease if not reinforced, then activity in the amygdala must be susceptible to natural decay or top-down modulation. However, it seems that the CAS should impede such decay or modulation, thereby prolonging negative emotions. In the long term, the CAS may produce more stable changes in the amygdala as it repeatedly presents threat-related information. More generally, reduction of threat-related processing activity in the amygdala should be sensitive to aspects of the CAS namely, worry, rumination, or threat monitoring. These processes may impede top-down control necessary for reducing activity.

What effects could MCT and strategies such as the ATT and DM have on amygdala activation and its interactions with other cortical areas? It can be assumed that effectively increasing metacognitive control should be detectable in the brain regions involved in executive functioning and working memory. Thus, ATT effects and DM should impact on areas of the prefrontal cortex implicated in control. Furthermore, they should diminish activity in the amygdala and/or increase the individual's ability to modulate levels of activity when exposed to or after exposure to salient emotional stimuli. Thus, the use of strategies and thinking styles can strengthen executive control and flexibility and influence subcortical processing.

MCT IN A WIDER CONTEXT

Consciousness

Much of human experience requires consciousness of the self. Human suffering is underpinned by disturbances in the way we know and regulate ourselves.

Metacognitions support the processes involved in developing and refining the self-image. They also allow us to see our thoughts as an observer, see ourselves seeing, hear ourselves hearing, and enable us to become the dispassionate watcher of all that we think, feel, and perceive. I'm not sure that we can hear ourselves hearing—that is probably wrong—but the point is we can try to do that because we have an inner mental model of what it is like to hear, just as we have inner models of what it is like to see or to think about the self.

Our inner mental model cannot be observed: it is part of the observer. The limits of inner consciousness are probably reached at the point of DM, that is, at the point of being the observer of cognition. There is probably no further regress to be experienced beyond the sense of self as observer of conscious products during DM. It is the definitive essence of what it is to be conscious. This inexorable link between metacognition and the ability to experience a definitive self suggests an important role of metacognitive theory in developing an account of human consciousness.

Hard and Soft MCT

In this book I have largely avoided detailed discussion of the primacy of cognition versus metacognition in the development of psychological disorder. That is because these levels undoubtedly interact in all but the most simple of cognitive enterprises. However, we could assume what might be termed a "hard" or a "soft" metacognitive approach that I briefly alluded to in the introduction to this book.

The "hard" MCT approach sees negative knowledge about the self and the world as a product of metacognitions. Dysfunctional thoughts and beliefs are the current construction in online processing guided by metacognition. For example, the belief "I'm worthless" may actually be the end product of a rumination response. It is an item of knowledge that is manufactured by the individual's thinking style. We might hypothesize that use of techniques such as the "*vertical arrow*" in cognitive therapy may be nothing more than encouraging the patient to ruminate out loud in response to a negative thought.

In contrast, a "soft" MCT approach might assert that metacognitive knowledge is stored separately from other negative social knowledge but they are both stable representations in memory. Thus, other knowledge is not situationally "manufactured" by the activities of online processing. The question of which approach to take is important because, if negative self-beliefs are repeatedly generated by metacognitions guiding information processing (hard MCT), then our patients who repeatedly claim that they "feel that they are bad" are probably expressing the fact that they have metacognitions that generate this output although they might be able to rationally appraise the belief as false. However, rational evaluation does not necessarily change the metacognitions and thinking process that generates this felt experience.

In "hard" MCT a dysfunctional felt sense suggests that the metacognitions that generate this item of information are still present, but the person has acquired the metacognitive ability to rationally reevaluate this output (i.e., "I know logically I'm not bad, but I still feel as if I'm bad"). Thus, cognitive challenging of a conviction evokes metacognitive appraisal but does not necessarily change the plans that guide processing and the mode in which a thought is experienced. Level of conviction or belief may not exist as a stable cognitive representation beyond the act of appraising a thought's validity or a feeling's meaning. Perhaps the thing that truly makes thoughts tangible and realistic is their intrusive quality and the mode in which they are experienced rather than any "belief" in them. Changing the intrusiveness of thoughts and the mode in which they are experienced (object vs. metacognitive) may well modify their realism. Thus, changing a patient's inner metacognitive model of his or her thoughts rather than changing his or her beliefs is likely to be where the action lies in effective psychotherapies.

To experience a thought in object mode is to fuse that thought with perceptions of reality, but to experience that thought in metacognitive mode is to see it as an event in the mind. The more traditional challenging of conviction in cognitions may simply offer an indirect means of partially inducing the metacognitive mode. When the person no longer believes a thought is true it implies that the person is able to see it as a nonveridical event in the mind. However, that does not mean that the actual experience of the thought is one of DM. It is possible to appraise a thought as unrealistic but still not experience the thought as a separate observer. Experiential awareness rather than conceptual analysis places the thought and the individual in relative perspective and is the deeper procedural change in metacognition that is required. It is evident that as humans we do not often stand back from our thoughts and observe them as we might stand back from an oil painting and survey the entire scene. But it is possible to acquire the ability to watch our thoughts and the outside world as a complete superimposed landscape separate from self. DM and the meta-cognitive mode encompass that process of standing back. It is a process that can be implemented independently of whether a thought is accurate. DM adds to the concept of standing back by introducing the suspension of motivated attempts to analyze, cope, or exert control in response to inner experiences. It also adds the concept of subjectively experiencing self as observer, as a core and indivisible consciousness. These experiences open up the way to acquire new plans for responding to internal and external events. In a broader context they provide ways of experiencing and developing a more flexible and holistic sense of self.

CLOSING REMARKS

At the beginning of this book I set out the aim of presenting a comprehensive treatment manual for the implementation of MCT.

MCT is a form of cognitive therapy in the sense that it modifies thinking. But, as we have seen, it differs significantly from the latter in its theoretical and conceptual underpinnings, in its disorder-specific models, in its focus on processes and metacognitive knowledge, and in many of the techniques it uses. The experience of using MCT in disorders such as generalized anxiety, depression, posttraumatic stress, obsessive–compulsive disorder, social phobia, and health anxiety suggest that it often has large and rapid effects. Focusing on processing styles, experiences, and metacognitive beliefs provides an alternative to traditional procedures of repeated and prolonged exposure and questioning the content and validity of ordinary cognitions.

I began this book with a statement: "Thoughts don't matter, but your response to them does." Throughout this book I have illustrated how these responses guided by metacognitions are at the hub of emotional and conscious experience of the self and the world. In time, a complete metacognitive theory might explain the architecture and dynamics of consciousness. Then we would be able to create it artificially, but for the time being we can settle for experimenting with our own. Metacognition makes this possible because it controls the nature of thinking and allows us to transcend the limitations and difficulties associated with ordinary thought and belief. Metacognition provides a world of subjective experience and change that remains to be explored by all of us.

Appendices

METACOGNITIONS QUESTIONNAIRE 30 (MCQ-30)
Adrian Wells and Samantha Cartwright-Hatton

This questionnaire is concerned with beliefs people have about their thinking. Listed below are a number of beliefs that people have expressed. Please read each item and say how much you *generally* agree with it by *circling* the appropriate number.

Please respond to all the items, there are no right or wrong answers.

Gender: _____   Age: _____

	Do not agree	Agree slightly	Agree moderately	Agree very much
1. Worrying helps me to avoid problems in the future.	1	2	3	4
2. My worrying is dangerous for me.	1	2	3	4
3. I think a lot about my thoughts.	1	2	3	4
4. I could make myself sick with worrying.	1	2	3	4
5. I am aware of the way my mind works when I am thinking through a problem.	1	2	3	4
6. If I did not control a worrying thought, and then it happened, it would be my fault.	1	2	3	4
7. I need to worry in order to remain organized.	1	2	3	4
8. I have little confidence in my memory for words and names.	1	2	3	4
9. My worrying thoughts persist, no matter how I try to stop them.	1	2	3	4
10 Worrying helps me to get things sorted out in my mind.	1	2	3	4
11. I cannot ignore my worrying thoughts.	1	2	3	4
12. I monitor my thoughts.	1	2	3	4
13. I should be in control of my thoughts all of the time.	1	2	3	4
14. My memory can mislead me at times.	1	2	3	4

(continued)

	Do not agree	Agree slightly	Agree moderately	Agree very much
15. My worrying could make me go mad.	1	2	3	4
16. I am constantly aware of my thinking.	1	2	3	4
17. I have a poor memory.	1	2	3	4
18. I pay close attention to the way my mind works.	1	2	3	4
19. Worrying helps me cope.	1	2	3	4
20. Not being able to control my thoughts is a sign of weakness.	1	2	3	4
21. When I start worrying, I cannot stop.	1	2	3	4
22. I will be punished for not controlling certain thoughts.	1	2	3	4
23. Worrying helps me to solve problems.	1	2	3	4
24. I have little confidence in my memory for places.	1	2	3	4
25. It is bad to think certain thoughts.	1	2	3	4
26. I do not trust my memory.	1	2	3	4
27. If I could not control my thoughts, I would not be able to function.	1	2	3	4
28. I need to worry in order to work well.	1	2	3	4
29. I have little confidence in my memory for actions.	1	2	3	4
30. I constantly examine my thoughts.	1	2	3	4

Please ensure that you have responded to all items. Thank you.

(continued)

MCQ-30: Scoring Key

Enter the number given by the subject for each item in the relevant box below and then sum the scores to produce a subscale total.

POS	NEG	CC	NC	CSC
1 ___	2 ___	8 ___	6 ___	3 ___
7 ___	4 ___	14 ___	13 ___	5 ___
10 ___	9 ___	17 ___	20 ___	12 ___
19 ___	11 ___	24 ___	22 ___	16 ___
23 ___	15 ___	26 ___	25 ___	18 ___
28 ___	21 ___	29 ___	27 ___	30 ___
Total ___	___	___	___	___

The subscales are:

POS = positive beliefs about worry
NEG = negative beliefs about uncontrollability and danger of worry
CC = cognitive confidence
NC = need for control
CSC = cognitive self-consciousness

An overall total MCQ score can be obtained by summing the subscale totals.

META-WORRY QUESTIONNAIRE (MWQ)
Adrian Wells

This questionnaire assesses thoughts and ideas about worrying. Listed below are some thoughts that you may have about worrying when you notice yourself worrying. Indicate how often each thought occurs by placing a circle around a number in the *left*-hand column.

WHEN I AM WORRYING I THINK:

Never	Sometimes	Often	Almost always		
1	2	3	4	I am going crazy with worrying.	_____
1	2	3	4	My worrying will escalate and I'll cease to function.	_____
1	2	3	4	I'm making myself ill with worry.	_____
1	2	3	4	I'm abnormal for worrying.	_____
1	2	3	4	My mind can't take the worrying.	_____
1	2	3	4	I'm losing out in life because of worrying.	_____
1	2	3	4	My body can't take the worrying.	_____

When you are worrying, how much do you believe each of these thoughts? Please rate your belief by choosing a number from the scale below and put the number on the line at the *right* of each thought.

0	10	20	30	40	50	60	70	80	90	100

I do not believe this thought at all	*I am completely convinced this thought is true*

THOUGHT FUSION INSTRUMENT (TFI)
Adrian Wells, Petra Gwilliam, and Samantha Cartwright-Hatton

People have different beliefs about the power of their thoughts and experiences. Listed below are a number of these beliefs. Please read each one and indicate how much you believe it by circling a number on the right-hand scale. There are no right or wrong answers. Do not think too much about each one, indicate how much you generally believe it.

	I do not believe this at all										I am completely convinced this is true
1. If I think about an unpleasant event, it will make it more likely to happen.	0	10	20	30	40	50	60	70	80	90	100
2. If I have thoughts about harming myself, I will end up doing it.	0	10	20	30	40	50	60	70	80	90	100
3. If I think I'm in danger, it must mean I am in danger.	0	10	20	30	40	50	60	70	80	90	100
4. Having bad thoughts means I will do something bad.	0	10	20	30	40	50	60	70	80	90	100
5. If I think about an unpleasant event, it means it must have happened.	0	10	20	30	40	50	60	70	80	90	100
6. If I have thoughts about harming someone, I will act on them.	0	10	20	30	40	50	60	70	80	90	100
7. If I think things are contaminated by other people's experiences, it means they are contaminated.	0	10	20	30	40	50	60	70	80	90	100
8. My thoughts alone have the power to change the course of events.	0	10	20	30	40	50	60	70	80	90	100
9. Some objects give off bad vibes.	0	10	20	30	40	50	60	70	80	90	100
10. When I have bad thoughts it must mean I want to have them.	0	10	20	30	40	50	60	70	80	90	100
11. My feelings can be transferred into objects.	0	10	20	30	40	50	60	70	80	90	100
12. If I think of harming someone, it will harm him or her.	0	10	20	30	40	50	60	70	80	90	100
13. My thoughts become reality. If I think something, it will come true.	0	10	20	30	40	50	60	70	80	90	100
14. My memories/thoughts can be passed into objects.	0	10	20	30	40	50	60	70	80	90	100

Attention Training Techniques Summary Sheet

You have practiced the attention training technique (ATT) with your therapist. In order for the technique to work you need to practice it yourself for homework. These notes are intended to help you and provide a means of monitoring your practice.

1. You will need to find a place to practice where you can introduce or identify a range of different sounds (at least three, but the more the better). Discuss this with your therapist. Potential sounds I can introduce and use are:
   a.
   b.
   c.
   d.
   e. Sounds that may occur outside in the near distance
   f. Sounds that may occur in the far distance
   g. Sounds that may occur on the left
   h. Sounds that may occur on the right

2. Practice for 10–12 minutes as follows: Approximately 5 minutes focusing on different individual sounds; 5 minutes rapidly shifting between them/locations; 2 minutes divided attention.

3. Please note the days you have practiced by placing an X in the table below.

	Mon.	Tues.	Wed.	Thurs.	Fri.	Sat.	Sun.
Week 1							
Week 2							
Week 3							
Week 4							

Self-Attention Rating Scale

At this moment in time how much is your attention focused on yourself or on your external environment?

Please indicate by giving me a number on the scale.

−3	−2	−1	0	+1	+2	+3
Entirely externally focused			Equal amounts			Entirely self-focused

CAS-1

1. How much time in the last week have you found yourself dwelling on or worrying about your problems? (Circle a number below.)

0	1	2	3	4	5	6	7	8

None of
the time

Half of
the time

All of the
time

2. How much time in the last week have you been focusing attention on the things you find threatening (e.g., symptoms, thoughts, danger)? (Circle a number below.)

0	1	2	3	4	5	6	7	8

None of
the time

Half of
the time

All of the
time

3. How often in the last week have you done the following in order to cope with your negative feelings or thoughts? (Place a number from the scale below next to each item.)

0	1	2	3	4	5	6	7	8

None of
the time

Half of
the time

All of the
time

Avoided situations ☐   Tried not to think ☐   Used alcohol/ ☐
                        about things   drugs

Asked for ☐   Tried to control ☐   Controlled ☐
reassurance   my emotions   my symptoms

4. Below are a number of beliefs people have. Indicate how much you believe each one by placing a number from the scale below next to each item.

0	10	20	30	40	50	60	70	80	90	100

I do not believe this at all

I'm completely convinced
this is true

Worrying too much ☐   Worrying helps me cope. ☐
could harm me.

Strong emotions ☐   Focusing on possible threat ☐
are dangerous.   can keep me safe.

I cannot control my thoughts. ☐   It is important to control my thoughts. ☐

Some thoughts could make me ☐   Analyzing my problems will help me ☐
lose my mind.   find answers.

Generalized Anxiety Disorder Scale—Revised
(GADS-R)

1. How distressing/disabling have your worries been in the last week? (Circle a number below.)

0	1	2	3	4	5	6	7	8

Not at all   Moderately   Extremely—the worst they have ever been

2. How much time in the last week have you been worrying about situations? (Circle a number below.)

0	1	2	3	4	5	6	7	8

None of the time   Half of the time   All of the time

3. How often have you done each of the following in order to cope with your worry in the last week? (Place a number from the scale below next to each item.)

0	1	2	3	4	5	6	7	8

None of the time   Half of the time   All of the time

Tried to distract myself ☐   Tried not to think about things ☐

Tried to control my thinking ☐   Looked for evidence ☐

Tried to reason things out ☐   Acted cautiously ☐

Asked for reassurance ☐   Planned how to cope ☐

Talked to myself ☐   if my worries were true

4. How often in the past week have you avoided the following in order to prevent worrying? (Place a number from the scale below next to each item.)

0	1	2	3	4	5	6	7	8

None of the time   Half of the time   All of the time

News items ☐   Thoughts of illness ☐

Social situations ☐   Thoughts of accidents/loss ☐

Uncertainty ☐   Other (specify): _____ ☐

(continued)

5. Below are a number of beliefs that people have about their worries. Indicate how much you believe each one by placing a number from the scale below next to each item.

0	10	20	30	40	50	60	70	80	90	100

I do not believe this at all

I'm completely convinced
this is true

I could go crazy with worry. ☐

Worrying could harm me. ☐

Worrying puts my body under stress. ☐

If I don't control my worry, ☐
it will control me.

My worrying is uncontrollable. ☐

If I worry too much I could ☐
lose control.

Worrying helps me cope. ☐

If I worry I'll be prepared. ☐

Worrying keeps me safe. ☐

Worrying helps me get things done. ☐

Something bad would happen ☐
if I didn't worry.

Worrying helps me solve problems. ☐

Posttraumatic Stress Disorder Scale (PTSD-S)

1. How distressing and disabling have your symptoms been in the last week? (Circle a number below.)

0	1	2	3	4	5	6	7	8

Not at all   Moderately   Extremely—the worst they have ever been

2. How much of the time in the last week have you responded to your thoughts about the trauma by analyzing what happened and why? (Circle a number below.)

0	1	2	3	4	5	6	7	8

None of the time   Half of the time   All of the time

3. How much time in the last week have you been worrying about what could happen in the future? (Circle a number below.)

0	1	2	3	4	5	6	7	8

None of the time   Half of the time   All of the time

4. How often have you done each of the following to cope with your symptoms in the last week? (Place a number from the scale below next to each item.)

0	1	2	3	4	5	6	7	8

None of the time   Half of the time   All of the time

Avoided reminders of the trauma	☐	Tried to distract myself	☐
Controlled my thoughts	☐	Used alcohol/drugs	☐
Controlled my emotions	☐	Tried to work things out	☐
Avoided places	☐	Checked that things were safe	☐
Acted cautiously	☐	Avoided certain activities	☐
Planned how to cope	☐		

5. How often have you found yourself focusing your attention on potential danger in the last week? (Circle a number below.)

0	1	2	3	4	5	6	7	8

Never   Often   Always

(continued)

6. Below are a number of beliefs people have. Indicate how much you believe each one by placing a number from the scale below next to each item.

0	10	20	30	40	50	60	70	80	90	100

I do not believe this at all

I'm completely convinced this is true

I must go over events to make sense of them. ☐

It is important not to have gaps in my memory. ☐

Thinking about threats in the future will help me cope. ☐

Worrying will keep me safe. ☐

Paying attention to danger will keep me safe. ☐

I must stop thinking about what happened. ☐

It's not normal to keep thinking about the trauma. ☐

I must be weak to respond like this. ☐

I could lose my mind if I continue to think this way. ☐

I'll never be normal again. ☐

My mind has been damaged by what happened. ☐

I have lost control of my thoughts. ☐

Obsessive–Compulsive Disorder Scale (OCD-S)

1. How distressing and disabling have your obsessional thoughts/urges been in the last week? (Circle a number below.)

0	I	2	3	4	5	6	7	8

Not at all   Moderately   Extremely—the worst they have ever been

2. How often in the past week have you done the following in order to cope with your obsessions? (Place a number from the scale below next to each item.)

0	I	2	3	4	5	6	7	8

None of the time   Half of the time   All of the time

Repeatedly checked	☐	Used a mental ritual	☐
Tried to control my thinking	☐	Looked for evidence	☐
Washed or cleaned	☐	Acted cautiously	☐
Asked for reassurance	☐	Tried to make things perfect	☐
Repeated my actions	☐		

3. How often in the past week have you avoided the following? (Place a number from the scale below next to each item.)

0	I	2	3	4	5	6	7	8

None of the time   Half of the time   All of the time

News items	☐	Certain thoughts	☐
Social situations	☐	Touching certain things	☐
Touching people	☐	Uncertainty	☐

(continued)

4. Below are a number of beliefs that people have about their obsessions and rituals. Indicate how much you believe each one by placing a number from the scale below next to each item.

0	10	20	30	40	50	60	70	80	90	100

I do not believe this at all   I'm completely convinced
                                                          this is true

Obsessional thoughts could change me as a person.   ☐

If I think something is contaminated, it probably is contaminated.   ☐

Obsessional thoughts could make me do bad things.   ☐

Obsessional thoughts increase the chance of negative events in the future.   ☐

If I think something bad has happened, it probably has happened   ☐
even though I can't remember it.

Some thoughts must always be controlled.   ☐

I cannot have peace of mind unless I perform my rituals.   ☐

My anxiety will persist if I don't perform my rituals.   ☐

Something bad will happen if I don't perform my rituals.   ☐

Neutralizing my thoughts keeps others/me safe.   ☐

Major Depressive Disorder Scale (MDD-S)

1. How severe and disabling has your depression been in the last week? (Circle a number below.)

0	1	2	3	4	5	6	7	8

Not at all   Moderately   Extremely—the
worst it has
ever been

2. How much time in the last week have you been thinking about and analyzing your thoughts and feelings and trying to understand why you are like this? (Circle a number below.)

0	1	2	3	4	5	6	7	8

None of   Half of   All of the
the time   the time   time

3. How often in the past week have you done the following in order to cope with your depression? (Place a number from the scale below next to each item.)

0	1	2	3	4	5	6	7	8

None of   Half of   All of the
the time   the time   time

Tried to rest more	☐	Punished myself	☐
Tried to reason things out	☐	Analyzed why I felt like this	☐
Used alcohol	☐	Got angry at myself	☐
Decreased my activities	☐	Increased my sleep	☐
Tried not to think about things	☐		

4. How often in the past week have you avoided the following? (Place a number from the scale below next to each item.)

0	1	2	3	4	5	6	7	8

None of   Half of   All of the
the time   the time   time

Interests/hobbies	☐	Making decisions	☐
Social situations	☐	Solving problems	☐
Getting on with work	☐	Planning ahead	☐

(continued)

5. Below are a number of beliefs that people have about their depressive thinking (called rumination). Indicate how much you believe each one by placing a number from the scale below next to each item.

0	10	20	30	40	50	60	70	80	90	100

I do not believe this at all   I'm completely convinced
this is true

I cannot control my depressive thoughts (rumination). ☐

My depressive thoughts are a sign I'm losing my mind. ☐

My depressive thoughts control me. ☐

I'm defective/abnormal for thinking like this. ☐

Ruminating helps me cope. ☐

If I analyze why I feel this way, I'll find answers. ☐

Ruminating helps me understand my depression. ☐

Ruminating helps me solve problems. ☐

GAD Case Formulation Interview

Introduction: I'd like to focus on the last time you had a significant and uncontrollable worry episode and you were distressed by it. I'm going to ask you a series of questions about that experience.

1. What was the initial thought that triggered your worrying?

2. When you had that thought, what did you then worry about?

3. When you worried about those things how did that make you feel emotionally? (**Probe:** Did you feel anxious? What symptoms did you have?)

4. When you had those feelings and symptoms, did you think something bad could happen as a result of worrying and feeling that way? (**Probe:** What is the worst that could happen if you continued to worry?)

5a. Do you believe that worrying is bad in any way? (**Probe:** Can worry be harmful?)

5b. Worrying appears to be a problem, so why don't you stop worrying? (**Probe:** Do you believe worrying is uncontrollable?)

6. Apart from negative beliefs about worrying, do you think that worrying can be useful in any way? (**Probes:** Can worrying help you cope? Does it help you foresee problems and avoid them? Are there any advantages to worrying?)

7. When you start worrying do you do anything to try and stop it? (**Probes:** Do you avoid situations, ask for reassurance, try to find out if there is really something to worry about, use alcohol or drugs?)

8a. Do you use more direct strategies to try and control your thoughts, such as trying not to think about things that may trigger worrying?

8b. Have you ever tried to interrupt a worry by deciding not to engage in it at the time?

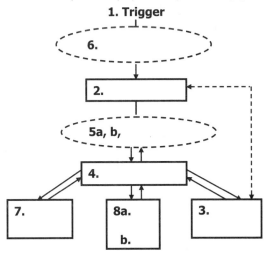

From Wells (2006). Copyright by Routledge. Reprinted by permission in Wells (2009). Permission to photocopy this appendix is granted to purchasers of this book for personal use only (see copyright page for details).

PTSD Case Formulation Interview

Introduction: I'm going to ask you about the symptoms that are causing you distress so we might explore what is maintaining them.

1. What symptoms have you repeatedly had in the last month?
   Any intrusive thoughts about the trauma, anxiety, nightmares, feeling startled, etc.?

2. When you have (specific symptoms) how do you cope or manage them?

      Probes: Do you do anything to avoid these symptoms?
               Are you trying to avoid or control thoughts?
               Are you paying attention to things differently?
               Are you going over what happened to make sense of it?
               Are you worrying about dangers in the future?
               Are you avoiding situations?
               Are you trying to control your emotions?
               Are you coping by drinking or using drugs?

3a. What are your concerns about your symptoms?
    What does it mean to you that you feel like this?
    What's the worst that could happen if you continue to have symptoms?

3b. Are there advantages to going over what happened?
    Are there advantages to worrying about danger?
    Are there advantages to focusing on danger?
    How does controlling your thoughts/emotions help?

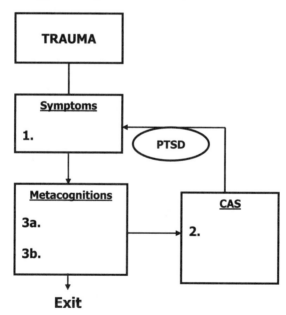

OCD Case Formulation Interview

Introduction: I'm going to ask you about the last time you were distressed by an obsessional thought and you felt compelled to respond to it. When was that?

1. What was the thought/image/impulse that triggered you?

2. When you had that thought, how did you feel emotionally (e.g., anxious/scared)?

3. What did having that thought mean? (What is the worst that could happen? What would happen if you did nothing to deal with the thought?)

4. Do you believe these thoughts mean something? What's the worst they could mean? How much did you believe that at the time?

5. Did you do anything to stop [insert negative belief about thought] from happening? Did you do anything to stop yourself doubting? Did you try to stop feeling anxious (What did you do?)? Did you engage in any rituals?

6. What are the advantages of engaging in those responses? What would happen if you no longer responded to your thoughts/doubts/feelings by doing these things? How do you know when it is safe to stop your rituals?

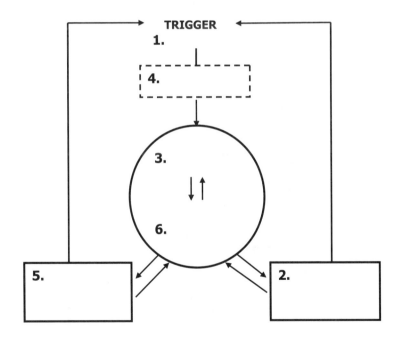

From Wells (2006). Copyright by Routledge. Reprinted by permission in Wells (2009). Permission to photocopy this appendix is granted to purchasers of this book for personal use only (see copyright page for details).

Depression Case Formulation Interview

Introduction: I'm going to ask you about a recent time when you found yourself dwelling on your problem and how bad you felt. Can you think of a recent time?

1. What was the initial negative thought that started off your dwelling?

2. What did you then think? Then what was the next thought? Then what did you think? How long did your thinking go on for?

3. When you were thinking like that what happened to your emotions? What happened to your depression? What did you end up thinking? How did it affect your behavior?

4a. It seems that rumination makes things worse. Is it something you can stop doing? How uncontrollable is it?

4b. Do you believe you can do anything about your symptoms? Do you think your depression is biological or psychological?

5. Are there any advantages to rumination or analyzing why you feel this way? Can dwelling on your feelings help you in any way?

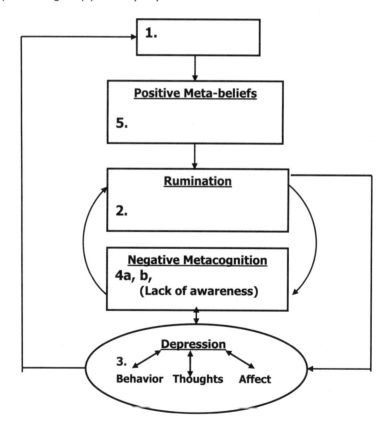

From Wells (2009). Copyright by The Guilford Press. Permission to photocopy this appendix is granted to purchasers of this book for personal use only (see copyright page for details).

GAD Treatment Plan

Yes	No	
		Session 1
☐	☐	Generate case formulation.
☐	☐	Socialize to model.
☐	☐	Run suppression experiment.
☐	☐	Begin challenging uncontrollability belief.
☐	☐	Practice detached mindfulness (DM).
☐	☐	Introduce worry postponement.
☐	☐	Homework: DM and worry postponement.
		Session 2
☐	☐	Review homework and GADS-R, especially uncontrollability beliefs.
☐	☐	Continue socialization if necessary.
☐	☐	Verbal and behavioral reattribution—uncontrollability.
☐	☐	Homework: Continue worry postponement and introduce loss-of-control experiment.
		Session 3
☐	☐	Review homework and GADS-R, especially uncontrollability beliefs.
☐	☐	Continue to challenge uncontrollability (counterevidence).
☐	☐	Run loss-of-control experiment in session.
☐	☐	Explore and ban maladaptive control/avoidance behaviors.
☐	☐	Homework: Continue worry postponement, reverse worry avoidance behaviors, loss-of-control experiment.
		Session 4
☐	☐	Review homework and GADS-R, especially uncontrollability *and* behaviors.
☐	☐	Continue challenging uncontrollability if necessary.
☐	☐	Begin challenging danger beliefs.
☐	☐	Try to go crazy, or damage self with worry experiment.
☐	☐	Homework: Push worry to test dangers.

(continued)

<u>Session 5</u>

☐ ☐ Review homework and GADS-R, especially danger belief.

☐ ☐ Continue challenging beliefs about danger.

☐ ☐ Run an in-session experiment to challenge danger.

☐ ☐ Homework: Behavioral experiments to challenge danger.

<u>Session 6</u>

☐ ☐ Review homework and GADS-R, especially danger beliefs and remaining unhelpful strategies.

☐ ☐ Continue challenging beliefs about danger.

☐ ☐ Focus on reversing any remaining maladaptive strategies.

☐ ☐ Homework: Behavioral experiments to challenge danger.

<u>Session 7</u>

☐ ☐ Review homework and GADS-R, especially danger.

☐ ☐ If negative beliefs are at zero, begin challenging positive beliefs.

☐ ☐ Homework: Mismatch strategy or other experiments to challenge positive beliefs.

<u>Session 8</u>

☐ ☐ Review homework and positive beliefs on GADS-R.

☐ ☐ Continue challenging positive beliefs.

☐ ☐ In-session mismatch strategy.

☐ ☐ Homework: Behavioral experiments (e.g., increase and decrease worry experiment).

<u>Session 9</u>

☐ ☐ Review homework and GADS-R. Check residual avoidance and maladaptive coping.

☐ ☐ Work on reversing residual symptoms.

☐ ☐ Continue challenging positive beliefs.

☐ ☐ Start work on new plan.

☐ ☐ Homework: Ask patient to write brief summary of treatment.

<u>Session 10</u>

☐ ☐ Review summary. Check GADS-R.

☐ ☐ Work on therapy blueprint (relapse prevention).

☐ ☐ Reinforce replacement plan and illustrate with example.

☐ ☐ Schedule booster sessions.

☐ ☐ Homework: Specify continued applications.

PTSD Treatment Plan

Yes	No	
		Session 1
☐	☐	Generate case formulation.
☐	☐	Socialize to model.
☐	☐	Use healing metaphor.
☐	☐	Challenge negative beliefs about symptoms.
☐	☐	Practice detached mindfulness (DM).
☐	☐	Introduce worry postponement.
☐	☐	Homework: Apply DM and worry postponement.
		Session 2
☐	☐	Review homework and PTSD-S, especially items 2 and 3.
☐	☐	Continue socialization if necessary.
☐	☐	Run advantages–disadvantages analysis of worry/rumination.
☐	☐	Practice DM.
☐	☐	Continue challenging negative beliefs about symptoms.
☐	☐	Homework: Continue DM and worry postponement.
		Session 3
☐	☐	Review homework and PTSD-S, especially items 2 and 3.
☐	☐	Challenge positive beliefs about worry and rumination.
☐	☐	Review worry postponement and broaden application.
☐	☐	Explore and ban thought suppression.
☐	☐	Homework: Continue DM and worry postponement with a broadening of application. Ban suppression.
		Session 4
☐	☐	Review homework and PTSD-S, especially items 2, 3, and 4.
☐	☐	Broaden application of worry/rumination postponement.
☐	☐	Challenge remaining positive beliefs about worry/rumination and negative beliefs about symptoms.
☐	☐	Explore and start elimination of other maladaptive coping strategies (see item 4 on PTSD-S).
☐	☐	Homework: Continue generalization of worry/rumination postponement. Ban specific maladaptive coping behaviors.

(continued)

Session 5

☐ ☐ Review homework and PTSD-S.

☐ ☐ Check the nature of any conceptual processing. Has it simply changed to another form and is still ongoing?
(More work if necessary.)

☐ ☐ Explore remaining avoidance and maladaptive coping and eliminate it.

☐ ☐ Work on residual beliefs about worry and rumination.

☐ ☐ Homework: Continue worry/rumination ban. Elimination of maladaptive coping, especially avoidance.

Session 6

☐ ☐ Review homework and PTSD-S.

☐ ☐ Run advantages–disadvantages analysis of threat monitoring.

☐ ☐ Challenge positive beliefs about threat monitoring.

☐ ☐ Ban threat monitoring. Suggest alternatives.

☐ ☐ Homework: Continue worry/rumination ban. Practice awareness and abandonment of threat monitoring.

Session 7

☐ ☐ Review homework and PTSD-S.

☐ ☐ Introduce attention refocusing.

☐ ☐ Challenge remaining positive and negative beliefs.

☐ ☐ Homework: Return to pretrauma routines and apply new strategies. Review remaining maladaptive coping.

Session 8

☐ ☐ Review homework and PTSD-S.

☐ ☐ Work on residual worry, rumination, beliefs, coping, attention.

☐ ☐ Work on residual beliefs.

☐ ☐ Begin work on therapy blueprint.

☐ ☐ Homework: Patient writes brief summary of treatment. Continue ban on worry/rumination, threat monitoring.

(continued)

<u>Session 9</u>

☐ ☐ Review homework and PTSD-S.

☐ ☐ Work on residual issues indicated on PTSD-S.

☐ ☐ Write out new plan for dealing with intrusions and symptoms.

☐ ☐ Complete therapy blueprint.

☐ ☐ Homework: Practice implementing new plan.

<u>Session 10</u>

☐ ☐ Review homework and PTSD-S.

☐ ☐ Reinforce new plan and illustrate with a hypothetical future example.

☐ ☐ Check for any residual beliefs.

☐ ☐ Schedule booster session.

☐ ☐ Homework: Specify continued application.

OCD Treatment Plan

Yes	No	
		Session 1
☐	☐	Generate case formulation.
☐	☐	Socialize to model.
☐	☐	Run suppression experiment.
☐	☐	Practice detached mindfulness (DM)—neutral thought.
☐	☐	Practice DM—obsessional thought.
☐	☐	Homework: Apply DM to intrusions.
		Session 2
☐	☐	Review homework and OCD-S.
☐	☐	Continue socialization—problem is beliefs about thoughts.
☐	☐	Further practice of DM.
☐	☐	Introduce exposure and response commission (ERC) or ritual postponement.
☐	☐	Homework: Apply ERC or ritual postponement.
		Session 3
☐	☐	Review homework and OCD-S, especially fusion beliefs.
☐	☐	Further practice of DM and ERC.
☐	☐	Verbal challenging of TEF, TAF, and TOF.
☐	☐	Run in-session behavioral experiments for TEF, TAF, and TOF.
☐	☐	Homework: Apply DM to intrusions. Run behavioral experiments.
		Session 4
☐	☐	Review homework and OCD-S, especially fusion beliefs.
☐	☐	Continue verbal challenging of TEF, TAF, and TOF.
☐	☐	Run in-session behavioral experiments for TEF, TAF, and TOF.
☐	☐	Homework: Continue DM. Run specific behavioral experiments.

(continued)

Session 5

☐ ☐ Review homework and OCD-S, especially fusion beliefs.

☐ ☐ Continue verbal challenging of TEF, TAF, and TOF.

☐ ☐ Run further behavioral experiments in session.

☐ ☐ Explore beliefs about rituals.

☐ ☐ Homework: Run specific behavioral experiments (e.g., exposure and response-prevention experiments).

Session 6

☐ ☐ Review homework and OCD-S, especially fusion beliefs and rituals.

☐ ☐ Continue challenging TEF, TAF, and TOF.

☐ ☐ Challenge beliefs about rituals.

☐ ☐ Homework: Ban rituals to test predictions about consequences. Increase exposure to thoughts.

Session 7

☐ ☐ Review homework and OCD-S, especially fusion beliefs and rituals.

☐ ☐ Continue work on TEF, TAF, and TOF (use exposure experiments).

☐ ☐ Continue modifying beliefs about rituals.

☐ ☐ Explore and begin to change stop signals.

☐ ☐ Homework: Ban rituals, practice alternative criteria for knowing, increase exposure.

Session 8

☐ ☐ Review homework and OCD-S, especially residual avoidance and beliefs.

☐ ☐ Continue work on TEF, TAF, and TOF (use exposure experiments).

☐ ☐ Continue to change stop signals and criteria for knowing.

☐ ☐ Devise new plan for dealing with intrusions.

☐ ☐ Homework: Implement new plan, increase exposure.

(continued)

Session 9

☐ ☐ Review homework and OCD-S, especially residual avoidance and rituals.

☐ ☐ Work on remaining fusion beliefs.

☐ ☐ Work on banning remaining rituals/avoidance.

☐ ☐ Begin therapy blueprint.

☐ ☐ Homework: Ask patient to work on blueprint. Implement new plan.

Session 10

☐ ☐ Review homework and OCD-S, especially any residual beliefs, avoidance, and rituals.

☐ ☐ Work on residual beliefs and behaviors.

☐ ☐ Relapse prevention: Consolidate new plan for dealing with obsessions in future.

☐ ☐ Finalize therapy blueprint.

☐ ☐ Schedule booster sessions.

☐ ☐ Homework: Specify continued application.

Depression Treatment Plan

Yes	No	
		Session 1
☐	☐	Generate case formulation.
☐	☐	Socialize to model.
☐	☐	Identify and label rumination episodes (enhancing meta-awareness).
☐	☐	Attention training technique (ATT) practice.
☐	☐	Complete ATT summary sheet.
☐	☐	Homework: ATT practice (two times per day), diary of ATT practice.
		Session 2
☐	☐	Review homework and MDD-S, especially rumination time and uncontrollability belief.
☐	☐	Introduce and practice detached mindfulness (DM).
☐	☐	Introduce rumination postponement as experiment to modify uncontrollability belief.
☐	☐	ATT practice.
☐	☐	Homework: ATT practice; apply DM and rumination postponement.
		Session 3
☐	☐	Review homework and MDD-S, especially rumination time and uncontrollability belief.
☐	☐	Identify triggers for rumination and practice DM (contrast active rumination with practice of rumination postponement in session).
☐	☐	Challenge uncontrollability metacognitions (e.g., modulation experiment).
☐	☐	ATT practice.
☐	☐	Explore activity levels and avoidant coping.
☐	☐	Homework: ATT practice; apply DM and rumination postponement (to all triggers). Increase activity levels.

(continued)

<u>Session 4</u>

☐ ☐ Review homework and MDD-S, especially rumination time, uncontrollability belief, activity levels, and unhelpful coping.

☐ ☐ Check that rumination postponement is being applied to at least 75% of triggers and rumination episodes last no longer than 2 minutes. (Reinforce greater application.)

☐ ☐ Challenge positive beliefs about rumination.

☐ ☐ ATT practice.

☐ ☐ Homework: Practice ATT, widen application of DM and rumination postponement, schedule activities.

<u>Session 5</u>

☐ ☐ Review homework and MDD-S, especially rumination time, positive beliefs, and activity level.

☐ ☐ Check consistent and wide application of DM.

☐ ☐ Continue challenging positive beliefs about rumination.

☐ ☐ Review activity levels and suggest enhancements (explore and ban other unhelpful coping, e.g., excessive sleep, alcohol).

☐ ☐ ATT practice.

☐ ☐ Homework: ATT practice, rumination postponement, increased activities.

<u>Session 6</u>

☐ ☐ Review homework and MDD-S, especially rumination time, positive beliefs, and activity level.

☐ ☐ Explore and challenge negative beliefs about emotion/depression.

☐ ☐ ATT practice (increase difficulty).

☐ ☐ Homework: ATT practice, rumination postponement, maintain activities.

<u>Session 7</u>

☐ ☐ Review homework and MDD-S, especially rumination time, beliefs, and unhelpful coping.

☐ ☐ Work on writing new plans (complete plan summary sheet and give copy to patient).

☐ ☐ Explore and modify fears of recurrence.

☐ ☐ ATT practice.

☐ ☐ Homework: Practice ATT, implement new plan, start work on therapy blueprint.

(continued)

<u>Session 8</u>

☐ ☐ Review homework and MDD-S.

☐ ☐ Relapse prevention: Complete blueprint.

☐ ☐ Work on residual metacognitive beliefs.

☐ ☐ Anticipate future triggers and discuss how new plan will be applied.

☐ ☐ Schedule booster sessions.

New Plan Summary Sheet

MY TRIGGERS:

Old plan	New plan
Old responses that contribute to my symptoms	*New responses that overcome my symptoms*
1. Thinking style (e.g., "If I have a negative thought, then I worry about the future")	1. Thinking style (e.g., "If I have a negative thought, then I postpone worry for a day")
2. Behaviors	2. Behaviors
3. Attention focus	3. Attention focus
	4. Reframe

Instructions: It is important to be aware of the triggers for your old way of coping, your "old plan." When you notice a trigger or aspects of your "old plan" in action, you must shift to using your "new plan," as described above. Under "Reframe," write a sentence summarizing what you have learned about your thoughts.

References

Abramowitz, J. S., Whiteside, S., Kalsky, S. A., & Tolin, D. A. (2003). Thought control strategies in obsessive–compulsive disorder: A replication and extension. *Behaviour Research and Therapy, 41,* 529–554.

Agras, W. S., & Berkowitz, R. (1980). Clinical research and behavior therapy: Halfway there? *Behavior Therapy, 11,* 472–487.

Allott, R., Wells, A., Morrison, A. P., & Walker, R. (2005). Distress in Parkinson's disease: Contributions of disease factors and metacognitive style. *British Journal of Psychiatry, 187,* 182–183.

American Psychiatric Association. (1994). *Diagnostic and statistical manual of mental disorders* (4th ed.). Washington, DC: Author.

American Psychiatric Association. (2000). *Diagnostic and statistical manual of mental disorders* (4th ed., text rev.). Washington, DC: Author.

Amir, N., Cashman, L., & Foa, E. B. (1997). Strategies of thought control in obsessive–compulsive disorder. *Behaviour Research and Therapy, 35,* 775–777.

Barlow, D. M. (2002). *Anxiety and its disorders: The nature and treatment of anxiety and panic* (2nd ed.). New York: Guilford Press.

Barsky, A. J., Wyshak, G., & Klerman, G. L. (1990). The Somatosensory Amplifical Scale and its relationship to hypochondriasis. *Journal of Psychiatric Research, 24,* 323–334.

Beck, A. T. (1967). *Depression: Causes and treatment.* Philadelphia: University of Pennsylvania Press.

Beck, A. T. (1976). *Cognitive therapy and the emotional disorders.* New York: International Universities Press.

Beck, A. T., Epstein, N., Brown, G., & Steer, R. A. (1988). An inventory for measuring depression. *Archives of General Psychiatry, 4,* 561–571.

Beck, A. T., Rush, A. J., Shaw, B. F., & Emery, G. (1979). *Cognitive therapy of depression.* New York: Guilford Press.

Beck, A. T., Steer, R. A., & Brown, G. K. (1996). *Beck Depression Inventory–II.* San Antonio: Psychological Corporation.

Bishop, S. R., Lau, M., Shapiro, S., Carlson, L., Anderson, N. D., Carmody, J., et al. (2004). Mindfulness: A proposed operational definition. *Clinical Psychology: Science and Practice, 11*, 230–241.

Bisson, J. L., Jenkins, P. L., Alexander, J., & Bannister, C. (1997). Randomized controlled trial of psychological debriefing for victims of acute burn trauma. *British Journal of Psychiatry, 171*, 78–81.

Borkovec, T. D., Robinson, E., Pruzinsky, T., & DePree, J. A. (1983). Preliminary exploration of worry: Some characteristics and processes. *Behaviour Research and Therapy, 21*, 9–16.

Bouman, T. K., & Meijer, K. J. (1999). A preliminary study of worry and metacognitions in hypochondriasis. *Clinical Psychology and Psychotherapy, 6*, 96–102. [Special issue: Metacognition and cognitive behaviour therapy]

Broadbent, D. E., Cooper, P. F., Fitzgerald, P., & Parkes, K. R. (1982). The Cognitive Failures Questionnaire (CFQ) and its correlates. *British Journal of Clinical Psychology, 21*, 1–16.

Brown, A. L. (1978). Knowing when, where, and how to remember: A problem of metacognition. In R. Glaser (Ed.), *Advances in instructional psychology* (pp. 367–406). Hillsdale, NJ: Erlbaum.

Brown, K. W., & Ryan, R. M. (2003). The benefits of being present: Mindfulness and its role in psychological wellbeing. *Journal of Personality and Social Psychology, 84*, 822–848.

Butler, G., Wells, A., & Dewick, H. (1995). Differential effects of worry and imagery after exposure to a stressful stimulus: A pilot study. *Behavioural and Cognitive Psychotherapy, 23*, 45–56.

Cartwright-Hatton, S., & Wells, A. (1997). Beliefs about worry and intrusions: The Meta-Cognitions Questionnaire and its correlates. *Journal of Anxiety Disorders, 11*, 279–296.

Carver, C. S., & Blaney, P. M. (1977). Perceived arousal, focus of attention and avoidance behaviour. *Journal of Abnormal Psychology, 86*, 154–162.

Cavanagh, M. J., & Franklin, J. (2000). *Attention training and hypochondriasis: Preliminary results of a controlled treatment trial.* Paper presented at the World Congress of Behavioral and Cognitive Therapies, Vancouver, Canada.

Clark, D. M., Ehlers, A., McManus, F., Hackmann, A., Fennell, M. J. V., Waddington, L., et al. (2003). Cognitive therapy versus fluoxetine in generalized social phobia: A randomized placebo-controlled trial. *Journal of Consulting and Clinical Psychology, 71*, 1058–1067.

Clark, D. M., & Wells, A. (1995). A cognitive model of social phobia. In R. G. Heimberg, M. R. Liebowitz, D. A. Hope, & F. R. Schneier (Eds.), *Social phobia: Diagnosis, assessment, and treatment* (pp. 69–93). New York: Guilford Press.

Colbear, J., & Wells, A. (2008). *Randomized controlled trial of metacognitive therapy for posttraumatic stress disorder.* Manuscript in preparation.

Davidson, J. (1996). *Davidson Trauma Scale.* New York: Multi-Health Systems Inc.

Davis, R. N., & Valentiner, D. P. (2000). Does meta-cognitive theory enhance our understanding of pathological worry and anxiety? *Personality and Individual Differences, 29*, 513–526.

Ellis, A. (1962). *Reason and emotion in psychotherapy.* New York: Lyle Stuart.

Ellis, A., & Harper, R. A. (1961). *A guide to rational living.* Englewood Cliffs, NJ: Prentice-Hall.

Eysenck, M. W. (1992). *Anxiety: The cognitive perspective.* Hove, UK: Erlbaum.

Fenigstein, A., & Vanable, P. A. (1992). Paranoia and self-consciousness. *Journal of Personality and Social Psychology, 62,* 129–138.

Fisher, P. L. (2006). The efficacy of psychological treatments for generalised anxiety disorder? In G. C. L. Davey & A. Wells (Eds.). *Worry and its psychological disorders: Theory, assessment and treatment* (pp. 359–377). Chichester, UK: Wiley.

Fisher, P. L., & Wells, A. (2005). Experimental modification of beliefs in obsessive–compulsive disorder: A test of the metacognitive model. *Behaviour Research and Therapy, 43,* 821–829.

Fisher, P. L., & Wells, A. (2008). Metacognitive therapy for obsessive–compulsive disorder: A case series. *Journal of Behavior Therapy and Experimental Psychiatry, 39,* 117–132.

Flavell, J. H. (1979). Metacognition and metacognitive monitoring: A new area of cognitive–developmental inquiry. *American Psychologist, 34,* 906–911.

Foa, E. B. (1995). *Posttraumatic Stress Diagnostic Scale manual.* Minneapolis, MN: NCS Pearson Systems.

Fresco, D. M., Frankel, A. N., Mennin, D. S., Turk, C. L., & Heimberg, R. G. (2002). Distinct and overlapping features of rumination and worry: The relationship of cognitive processes to negative affective states. *Cognitive Therapy and Research, 26,* 179–188.

Goodman, W. K., Price, L. H., Rasmussen, S. A., Mazure, C., Delgado, P., Heninger, G. R., et al. (1989). The Yale–Brown Obsessive Compulsive Scale: II. Validity. *Archives of General Psychiatry, 46,* 1012–1016.

Goodman, W. K., Price, L. H., Rasmussen, S. A., Mazure, C., Fleischmann, R. L., Hill, C. L., et al. (1989). The Yale–Brown Obsessive Compulsive Scale: I. Development, use and reliability. *Archives of General Psychiatry, 46,* 1006–1011.

Gotlib, I. H., & Cane, D. B. (1987). Construct accessibility and clinical depression: A longitudinal investigation. *Journal of Abnormal Psychology, 96,* 199–204.

Gwilliam, P., Wells, A., & Cartwright-Hatton, S. (2004). Does meta-cognition or responsibility predict obsessive–compulsive symptoms: A test of the metacognitive model. *Clinical Psychology and Psychotherapy, 11,* 137–144.

Hammarberg, M. (1992). Penn Inventory for Posttraumatic Stress Disorder: Psychometric properties. *Psychological Assessment, 4,* 67–76.

Hayes, S. C., Strosahl, K. D., & Wilson, K. G. (1999). *Acceptance and commitment therapy: An experiential approach to behavior change.* New York: Guilford Press.

Hazlett-Stephens, H. (1997). *The role of relaxation in the reduction of fear: An investigation of speech anxiety.* Paper presented at the annual meeting of the Association for Advancement of Behavior Therapy, Miami, FL.

Hermans, D., Martens, K., De Cort, K., Pieters, G., & Eelen, P. (2003). Reality monitoring and metacognitive beliefs related to cognitive confidence in obsessive–compulsive disorder. *Behaviour Research and Therapy, 41,* 383–401.

Hodgson, R. J., & Rachman, S. (1977). Obsessive–compulsive complaints. *Behaviour Research and Therapy, 15,* 389–395.

Holeva, V., Tarrier, N., & Wells, A. (2001). Prevalence and predictors of acute PTSD following road traffic accidents: Thought control strategies and social support. *Behavior Therapy, 32,* 65–83.

Horowitz, M. J., Wilner, N., & Alvarez, W. (1979). Impact of Event Scale: A measure of subjective stress. *Psychosomatic Medicine, 41,* 209–218.

Ingram, R. E. (1990). Self-focused attention in clinical disorders: Review and a conceptual model. *Psychological Bulletin, 107,* 156–176.

Janeck, A. S., Calamari, J. E., Riemann, B. C., & Heffelfinger, S. K. (2003). Too much thinking about thinking?: Metacognitive differences in obsessive–compulsive disorder. *Journal of Anxiety Disorders, 17,* 181–195.

Kabat-Zinn, J. (1990). *Full catastrophe living: The program of the Stress Reduction Clinic at the University of Massachusetts Medical Center.* New York: Dell.

Kabat-Zinn, J. (1994). *Mindfulness meditation for everyday life.* New York: Hyperion.

Kaspi, S. P., McNally, R. J., & Amir, N. (1995). Cognitive processing of emotional information in posttraumatic stress disorder. *Cognitive Therapy and Research, 19,* 433–444.

Knight, A. (2004). *Prevalence and predictors of post-traumatic stress disorder following intensive care unit treatment.* Unpublished thesis submitted, University of Manchester, Faculty of Medicine, UK.

Lavy, E. H., & van den Hout, M. (1990). Thought suppression induces intrusions. *Behavioural Psychotherapy, 18,* 225–238.

Lobban, F., Haddock, G., Kinderman, P., & Wells, A. (2002). The role of metacognitive beliefs in auditory hallucinations. *Personality and Individual Differences, 32,* 1351–1363.

Lyubomirsky, S., & Tkach, C. (2004). The consequences of dysphoric rumination. In C. Papageorgiou & A. Wells (Eds.), *Depressive rumination: Nature, theory and treatment* (pp. 21–41). Chichester, UK: Wiley.

Martin, L. L., & Tesser, A. (1989). Toward a motivational and structural theory of ruminative thought. In J. S. Uleman & J. A. Bargh (Eds.), *Unintended thought* (pp. 306–326). New York: Guilford Press.

Martin, L. L., & Tesser, A. (1996). Some ruminative thoughts. In R. S. Wyer (Ed.), *Advances in social cognition* (Vol. 9, pp. 1–47). Mahwah, NJ: Erlbaum.

Mathews, A., & MacLeod, C. (1985). Selective processing of threat cues in anxiety states. *Behaviour Research and Therapy, 23,* 563–569.

Matthews, G., & Harley, T. A. (1996). Connectionist models of emotional distress and attentional bias. *Cognition and Emotion, 10,* 561–600.

Matthews, G., & Wells, A. (1999). The cognitive science of attention and emotion. In T. Dalgleish & M. Power (Eds.), *Handbook of cognition and emotion* (pp. 171–192). New York: Wiley.

Matthews, G., & Wells, A. (2000). Attention, automaticity, and affective disorder. *Behaviour Modification, 24,* 69–93.

Matthews, G., & Wells, A. (2004). Rumination, depression and metacognition: The S-REF model. In C. Papageorgiou & A. Wells (Eds.), *Depressive rumination: Nature, theory and treatment* (pp. 125–151). Chichester, UK: Wiley.

Mellings, T. M. B., & Alden, L. E. (2000). Cognitive processes in social anxiety: The effects of self-focus, rumination and anticipatory processing. *Behaviour Research and Therapy, 38,* 243–257.

Merckelbach, H., Muris, P., van den Hout, M., & de Jong, P. (1991). Rebound effects of thought suppression: Intrusion-dependent? *Behavioural Psychotherapy, 19,* 225–238.

Metcalfe, J., & Shimamura, A. P. (1994). *Metacognition.* Cambridge, MA: MIT Press.

Morrison, A., & Wells, A. (2000). Thought control strategies in schizophrenia: A comparison with non-patients. *Behaviour Research and Therapy, 38,* 1205–1209.

Morrison, A. P., Wells, A., & Nothard, S. (2000). Cognitive factors in predisposition to auditory and visual hallucinations. *British Journal of Clinical Psychology, 39,* 67–78.

Morrison, A. P., Wells, A., & Nothard, S. (2002). Cognitive and emotional predictors of predisposition to hallucinations in non-patients. *British Journal of Clinical Psychology, 41,* 259–270.

Muris, P., Merckelbach, H., van den Hout, M. A., & de Jong, P. (1992). Suppression of emotional and neutral material. *Behaviour Research and Therapy, 30,* 639–642.

Myers, S., Fisher, P. L., & Wells, A. (2007, July). *The metacognitive model of obsessional–compulsive symptoms: An empirical model.* Paper presented at the World Congress of Cognitive and Behaviour Therapy, Barcelona, Spain.

Myers, S., & Wells, A. (2005). Obsessive–compulsive symptoms: The contribution of metacognitions and responsibility. *Journal of Anxiety Disorders, 19,* 806–817.

Nassif, Y. (1999). *Predictors of pathological worry.* Unpublished M. Phil. thesis, University of Manchester, UK.

Nelson, T. O., & Dunlosky, J. (1991). When people's judgments of learning (JOLs) are extremely accurate at predicting subsequent recall: The "delayed JOL effect." *Psychological Science, 2,* 267–270.

Nelson, T. O., Gerler, D., & Narens, L. (1984). Accuracy of feeling of knowing judgments for predicting perceptual identification and relearning. *Journal of Experimental Psychology: General, 113,* 282–300.

Nelson, T. O., & Narens, L. (1990). Metamemory: A theoretical framework and some new findings. In G. H. Bower (Ed.), *The psychology of learning and motivation* (pp. 125–173). New York: Academic Press.

Nelson, T. O., Stuart, R. B., Howard, G., & Crawley, M. (1999). Metacognition and clinical psychology: A preliminary framework for research and practice. *Clinical Psychology and Psychotherapy, 6,* 73–80. [Special issue: Metacognition and cognitive behaviour therapy]

Nolen-Hoeksema, S. (1991). Responses to depression and their effects on the duration of depressive episodes. *Journal of Abnormal Psychology, 100,* 569–582.

Nolen-Hoeksema, S. (2000). The role of rumination in depressive disorders and mixed anxiety/depressive symptoms. *Journal of Abnormal Psychology, 109,* 504–511.

Noelen-Hoeksema, S. (2004). The response styles theory. In C. Papageorgiou & A. Wells (Eds.), *Depressive rumination: Nature, theory and treatment* (pp. 107–123). Chichester, UK: Wiley.

Nolen-Hoeksema, S., & Larsen, J. (1999). *Coping with loss.* Mahwah, NJ: Erlbaum.

Nolen-Hoeksema, S., & Morrow, J. (1991). A prospective study of depression and posttraumatic stress symptoms after a natural disaster: The 1989 Loma Prieta earthquake. *Journal of Personaliy and Social Psychology, 61,* 115–121.

Nolen-Hoeksema, S., & Morrow, J. (1993). Effects of rumination and distraction on naturally occurring depressed mood. *Cognition and Emotion, 7,* 561–570.

Nuevo, R., Montorio, I., & Borkovec, T. D. (2004). A test of the role of metaworry in the prediction of worry severity in an elderly sample. *Journal of Behavior Therapy and Experimental Psychiatry, 35,* 209–218.

Papageorgiou, C., & Wells, A. (1998). Effects of attention training in hypochondriasis: An experimental case series. *Psychological Medicine, 28,* 193–200.

Papageorgiou, C., & Wells, A. (1999a). Process and metacognitive dimensions of depressive and anxious thoughts and relationships with emotional intensity. *Clinical Psychology and Psychotherapy, 2,* 156–162.

Papageorgiou, C., & Wells, A. (1999b). *Dimensions of depressive rumination and anxious worry: A comparative study.* Paper presented at the 33rd annual convention of the Association for Advancement of Behavior Therapy, Toronto, Canada.

Papageorgiou, C., & Wells, A. (2000). Treatment of recurrent major depression with attention training. *Cognitive and Behavioural Practice, 7,* 407–413.

Papageorgiou, C., & Wells, A. (2001a). Metacognitive beliefs about rumination in recurrent major depression. *Cognitive and Behavioral Practice, 8,* 160–164.

Papageorgiou, C., & Wells, A. (2001b). Positive beliefs about depressive rumination: Development and preliminary validation of a self-report scale. *Behavior Therapy, 32,* 13–26.

Papageorgiou, C., & Wells, A. (2001c). *Metacognitive vulnerability to depression: A prospective study.* Paper presented at the 35th annual convention of the Association for Advancement of Behavior Therapy, Philadelphia.

Papageorgiou, C., & Wells, A. (2003). An empirical test of a clinical metacognitive model of rumination and depression. *Cognitive Therapy and Research, 27,* 261–273.

Papageorgiou, C., & Wells, A. (Eds.). (2004). *Depressive rumination: Nature, theory, and treatment.* Chichester, UK: Wiley.

Papageorgiou, C., Wells, A., & Meina, L. J. (2008). *Development and preliminary validation of the Negative Beliefs about Rumination Scale.* Manuscript in preparation.

Patmore, A. (2006). *The truth about stress.* London: Atlantic Books.

Purdon, C. (1999). Thought suppression and psychopathology. *Behaviour Research and Therapy, 37,* 1029–1054.

Purdon, C. (2000, July). *Metacognitive and the persistence of worry.* Paper presented at the annual conference of the British Association of Behavioural and Cognitive Psychotherapy, Institute of Education, London.

Rachman, S. (1980). Emotional processing. *Behaviour Research and Therapy, 18,* 51–60.

Rachman, S. (1993). Obsessions, responsibility and guilt. *Behaviour Research and Therapy, 31,* 149–154.

Rachman, S., & deSilva, P. (1979). Abnormal and normal obsessions. *Behaviour Research and Therapy, 3,* 89–99.

Rassin, E., Merckelbach, H., Muris, P., & Spaan, V. (1999). Thought–action fusion as a causal factor in the development of intrusions. *Behaviour Research and Therapy, 37,* 231–237.

Rees, C. S., & van Koesveld, K. E. (2008). An open trial of group metacognitive therapy for obsessive–compulsive disorder. *Journal of Behavior Therapy and Experimental Psychiatry,* doi: 10.1016/j.jbtep.2007.11.004

Reynolds, M., & Wells, A. (1999). The Thought Control Questionnaire: Psychometric properties in a clinical sample, and relationships with PTSD and depression. *Psychological Medicine, 29,* 1089–1099.

Richards, A., & French, C. C. (1992). An anxiety-related bias in semantic activation when processing threat/neutral homographs. *Quarterly Journal of Experimental Psychology, 40,* 503–528.

Richards, A., French, C. C., Johnson, W., Naparstek, J., & Williams, J. (1992). Effects of mood manipulation and anxiety on performance of an emotional Stroop task. *British Journal of Psychology, 8,* 479–491.

Roemer, L., & Borkovec, T. D. (1994). Effects of suppressing thoughts about emotional material. *Journal of Abnormal Psychology, 103,* 467–474.

Roleofs, J., Papageorgiou, C., Gerber, R. D., Huibers, M., Peeters, F., & Arntz, A. (2007). On the links between self-discrepancies, rumination, metacognitions, and symptoms of depression in undergraduates. *Behaviour Research and Therapy, 45,* 1295–1305.

Roussis, P. (2007). Metacognitive factors in post-traumatic stress disorder (PTSD). Unpublished Ph.D. thesis. University of Manchester, Faculty of Medical and Human Sciences.

Roussis, P., & Wells, A. (2006). Post-traumatic stress symptoms: Tests of relationships with thought control strategies and beliefs as predicted by the metacognitive model. *Personality and Individual Differences, 40,* 111–122.

Roussis, P., & Wells, A. (2008). Psychological factors predicting stress symptoms: Metacognition, thought control and varieties of worry. *Anxiety, Stress & Coping, 21,* 213–225.

Ruscio, A. M., & Borkovec, T. D. (2004). Experience and appraisal of worry among high worriers with and without generalized anxiety disorder. *Behaviour Research and Therapy, 42,* 1469–1482.

Sanavio, E. (1988). Obsessions and compulsions: The Padua Inventory. *Behaviour Research and Therapy, 26,* 169–177.

Sarason, I. G. (1984). Test anxiety, stress, and cognitive interference: Reactions to tests. *Journal of Personality and Social Psychology, 46,* 929–938.

Schneider, W., Dumais, S. T., & Shiffrin, R. M. (1984). Automatic and control processing and attention. In R. Parasuraman & D. R. Davies (Eds.), *Varieties of attention.* New York: Academic Press.

Segal, Z. V., & Vella, D. D. (1990). Self-schema in major depression: Replication and extension of a priming methodology. *Cognitive Therapy and Research, 14,* 161–176.

Segerstrom, S. C., Tsao, J. C. I., Alden, L. E., & Craske, M. G. (2000). Worry and rumination: Repetitive thought as a concomitant and predictor of negative mood. *Cognitive Therapy and Research, 24,* 671–688.

Shiffrin, R. M., & Schneider, W. (1977). Controlled and automatic human information processing: II. Perceptual learning, automatic attending, and a general theory. *Psychological Review, 84,* 127–190.

Siegle, G. J., Ghinassi, F., & Thase, M. E. (2007). Neurobehavioral therapies in the 21st century: Summary of an emerging field and an extended example of cognitive control training for depression. *Cognitive Therapy and Research, 31,* 235–262.

Simons, M., Schneider, S., & Herpertz-Dahlmann, B. (2006). Metacognitive therapy versus exposure and response prevention for pediatric obsessive–compulsive disorder. *Psychotherapy and Psychosomatics, 75,* 257–264.

Spada, M. M., Mohiyeddini, C., & Wells, A. (2008). Measuring metacognitions associated with emotional distress: Factor structure and predictive validity of the Metacognitions Questionnaire 30. *Personality and Individual Differences, 45,* 238–242.

Spada, M. M., Moneta, G. B., & Wells, A. (2007). The relative contribution of metacognitive beliefs and alcohol expectancies to drinking behaviour. *Alcohol and Alcoholism, 42,* 567–574.

Spada, M. M., Nikcevic, A. V., Moneta, G. B., & Wells, A. (2007). Metacognition as a mediator of the relationship between emotion and smoking dependence. *Addictive Behaviors, 36,* 2120–2129.

Spada, M. M., & Wells, A. (2005). Metacognitions, emotion and alcohol use. *Clinical Psychology and Psychotherapy, 12,* 150–155.

Spada, M., & Wells, A. (2006). Metacognitions about alcohol use in problem drinkers. *Clinical Psychology and Psychotherapy, 13,* 138–143.

Spada, M. M., & Wells, A. (2008a). Metacognitive beliefs about alcohol use: Development and validation of two self-report scales, *Addictive Behaviors, 33,* 515–527.

Spada, M. M., & Wells, A. (2008b). *An empirical test of a metacognitive model of problem drinking.* Manuscript in preparation.

Spada, M. M., Zandvoort, M., & Wells, A. (2007). Metacognitions in problem drinkers. *Cognitive Therapy and Research, 31,* 709–716.

Spasojevic, J., Alloy, L. B., Abramson, L. Y., Maccoon, D., & Robinson, M. S. (2004). Reactive rumination: Outcomes, mechanisms, and developmental antecedents. In C. Papageorgiou & A. Wells (Eds.), *Depressive rumination: Nature, theory and treatment* (pp. 43–58). Chichester, UK: Wiley.

Stirling, J., Barkus, E., & Lewis, S. (2007). Hallucination proneness, schizotypy and metacognition. *Behaviour Research and Therapy, 45,* 1401–1408.

Valmaggia, L., Bouman, T. K., & Schuurman, L. (2007). Attention training with auditory hallucinations: A case study. *Cognitive and Behavioral Practice, 14,* 127–133.

van den Hout, M., & Kindt, M. (2003a). Repeated checking causes memory distrust. *Behaviour Research and Therapy, 41,* 301–316.

van den Hout, M., & Kindt, M. (2003b). Phenomenological validity of an OCD memory model and the remember/know distinction. *Behaviour Research and Therapy, 41,* 369–378.

Warda, G., & Bryant, R. A. (1998). Cognitive bias in acute stress disorder. *Behaviour Research and Therapy, 36,* 1177–1183.

Wegner, D. M., Schneider, D. J., Carter, S. R., III, & White, T. L. (1987). Paradoxical effects of thought suppression. *Journal of Personality and Social Psychology, 53,* 5–13.

Wells, A. (1985). Relationship between private self-consciousness and anxiety scores in threatening situations. *Psychological Reports, 57,* 1063–1066.

Wells, A. (1990a). Effects of dispositional self-focus, appraisal, and attention instructions on responses to a threatening stimulus. *Anxiety Research, 3,* 291–301.

Wells, A. (1990b). Panic disorder in association with relaxation induced anxiety: An attention training approach to treatment. *Behaviour Therapy, 21,* 273–280.

Wells, A. (1994). A multidimensional measure of worry: Development and preliminary validation of the Anxious Thoughts Inventory. *Anxiety, Stress and Coping, 6,* 289–299.

Wells, A. (1995). Meta-cognition and worry: A cognitive model of generalised anxiety disorder. *Behavioural and Cognitive Psychotherapy, 23,* 301–320.

Wells, A. (1997). *Cognitive therapy of anxiety disorders: A practice manual and conceptual guide.* Chichester, UK: Wiley.

Wells, A. (2000). *Emotional disorders and metacognition: Innovative cognitive therapy.* Chichester, UK: Wiley.

Wells, A. (2005a). The metacognitive model of GAD: Assessment of meta-worry and relationship with DSM-IV generalized anxiety disorder. *Cognitive Therapy and Research, 29,* 107–121.

Wells, A. (2005b). Detached mindfulness in cognitive therapy: A metacognitive analysis and ten techniques. *Journal of Rational-Emotive and Cognitive-Behavior Therapy, 23,* 337–355.

Wells, A. (2006). Cognitive therapy case formulation in anxiety disorders. In N. Tarrier (Ed.), *Case formulation in cognitive behaviour therapy: The treatment of challenging and complex cases* (pp. 52–80). Hove, UK: Routledge.

Wells, A., & Carter, C. (1999). Preliminary tests of a cognitive model of generalised anxiety disorder. *Behaviour Research and Therapy, 37,* 585–594.

Wells, A., & Carter, K. (2001). Further tests of a cognitive model of generalized anxiety disorder: Metacognitions and worry in GAD, panic disorder, social phobia, depression, and nonpatients. *Behavior Therapy, 32,* 85–102.

Wells, A., & Cartwright-Hatton, S. (2004). A short form of the Metacognitions Questionnaire: Properties of the MCQ 30. *Behaviour Research and Therapy, 42,* 385–396.

Wells, A., & Davies, M. (1994). The Thought Control Questionnaire: A measure of individual differences in the control of unwanted thought. *Behaviour Research and Therapy, 32,* 871–878.

Wells, A., Fisher, P. L., Myers, S., Wheatley, J., Patel, T., & Brewin, C. (in press). Metacognitive therapy in recurrent and persistent depression: A multiple-baseline study of a new treatment. *Cognitive Therapy and Research.*

Wells, A., Fisher, P. L., Myers, S., Wheatley, J., Patel, T., & Brewin, C. (2008). *An open trial of metacognitive therapy in the treatment of major depressive disorder.* Manuscript in preparation.

Wells, A., Gwilliam, P., & Cartwright-Hatton, S. (2001). *The Thought Fusion Instrument.* Unpublished self-report scale, University of Manchester, UK.

Wells, A., & King, P. (2006). Metacognitive therapy for generalized anxiety disorder: An open trial. *Journal of Behavior Therapy and Experimental Psychiatry, 37,* 206–212.

Wells, A., & Matthews, G. (1994). *Attention and emotion: A clinical perspective.* Hove, UK: Erlbaum.

Wells, A., & Matthews, G. (1996). Modelling cognition in emotional disorder: The S-REF model. *Behaviour Research and Therapy, 32,* 867–870.

Wells, A., & Morrison, A. (1994). Qualitative dimensions of normal worry and normal obsessions: A comparative study. *Behaviour Research and Therapy, 32,* 867–870.

Wells, A., & Papageorgiou, C. (1995). Worry and the incubation of intrusive images following stress. *Behaviour Research and Therapy, 33,* 579–583.

Wells, A., & Papageorgiou, C. (1998a). Social phobia: Effects of external attention focus on anxiety, negative beliefs and perspective taking. *Behavior Therapy, 29,* 357–370.

Wells, A., & Papageorgiou, C. (1998b). Relationships between worry, obsessive–compulsive symptoms, and meta-cognitive beliefs. *Behaviour Research and Therapy, 39,* 899–913.

Wells, A., & Papageorgiou, C. (2001). Brief cognitive therapy for social phobia: A case series. *Behaviour Research and Therapy, 39,* 713–720.

Wells, A., & Sembi, S. (2004a). Metacognitive therapy for PTSD: A core treatment manual. *Cognitive and Behavioral Practice, 11,* 365–377.

Wells, A., & Sembi, S. (2004b). Metacognitive therapy for PTSD: A preliminary investigation of a new brief treatment. *Journal of Behavior Therapy and Experimental Psychiatry, 35,* 307–318.

Wells, A., Welford, M., Fraser, J., King, P., Mendel, E., Wisely, J., et al. (2008). Chronic PTSD treated with metacognitive therapy: An open trial. *Cognitive and Behavioral Practice, 15,* 85–92.

Wells, A., Welford, M., King, P., Papageorgiou, C., Wisely, J., & Mendel, E. (2008). *A randomised trial of metacognitive therapy versus applied relaxation in the treatment of generalised anxiety disorder.* Manuscript in preparation.

Wells, A., White, J., & Carter, K. (1997). Attention training: Effects on anxiety and beliefs in panic and social phobia. *Clinical Psychology and Psychotherapy, 4,* 226–232.

Wenzlaff, R. M., & Wegner, D. M. (2000). Thought suppression. *Annual Review of Psychology, 51,* 59–91.

Williams, J. M. G., Watts, F. N., MacLeod, C., & Mathews, A. (1988). *Cognitive psychology and emotional disorders.* Chichester, UK: Wiley.

Wine, J. D. (1971). Test anxiety and the direction of attention. *Psychological Bulletin, 76,* 92–104.

Yilmaz, E. A., Gencoz, T., & Wells, A. (2007a, July). *The causal role of metacognitions in the development of anxiety and depression: A prospective study.* Paper presented at the World Congress of Cognitive and Behaviour Therapy, Barcelona, Spain.

Yilmaz, E. A., Gencoz, T., & Wells, A. (2007b, July). *The unique contribution of cognitions and metacognitions to depression.* Paper presented at the World Congress of Cognitive and Behaviour Therapy, Barcelona, Spain.

Index

Page numbers followed by *f* or *t* indicate figures or tables.

selective attention link, evidence,
225–227
Socratic dialogue approach, 43, 45–47
strategic processing in, 226
Tiger task, 82, 142
Tip-of-the-tongue effect, 6
Transdiagnostic treatment
cognitive attentional syndrome target,
250–251
specifications, 250
universal case formulation in, 251–255,
252*f*, 253*f*
Trauma. *See* Posttraumatic stress disorder
"Trauma-lock," 129
Treatment outcome
rating scales, 33–34
studies, 239–246
Triggers
alternative processing plans, 220, 292
attention training, 211
in depression, 200, 211–213, 220
detached mindfulness, 211–213
elicitation of, 168
obsessive–compulsive disorder, 162*f*,
163
case formulation, 164, 165*f*, 168
posttraumatic stress disorder, 151
Two-minds strategy, and worry, 103
Type 1 worry
and generalized anxiety disorder, 92,
95
metacognitive model, 92, 93*f*, 95
Type 2 worry. *See* Meta-worry

U

Uncontrollability beliefs
in depression, 213–217
elicitation, 101–102
in generalized anxiety disorder, 92,
94*t*, 105–110
studies, 235
loss-of-control experiment in, 109–110
in obsessive–compulsive disorder,
studies, 228–229
rumination modulation experiment,
214–217
verbal challenges, 108–109

verbal reattribution, 105–106, 215
worry postponement technique,
107–108
Universal case formulation, 251–255,
252*f*, 253*f*
health anxiety/panic example,
252–253, 253*f*
self-regulatory executive function
model, 251–252, 252*f*

V

Verbal loop technique, 84–85
Verbal reattribution techniques, 48–50
case examples, 49–50
depression, 215–217
generalized anxiety disorder, 105–110,
117–119
metacognitive beliefs modification,
48–50
obsessive–compulsive disorder, 180–182
uncontrollable beliefs exploration,
105–106, 215–217
"Vertical arrow" technique, 257

W

Worry
alternative processing plan, 121–122,
122*f*
behavioral experiments, 115–117
case vignettes, 11–13
and cognitive attentional syndrome,
11–13
consequences, 13–14
controllability question, 91–92
counterevidence on effects of, 111–115
definition, 89–91
detached mindfulness, 106–108
detection of, 39–41, 44–45
evidence for negative effects, 223–225,
233–234
in generalized anxiety disorder, 89–96
treatment structure, 96–123
habit strength link, 14
harmfulness question, 110–115
behavioral experiments, 115–117